When Strangers Become Family

As the 21st Century unfolds, the traditional welfare state that evolved during the 20th Century faces serious threats to the solidarity that social programs were meant to strengthen. The rise of populist and nationalist parties reflects the decline of a sense of belonging and inclusiveness that mass education and economic progress were meant to foster, as traditional politics and parties are rejected by working- and middle-class individuals who were previously their staunchest supporters. Increasingly, these groups reject the growing gaps in income, power, and privilege that they perceive between themselves and highly educated and cosmopolitan business, academic, and political elites.

When Strangers Become Family examines the potential role of civil society organizations in guaranteeing the rights and addressing the needs of vulnerable groups, paying particular attention to their role in advocacy for and service delivery to older people. The book includes a discussion of the origins and functions of this sector that focuses on the relationship between the state and non-governmental organizations, as well as a close examination of Mexico – a middle-income nation with a rapidly aging population and limited state welfare for older people. The data reveals important aspects of the relationship among government actors, civil society organizations, and political parties. Ronald Angel and Verónica Montes-de-Oca Zavala ask the fundamental question about the extent to which civil society organizations represent a potential mechanism whereby vulnerable individuals can join together to further their own interests and exercise their individual and group autonomy.

Ronald J. Angel is Professor of Sociology at the University of Texas-Austin and coauthor, along with Jacqueline L. Angel, of *Family, Intergenerational Solidarity, and Post-Traditional Society* and *Latinos in an Aging World*.

Verónica Montes-de-Oca Zavala is Professor of Sociology and Demography at the Universidad Nacional Autónoma de México (UNAM). She is the author of *Envejecimiento en América Latina y el Caribe*.

Aging and Society

Edited by Carroll L. Estes and Assistant Editor Nicholas DiCarlo

This pioneering series of books creatively synthesizes and advances key, inter-sectional topics in gerontology and aging studies. Drawing from changing and emerging issues in gerontology, influential scholars combine research into human development and the life course; the roles of power, policy, and parti-sanship; race and ethnicity; inequality; gender and sexuality; and cultural studies to create a multi-dimensional and essential picture of modern aging.

Aging A – Z:
Concepts toward Emancipatory Gerontology (2019)
Carroll L. Estes with Nicholas DiCarlo

The Privatization of Care:
The Case of Nursing Homes (2020)
Pat Armstrong, Hugh Armstrong et al.

Age and the Research of Sociological Imagination:
Power, Ideology, and the Life Course (2021)
Dale Dannefer

When Strangers Become Family:
The Role of Civil Society in Addressing the Needs of Aging
Populations (2021)
Ronald Angel and Verónica Montes-de-Oca Zavala

For more information about this series, please visit:
https://www.routledge.com/Aging-and-Society/book-series/AGINGSOC

When Strangers Become Family

The Role of Civil Society in Addressing the Needs of Aging Populations

Ronald J. Angel and Verónica Montes-de-Oca Zavala

Routledge
Taylor & Francis Group
NEW YORK AND LONDON

First published 2022
by Routledge
52 Vanderbilt Avenue, New York, NY 10017

and by Routledge
2 Park Square, Milton Park, Abingdon, Oxon OX14 4RN

*Routledge is an imprint of the Taylor & Francis Group, an informa
business*

Library of Congress Cataloging-in-Publication Data
Names: Angel, Ronald, author. | Montes de Oca Zavala, Verónica,
author.
Title: When strangers become family : the role of civil society in
addressing the needs of aging populations / Ronald Angel, Verónica
Montes-de-Oca Zavala.
Description: New York, NY : Routledge, 2021. |
Series: Aging and society | Includes bibliographical references.
Identifiers: LCCN 2021012634 | ISBN 9781032071466 (hardback) |
ISBN 9780367459994 (paperback) | ISBN 9781003205609 (ebook)
Subjects: LCSH: Older people--Services for. | Older people--Services
for--Mexico. | Older people--Services for--United States. |
Population aging--Social aspects--Mexico. | Population aging--Social
aspects--United States. | Non-governmental organizations--Mexico. |
Non-governmental organizations--United States.
Classification: LCC HV1451 .A6746 2021 | DDC 362.60972--dc23
LC record available at https://lccn.loc.gov/2021012634

ISBN: 978-1-032-07146-6 (hbk)
ISBN: 978-0-367-45999-4 (pbk)
ISBN: 978-1-003-20560-9 (ebk)

DOI: 10.4324/9781003205609

Typeset in Garamond
by Taylor & Francis Books

MIX
Paper from
responsible sources
FSC
www.fsc.org
FSC™ C013985

Printed in the United Kingdom
by Henry Ling Limited

Contents

Illustrations

Figures

Table

Acknowledgements

We want to thank the large number of individuals who make this project possible. Primarily, we thank the older individuals who shared their life experiences and who contributed their time. We also thank the leaders and members of the civil society organizations and other groups who volunteered their time and recounted their struggles for human rights and shared with us their dedication to fighting for the rights and satisfying the political, material, and psychological needs of older people. From them we learned that a society that dignifies old age is a society that ensures the dignity of everyone and insures its future.

In addition, we are grateful for the financial support of the National Autonomous University of Mexico (UNAM) through the General Directorate of Academic Personnel Affairs (DGAPA) and the Support Program for Research and Technological Innovation Projects (PAPIIT) with project number IG300517 "Active aging and citizenship. Government mechanisms for social inclusion, poverty reduction and inequality in older adults in Mexico" (2017–2019). Additional funding for data analysis was provided by the Policy Research Institute-International Program, LBJ School of Public Affairs, and the Research Center for Minority Aging Research (NIA grant number 5P30AG059301–02) at the University of Texas, Austin. The Instituto de Investigaciones Sociales of UNAM (IISUNAM) provided invaluable administrative support to the project.

We are particularly grateful to dedicated members of the research team, whose insights and close attention to detail made the field experience a success. They conducted the interviews with great skill. We appreciate their time and dedication, as well as their valuable intellectual and practical input. We wish to give special thanks to the following individuals: María Del Pilar Alonso Reyes (Faculty of Sciences (FC-UNAM)); José Antonio Flores Diaz (FC-UNAM); Alma Miriam Bermúdez Espinosa (National School of Social Work (ENTS-UNAM)); Gina Irene Villagómez Valdés (Autonomous University of Yucatán (UADY-Yucatán, Mexico)); Feliciano Villar Posada (Barcelona University (UB-Spain)); Rodrigo Serrat Fernández (UB-Spain); María Del Rocío Enríquez Rosas (ITESO-Mexico);

Rosaura Avalos Pérez (ENTS-UNAM); Fermina Rojo Pérez (Consejo Superior de Investigaciones Científicas (CSIC-Spain)); Gloria Fernández-Mayoralas Fernández (CSIC-Spain); Vicente Rodríguez Rodríguez (CSIC-Spain); María Concepción Arroyo Rueda (UJED-Mexico); Paola Carmina Gutiérrez Cuellar (Instituto de Investigaciones Sociales de la Universidad de Baja California-Mexico); Patricia Rea Ángeles (IISUNAM-Conacyt Chairs-Mexico); Sagrario Garay Villegas (Universidad Autónoma de Nuevo León (UANL-Mexico)); Ana Fidelia Aparicio Trejo (Seminario Universitario Interdisciplinario sobre Envejecimiento y Vejez (SUIEV-UNAM)); Edith Hernández (SUIEV-UNAM); Karla Pérez Guadarrama (SUIEV-UNAM); and Paola Magdaleno (SUIEV-UNAM).

Chapter 1

Struggling Collectively for Truth and Justice

Since the end of the repressive dictatorships and political violence that gripped Latin America during the second half of the 20th Century, the subcontinent has engaged in an ongoing process of recovery that involves coming to terms with that violent past (Monsiváis 1987; Poniatowska 1980; Villalón 2017). Individual identities, as well as collective identities, require that distorted and false images of the past be corrected (Garrard 2017; Jelin and Kaufman 2006). Memories and narratives structure the past, which determine the possibilities for the present and future (Hancock 2016; Lechner and Güell 2006). Forgetting the past does not negate or even diminish its power over the present, it simply allows that influence to remain invisible, as in Gabriel Garcia Marquez' fictional rendition in *Cien Años de Soledad* (One Hundred Years of Solitude) of the actual Banana Strike Massacre that took place in Ciénaga, Colombia in 1928 (Márquez 1993 pp. 257–267).

The tale, which takes place in the fictional town of Macondo, poignantly captures the reality of historical denial. The massacre occurred when striking workers, who were demanding better working conditions, were fired upon by the military. In Marquez' fictional account, José Arcadio Segundo, one of the several generations of the Buendía family whose lives unfold in the novel, is the sole survivor of the massacre and awakens in a train filled with corpses that are being taken to be thrown into the sea to destroy the evidence. José Arcadio escapes and returns to Macondo where everyone assures him that nothing has happened; he is unable to convince anyone that the government's account that the strike ended peacefully and that the strikers simply went home is untrue. Denial and propaganda wiped the events from living memory, or at least from public discourse, but with reference to the real massacre not everyone forgot.

Today as the result of demands by civil society organizations, memory and truth commissions have been set up in many nations to keep the memories of past atrocities alive and to demand redress. Early efforts met with resistance from the state and were often unable to immediately determine the truth. One such case was the Matanza de Tlatelolco (Tlatelolco massacre) that took

DOI: 10.4324/9781003205609-1

place in the Tlatelolco plaza in Mexico City on October 2, 1968 when hundreds of students who were protesting the Olympics being held in Mexico City were murdered by the military (Rodda 1968). Thousands more were injured, missing, or taken into custody. The world paid little attention. Unmoved by the events, the International Olympic Committee announced that the games, which were to take place a few days later, would go on as scheduled. Immediate and even later attempts to determine what happened and who was responsible were largely unsuccessful. It was only many years later that the truth slowly came out, despite continued resistance by the government (Dillon 1998).

Other state-sponsored human rights violations have ultimately been brought to light and their perpetrators punished, if not immediately. Following a military coup in March 1976, Argentina was ruled by a series of military juntas. For seven years the military waged a dirty war against a growing leftist guerrilla movement and anyone the military judged to be subversive. During the dirty war thousands of supposed enemies of the state disappeared. Increasing domestic and international pressure, in conjunction with Argentina's defeat by Britain in the Malvinas/Falklands war, forced President Reynaldo Benito Bignone, a general who was later condemned to many years in prison on several charges including crimes against humanity, to hold elections in 1983. Raúl Alfonsín was elected President. During his first week in office Alfonsín created the Comisión Nacional sobre la Desaparición de Personas, CONADEP (National Commission on Disappeared Persons). In addition, the amnesty for atrocities that the military had granted itself was revoked. The introduction to the Commission's full report states the following:

> Our Commission was set up not to sit in judgment, because that is the task of the constitutionally appointed judges, but to investigate the fate of the people who disappeared during those ill-omened years of our nation's life. However, after collecting several thousand statements and testimonies, verifying or establishing the existence of hundreds of secret detention centres, and compiling over 50,000 pages of documentation, we are convinced that the recent military dictatorship brought about the greatest and most savage tragedy in the history of Argentina. Although it must be justice which has the final word, we cannot remain silent in the face of all that we have heard, read and recorded. This went far beyond what might be considered criminal offences, and takes us into the shadowy realm of crimes against humanity. Through the technique of disappearance and its consequences, all the ethical principles which the great religions and the noblest philosophies have evolved through centuries of suffering and calamity have been trampled underfoot, barbarously ignored.

> (CONADEP 1984)

More than forty years after the events that led to the creation of the Argentinian commission on the disappeared took place, Las Madres de Plaza de Mayo (the Mothers of the Plaza de Mayo) continue to protest regularly outside of the Casa Rosada (the residence and executive offices of the President) demanding a full accounting of what happened to their children. These women are by now quite old, but they are still active, and their mission has expanded beyond its original focus. This group serves as an example of what we deal with in this book. It illustrates the power of elderly women who have discovered that they can act collectively to change the existing reality. Initially, the mothers were focused exclusively on their own terrible loss, but as they have aged their mission has expanded, and they have become a voice against the socially damaging aspects of neoliberalism and other injustices (Borland 2006; Escalante Gonzalbo 2016). Their redefined and larger mission focuses on poverty, unemployment, hunger, corruption, and more. As is the case for other groups, their new vision of human rights includes social rights.

Guatemala, an impoverished Central American nation, was subjected to an extreme level of violence from the 1950s through the 1970s carried out by the government and various militia groups (Garrard 2017; United States Institute for Peace 1997). In 1982 the Guatemalan military conducted a scorched earth campaign against the newly formed revolutionary group, the Unidad Revolucionaria Nacional Guatemalteca, URNG (Guatemalan National Revolutionary Unit), resulting in a huge number of deaths. The indigenous Maya were singled out as enemies of the state and thousands were killed. In the 1990s the United Nations sponsored negotiations between the URNG and the government which took place in Spain. A peace agreement was finally signed in 1996. As part of the peace process a Comisión para el Esclarecimiento Histórico (Commission for Historical Clarification) was created to document human rights violations that occurred during the conflict and to preserve the memory of the victims, as well as to reduce the probability of further conflict. Among the Commission's findings was the following:

> The commission found that repressive practices were perpetrated by institutions within the state, in particular the judiciary, and were not simply a response of the armed forces. The report stated that in the four regions most affected by the violence, "agents of the state committed acts of genocide against groups of Mayan people."
> (United States Institute for Peace 1997, para. 122)

Yet atrocities and serious violations of human rights continue to occur, to such an extent that, as we discuss in Chapter three, even certain human rights activists have become discouraged and wonder if any real progress is being made. One recent example that captured international attention serves as a discouraging example. On September 26, 2014, forty-three students from the Ayotzinapa Rural Teachers' College disappeared in Iguala, Guerrero, Mexico. They were allegedly taken into custody by local police in cooperation with local gangs. Although it is unclear exactly what happened, it is clear that the students have disappeared. Unlike the Tlatelolco massacre, though, news of the event was immediately broadcast widely and civil society organizations and others brought pressure on the government for an accounting. Unfortunately, a complete accounting has yet to be made, but it is clear that events of this sort will no longer be immediately forgotten or suppressed as they might have been in the past. This elevated visibility of human rights violations, which is clearly facilitated by technology, is changing the ways in which individuals interact with one another, as well as with government at local, regional, national, and international levels.

Civil Society and the End of Silence

We could mention many more such examples of citizen efforts to redefine the past and expose serious violations of human rights in many parts of the world. These few examples from Latin America are only a small fraction of the efforts by human rights activists, lawyers, journalists, citizens groups, and others to expose and end state-sponsored human rights violations. One might conceive of these efforts as emerging from a growing international social movement focused on human and social rights that reflects a new consciousness and a growing willingness and ability of individuals acting collectively at various levels to foster human rights on a global scale. Truth commissions, though, are only one manifestation of civil society efforts to make basic changes to existing social, economic, and political arrangements.

The grand hope for civil society organizations is that they can serve as venues in which traditional social arrangements are questioned and contested, leading ultimately to change. Through these new venues various aspects of the welfare of marginalized groups, defined by the intersection of various identities including age, race, ethnicity, religion, gender, sexual preference, poverty, minority group status, social and political marginalization, and more can be brought to the public's attention and challenged. A major objective of these civil society actions is to alter the perceptions of excluded groups themselves of the reasons for their oppression. Rather than viewing their marginalization as inevitable, the objective is for the victims of injustice to recognize their situation as the result of social structures that must be altered through collective action.

Such objectives define political parties, but as we discuss in later chapters, traditional political parties have not brought about genuine democracy in many parts of the world, including Latin America and the Caribbean where labor parties have been weak. As we also discuss, in recent years we have witnessed a growing disillusionment with grand class-based theories focused on revolutionary change. Such theories and the movements they foster are increasingly irrelevant since they provide no truly viable theoretical or practical mechanisms for radical change. As we note, newer philosophies of horizontalism reject hierarchy and traditional political mobilization in favor of more local, non-hierarchical direct democracy. Whether such philosophies and the politics they give rise to can ultimately lead to changes in established structures of oppression remains an open question.

In addition to human rights, civil society organizations (CSOs), a label we use to refer to secular non-governmental, as well as faith-based organizations, work to protect the environment, to eliminate domestic violence, to educate children and adults, to assure adequate nutrition and health care, and much more. In Mexico civil society organizations were central in the struggle for open and fair elections during the last decades of the 20th Century (Olvera 2001; Olvera 2004; Olvera 2010). Prior to these efforts, elections were often stolen. Monitoring by civic groups, with the cooperation of international observers, resulted in the creation of the Instituto Nacional Electoral, INE (Federal Elections Institute), an autonomous agency that certifies federal elections (Issacharoff 2015, pp. 206–207). The focus on open and honest elections is clearly important, but elections alone do not guarantee full democracy. Our investigation goes beyond electoral reform to better understand the specific dimensions of the social movements of which civil society organizations are a part, as well as to document the extent to which they are redefining citizenship in ways that increase individuals' and groups' agency and civic consciousness.

In addition to documenting the successes and positive aspects of civil society organizations, we also examine their shortcomings and even their potentially negative effects. In this book we focus specifically on non-governmental and faith-based organizations that deal with issues that affect older people, a segment of the population that has historically suffered high rates of marginalization, poverty, and discrimination (Montes de Oca Zavala 2013; Montes de Oca Zavala and Gutiérrez Cuellar 2018). As we show, in recent years older individuals and their supporters have worked to alter the image of old age from that of a period during which one loses one's physical and mental capacities and becomes a burden, to that of a period when one is potentially active, engaged, and productive, and during which one is capable of acting in collaboration with others to further one's own and others' interests. Although we focus heavily on organizations composed of and operating in the interests of older individuals, the challenges these groups confront are similar to those faced by organizations that address the needs and rights of other groups.

Neoliberal Democratization

The context in which we develop our presentation is largely defined by the rise of neoliberalism and the response to it. The final decades of the 20th Century witnessed the election of conservative governments in North America and western Europe (Campbell and Pedersen 2001a; Escalante Gonzalbo 2016; Estes 2001b; Estes 2011). In the United States, Ronald Regan represented a profound rejection of traditional liberal government-led control of the economy, as did Margaret Thatcher in Great Britain. In these and other nations' market-based neoliberal political and economic policies, including market deregulation, decentralization of state functions, and a general reduction of state interventions in the economy replaced older state-directed economic approaches (Campbell 2004; Campbell and Pedersen 2001a). Neoliberalism represented a political as well as an economic philosophy that altered many of the most basic postwar social and economic arrangements, including labor market accords, industrial relations systems, redistributive tax structures, and social welfare programs (Bayón 2019; Estes 2001a; Estes 2001b). These radical shifts entailed a rejection of Keynesian-style management of aggregate demand and the affirmation of monetarist, supply-side, market-based policies, all of which represented a weakening of the traditional welfare-state social support mission (Campbell and Pedersen 2001b; Escalante Gonzalbo 2016).

This neoliberal philosophy was exported widely as part of what was known as the "Washington Consensus," a policy agenda that included an attempt to impose market-based economic systems in Latin America (Babb 2013; Stiglitz 2008; Williamson 2004). The Washington Consensus, and neoliberalism more generally, were promoted by international financial institutions including the World Bank, the International Monetary Fund, and the U.S. Treasury Department in the hope of fostering greater economic efficiency and growth (Babb and Kentikelenis 2018). As has been widely documented, while the new market-based policies might have had some positive effects on economic growth, that growth largely benefitted the wealthy and powerful. For the most part, though, the results were disappointing and reductions in social expenditures played havoc on the most marginal segments of the population (MacDonald and Ruckert 2009a; Shefner, Paskirtz, and Blad 2006; Stiglitz 2008). Neoliberal trickle-down policies promoted by the IMF and others were fundamentally ineffective and led to serious suffering even among the middle class. These negative impacts, in conjunction with the democratization of Latin American nations, provided the motivation and a venue for the emergence of various social movements to struggle against the inequities and deprivations of neoliberal policies.

Largely as a reaction to the disappointments and negative effects of neoliberal policies, the end of the 20th and early part of the 21st Centuries witnessed the reversal or weakening of many of the original neoliberal initiatives in most Latin American and Caribbean nations, ushering in a policy regime referred to as post-neoliberalism (MacDonald and Ruckert 2009a; Macdonald and Ruckert 2009b; Stiglitz 2008). The new policies were accompanied by a continent-wide shift to the left, frequently referred to as the "Pink Tide," with a greater focus on the needs of the poor and marginalized. This tide began in 1998 with Hugo Chávez' landslide presidential victory in Venezuela. His platform included an end to corruption, increased social spending, and a redistribution of oil wealth (Nelson 2019). As we know today, the initial hopes that brought Chávez to power have been long dashed and the nation's economy, as well as its political system, lie in ruins.

During this period other Latin American nations elected more progressive governments, most of which promised to reverse the most negative effects of the previous neoliberal policies (Cameron 2009; Macdonald and Ruckert 2009b). In 2000 Ricardo Lagos, leader of the Partido Socialista de Chile (Socialist Party of Chile), was elected President. In 2002 Luis Inácio "Lula" da Silva of the Partido dos Trabalhadores (Workers' Party) was elected President of Brazil. In 2003 Néstor Kirchner, a left-wing Peronist was elected President of Argentina. In 2004 Tabaré Vásquez, leader of the Frente Amplio (Broad Front) came to power in Uruguay. In 2005, a former coca union leader, Evo Morales, ran as the candidate of the Movimiento al Socialismo, MAS (Movement towards Socialism) and won the presidency in Bolivia. In 2006 Socialist Michelle Bachelet followed Ricardo Lagos to become President of Chile. In 2007 Rafael Correa became President of Ecuador. In that same year Daniel Ortega, the leader of the Sandinistas, won the presidential election in Nicaragua.

Left-wing leaders also mounted impressive electoral challenges in Peru and Mexico. In 2006 Andres Manuel López Obrador, the current President of Mexico, ran as the presidential candidate of the left-leaning Partido de la Revolución Democratica, PRD (Party of the Democratic Revolution) and came close to winning. All of these candidates ran on platforms that rejected many neoliberal policies that harmed the poor and vulnerable. In the long run, though, many neoliberal policies remained, if altered sufficiently to dampen their most serious negative effects.

Post-neoliberalism, though, is certainly not the end of the story. Life and history go on and the recent resurgence of populist nationalism in many nations around the world, often with a conservative and anti-civil society bias, suggests that the struggle for human and social rights is far from over. Following left-leaning administrations, the three largest economies in South America elected right-wing administrations (Encarnación 2018). In 2017 Miguel Juan Sebastián Piñera Echenique of the National Renewal Party won a second non-consecutive term as President in Chile, following Michelle Bachelete. In 2015 Mauricio Macri became President of Argentina replacing the administration of Cristina Fernández de Kirchner, and in 2019 Jair Bolsonaro was elected President of Brazil. These elections represent a significant weakening and maybe even an eventual reversal of the Pink Tide that installed so many left-wing governments on the continent.

The shift to the right, though, has not been universal nor has it swept the continent. In fact, in 2019 Argentina rejected conservative Mauricio Macri and returned Cristina Fernández de Kirchner to power as vice president with Alberto Fernández (no relation) serving as President. Kirchner will clearly be an influential advisor, and many expect Argentina to return to the policies that defined her presidency. Only time will tell. In 2018 Andres Manuel López Obrador, the left-wing populist who came close to winning the presidency in Mexico in 2006, was finally elected President. It is difficult to know how far and wide any shift toward the right or left might go, but it is also difficult to imagine that conservative governments would or could undo the progress in extending social rights that was part of the Pink Tide. In fact, right-wing populist parties could end up supporting such policies in their attempts to garner support. Such actions are traditional populist tactics of both the left and right.

A vibrant civil society is part of and contributes to the opening of the nations of Latin America (Olvera 2001; Olvera 2004). To the extent that the organizations of civil society foster democracy they contribute to reductions in inequality in the region (Huber and Stephens 2012). Numerous social movements have changed many individuals' and groups' conceptions of what is possible and what is right (Monsiváis 1987; Poniatowska 1980; Stahler-Sholk 2014; Stahler-Sholk, Vanden and Kuecker 2008). Women's groups, indigenous groups, LGBTQ organizations, and older persons have been mobilized and are not likely to fade back into obscurity and silence. Given the democratic openness of contemporary Latin American societies it seems unlikely that they are in any real danger of reverting to the old regimes of stolen elections and uncontested political oppression. Neoliberalism itself requires a national and international openness that would be almost impossible to reverse. Nonetheless, anything is possible and defenders of human and social rights must remain diligent.

The history of neoliberalism and its consequences have been widely analyzed and debated and we will not review those discussions in any detail. Our objective and our focus on Latin America and Mexico lead us to examine the detrimental aspects that these policies have had on vulnerable segments of those populations, including older individuals, and to investigate how civil society organizations have responded to counter those detrimental effects. The aspects of neoliberalism that specific nations adopted of course reflect local political, economic, and historical factors. Yet the general characteristics are fairly common, as are their consequences. Fiscal crises and calls for reductions in public spending pose serious challenges to all nations, and the retrenchment that results rarely has equal consequences for all segments of society. Even in highly developed European welfare states serious fiscal crises and the policies introduced to deal with them have led to an increase in marginalization among individuals who are often members of disadvantaged and stigmatized groups (Huber and Stephens 2001; Korpi 2003; O'Cinneide 2014).

Social Movements and Civil Society

Our focus on civil society responses to neoliberalism leads us immediately to the rise of social movements which have become a major force in many parts of the world, no more so though than in Latin America and the Caribbean (Stahler-Sholk, Vanden, and Becker 2014; Stahler-Sholk, Vanden, and Kuecker 2008). Neoliberal policies in Latin America have accompanied the rapid democratization of the continent and the rise of oppositional social movements. Fairly closed societies in which populations were severely repressed are now far more open, although oppositional civil society organizations continue to be harassed. The democratization and the greater openness of Latin American societies has provided venues in which individuals can come together to define their common agendas and demand justice and their basic human and social rights. Just a few years ago local, state, and national victories by Mexico's *Partido Revolucionario Institucional* PRI (Institutional Revolutionary Party), which ruled uninterrupted for over seventy years before its defeat in 2000, were suspect, and it was clear that many were stolen. Today Mexican elections are far more open and honest.

Truth commissions, as well as other organizations and groups that work to support and extend human rights and improve peoples' lives are examples of attempts by civil society organizations and the social movements of which they are a part to make fundamental changes in governance, economic hierarchies, political exclusion, human rights, and more. One might think of them as representing a form of direct democracy that involves more than simply voting, and includes collective attempts to directly shape public policies in many areas (Motta 2009; Motta 2014; Sitrin 2006). The general intent of those we deal with in this book is to improve the quality of life of individuals with few resources and little human or social capital, with the ultimate objective of empowering them to act as effective agents in furthering their own interests (Motta 2014). This objective clearly involves overthrowing entrenched power structures and systems of social stratification and ultimately gaining control of the state. Such an objective implies gaining power, as has been the objective of traditional revolutionary movements. Revolutionary movements, including Latin American and Caribbean revolutionary movements, though, have often been disappointing in terms of furthering democratic inclusion, even as they have improved the material and social conditions of the poor (Young and Schwartz 2012). For that reason, certain social movement activists reject striving to gain power, which they see as inevitably inimical to the objectives of greater social justice and inclusion (Holloway 2002; Holloway 2010).

Changing Society Without Taking Power

The rejection of power brings us immediately to one of the major dilemmas that confront civil society organizations and social movements of all sorts. How does one bring about change in basic power relations without assuming power? One alternative to gaining or even striving for power, with the tendencies to oligarchy that such a process risks, is summarized by a philosophy labeled "horizontalidad," or horizontalism in English. The term is employed by Mariana Sitrin and others to emphasize the highly democratic and participatory philosophies of certain organizations and the social movements they embody (Sitrin 2006; Sitrin 2014). Referring specifically to the riots that resulted from the economic crisis in Argentina in 2001 that forced President Fernando de la Rua out of office, Sitrin characterizes horizontalism as a new way of interacting that has become a hallmark of many autonomous movements (Motta 2009; Motta 2014). This new way of interacting is based on direct democracy and a rejection of authority and hierarchy, a philosophy which it shares with traditional anarchism. This position is in stark contrast to Peronism and other authoritarian regimes to be sure, but also to traditional political parties.

Of course, not all social movements embrace horizontalism. Indeed, many are quite hierarchical depending on their objectives and the context in which they operate. Revolutionary groups are of necessity vertical and hierarchical. Yet many new social movements are remarkably horizontal, which increases the ability of members to participate and engage in collective decisions, but which also has negative consequences in terms of the ability to develop wide collaborations and engage in effective political action (Stahler-Sholk 2014; Young and Schwartz 2012). One of the best known horizontal social movements emerged from the Zapatista uprising in Chiapas, Mexico in 1994 (Mora 2008; Olvera 2004; Olvera 2010; Stahler-Sholk 2014). The movement's philosophy emphasizes democracy and inclusion and rejects cooperation with the State, as well as political parties (Swords 2008).

Another example is the Movimiento de Trabajadores Desocupados de Solano (Movement of Unemployed Workers) in Argentina, one of the piquetero groups that was active during the 1990s (Motta 2009). Like the Zapatistas, this group rejected hierarchy and refused to cooperate with the government. Rather than organized political action they employed the "piquete," (picket), or in their case roadblocks, to force the government to meet their demands. Again, though, the ideal of optimal inclusion created problems of coordination with other groups. This approach, which is embodied in the title of John Holloway's book *Change the World Without Taking Power*, may seem naïve or simplistic, as Holloway concedes (Holloway 2002). Change is always resisted, often violently, by those who stand to lose power. How the rejection of power and affiliations with powerful groups can lead to meaningful change or the empowerment of marginalized groups remains unclear. Perhaps there is a lesson in Martin Luther King Jr.'s non-violent civil rights philosophy which in rejecting violence drew attention to the struggle of the innocent victims of racism for basic civil rights.

This horizontal and leveling focus that rejects hierarchy and is suspicious of formal organizations, governmental bureaucracies, and political parties, all of which imply authority, expertise, rank, and hierarchy has been criticized specifically because of its failure to engage in formal party-based political action (Pearce 2004; Young and Schwartz 2012). While local collective action represents a useful form of direct democratic engagement, there are no convincing theoretical arguments for the possibility of, and no real-world examples of how and under what circumstances large-scale systemic change can be brought about without access to traditional sources of power. As Holloway points out, though, revolutionary movements and leftist parties have for the most part been unsuccessful in bringing about radical democratic reform (Holloway 2002). When such parties achieve power, they often become oppressive and undemocratic. Unfortunately, though, the reality is that local community efforts, or even uncoordinated larger-scale efforts cannot, almost by definition, dismantle established structural sources of the extreme inequality that is typical of Latin America and the Caribbean.

This reality fuels a serious criticism of democratic social movements, and center and left parties more generally, which is that although they have mounted serious critiques of neoliberal economics and politics, they offer no viable alternatives to limited direct democracy and underdevelopment (Panizza 2005). This reality requires a reassessment of the extent of change that civil society organizations or the social movements of which they are a part can bring about, at least in the short term. The reality may be far more limited than the ideal. Even short-term and limited successes, though, can have important longer-term effects, again as was the case with the civil rights movement in the United States. When individuals realize that they can collectively demand and bring about change, the result could be an increase in civic consciousness and, eventually, more effective political involvement leading to meaningful reform.

Growth in the Number of CSOs since World War II

Charitable and non-governmental organizations have existed since antiquity, but their number began to increase significantly during the 19th Century as globalization increased and as weights and measures needed to be standardized, international travel and communication increased, and other aspects of international commerce and interaction required coordination. International non-governmental professional and charitable organizations were an important part of that process (Ehrenberg 2017). During the 20th Century, and especially after World War II, the growth in their number in both developing and developed countries has accelerated (Bebbington, Hickey, and Mitlin 2008; Boli and Thomas 1997; Boli and Thomas 1999; DeMars and Dijkzeul 2015; Eade 2000; Edwards 2014; Mendelson and Glenn 2002; Salamon and Anheier 1998; Salamon et al. 1999). CSOs have become a core aspect of civic life in most countries including those of Latin America and the Caribbean (Meyer 1999).

Civil society organizations are an increasingly important aspect of governance at all levels, and consist of a wide range of entities from universities to private clubs, professional organizations, advocacy groups, sports teams, museums, foundations, and more (Chambers and Kymlicka 2002; Edwards 2014; Salamon 2003; Salamon and Anheier 1998). An important subset consists of faith-based organizations, many of which engage in significant social action (Adkins, Occhipinti, and Heferan 2010; Ammerman 2005; Herbert 2003; Wuthnow 1996). The growth in their number reflects a general public acceptance of a more local way of addressing important social issues. Data from the Edelman Trust Barometer for 2018 indicates that trust in NGOs is high in many nations, including Mexico, where trust in these organizations far exceeds trust in the government (Edelman 2018).

Today CSOs are involved in health, education, human rights, women's issues, the environment, sustainable development, and much more (Boli and Thomas 1997; Boli and Thomas 1999a; Carroll 1992; Hall-Jones 2006; Hudock 1999; Keck and Sikkink 1998; Lee 2010; Robinson and Riddell 1995; Salamon 2003; Salamon and Anheier 1996b). They have assumed important and influential roles as advisors to the United Nations, other multilateral agencies, and national and local governments (Global Policy Forum 2010). Their numbers have increased rapidly in Latin America and the Caribbean where they have responded to states' inability to provide essential public services (Meyer 1999).

Many observers see CSOs as local manifestations of new social movements (Albrow et al. 2008; Boli and Thomas 1999a; Keck and Sikkink 1998; Pichardo 1997). Others view the rapid growth of these organizations as reflecting the spread of a global culture that is supranational in character and largely Western in values (Boli and Thomas 1997; Boli and Thomas 1999b). Boli and Thomas characterize world culture in the following way:

> When we speak of culture as global, we mean that definitions, principles, and purposes are cognitively constructed in similar ways throughout the world. The existence, general nature, and purposes of states, school systems, and transnational corporations are known everywhere. They are Durkheimian social facts, whether revered or

reviled. Thus, even though many of the world-cultural principles we discuss are contested and generate considerable conflict, their reification is enhanced by this very contestation.

(Boli and Thomas 1997, p. 173)

As Boli and Thomas clearly note, the content of this "world culture" remains contested. For many critics it represents a western European or American world view that is imposed upon other nations and cultures (Wright 2012). The homology in institutions that Boli and Thomas observe may result less from functional prerequisites and more from Western cultural hegemony. Clearly, we must retain a critical position as we explore the possibilities for civil society's ability to foster individual and group agency.

Not everyone accepts the world culture argument. Some observers locate the motivation for the growth in CSOs in the growing discontent of the impoverished and powerless segments of humanity. From this perspective civil society organizations are part of the global demand by poor people for greater social justice and a fairer distribution of global wealth (Bendaña 2006; Grzybowski 2000). Whatever the causes of the increase in the number and role of CSOs, they are important actors internationally and locally and their presence calls for a more sophisticated approach to understanding how they influence governance at all levels (Fisher 1997; Ruggie 1998). Most likely, explanations focused on world culture and the demands of poor people are to at least some degree correct. Yet different political and cultural contexts give rise to different civil society initiatives. Traditional realist perspectives that hold that only states matter in addressing development and other issues, or liberal perspectives that focus only on formal institutions miss a major dimension of political action and force for change. These explanations must be combined with constructivist perspectives that emphasize beliefs and ideas as they affect the actions of individuals and groups in demanding and bringing about change (DeMars and Dijkzeul 2015).

For many observers, in addition to serving as vehicles for the transmission of world culture, these organizations potentially serve as venues in which individuals can engage in dialog that can foster a sense of collective agency and the belief that significant change is possible. We discuss this possibility further in Chapter four as part of our examination of Antonio Gramsci's influence on civil society in Latin America. Such dialog takes place in several regional CSO forums on aging and human rights that are organized by the Economic Commission for Latin America and the Caribbean (ECLAC) and other regional actors. These allow various groups of older people to discuss issues that they feel are important and relevant and they provide a mechanism for the resolutions discussed to be conveyed back to ECLAC (CEPAL 2017). Such activities empower individuals and groups who have been silent to speak up, potentially fostering greater civic consciousness. As we discuss in great detail in Chapter three, civil society organizations are central in furthering the new human rights agenda as it applies to older people and other vulnerable groups.

Mexico: An Accelerated Demographic Transition

At the beginning of the 20th Century life expectancy at birth was 30 in Mexico and 50 in the United States (Kinsella 1992; Partida-Bush 2002, Figure 3). By the beginning of the 21st Century the gap in life expectancy between the two nations had nearly disappeared. In 2010 the median age of the Mexican population was 26; by 2050 it is projected to rise to 42, making it older than the United States in which the median age is projected to be 41 (Kochhar 2014). This rapid increase in life spans in Mexico reflects the astonishing pace of the demographic transition in that country. Although Mexico is still a young nation, it will not be for long (Angel, Vega, and López-Ortega 2017). In Mexico, individuals 60 and over make up the fastest growing segment of the population. The 2010 Mexican Census identified more than 10 million people, or 9% of the population, who were 60 or older. Fifteen percent of those individuals were 80 or older (INEGI 2010).

A rapidly aging population presents any nation, and especially low and middle-income nations, with serious short and long-term challenges since, as is the case in Mexico, relatively few individuals have formal retirement plans or significant savings (Aguila et al. 2016; Cotlear 2011; Hujo 2014; Mesa-Lago 2008; Willmore 2014). Although health care access is formally universal through the Instituto Nacional de Salud para el Bienestar, INSABI (National Institute of Health for Wellbeing), and non-contributory pensions have become universal, Mexico's old-age welfare state lags behind those of developed nations in terms of adequacy. The nation faces serious challenges in addressing the needs of a rapidly aging population given the reality of serious fiscal, organizational, and political constraints.

This changing demographic reality forms the background for our investigation of the potential role of civil society organizations in advocating for and providing services and assistance to a growing population of older persons. As we elaborate, such factors as greatly increased life spans that often include long periods of frailty and functional incapacity, the migration of children away from their parent's communities, the need for women to work, increasing divorce rates, and smaller families are undermining the capacity of the family to provide all of the care and support that frail aging parents need. Given the fact that federal, state, and municipal governments are limited in what they can provide, the potential complementary role of CSOs could be significant. As of yet we know little of how these organizations frame their missions, who they serve, how they are organized, and whether or not they are effective. Yet given the magnitude of the need, exploring their potential role is becoming more imperative.

The Support of Older People: A Universal Challenge

For all nations aging populations translate directly into rising expenditures for the financial support and health care of older people (CEPAL 2007; Cotlear 2011; Hujo 2014; Mesa-Lago 2008). In the high-income nations of Europe, the United States, and other developed nations the demographic transition that is proceeding so rapidly in less-developed nations began earlier and proceeded at a much slower pace. That slower pace, in conjunction with higher economic productivity, provided time to develop more extensive old age support systems. The vacuum that inadequate old age support systems create provides the impetus for CSO involvement. Yet debates over the nature, objectives, and effectiveness of civil society organizations in terms of the care of vulnerable segments of the population are ongoing. Some organizations effectively further the interests of their membership and benefit non-members, while others are largely ineffective and do little for the community at large. Our objective is not to arrive at some general assessment of the overall effectiveness of this confusing and complex network of organizations with multiple objectives, structures, and outcomes. Rather, our aim is to investigate variation in the objectives, membership, political activity, and explanatory frames, a phrase, as we explain below, we use to refer to the stated causes of the problems they address and their potential solutions, of different organizations that claim as at least part of their objectives addressing the rights and needs of older persons.

What Exactly Are Civil Society Organizations?

Debates over the extent of the civil society sector and the appropriate label to use in referring to the organizations that make it up continue endlessly. Whether one can draw clear and meaningful distinctions among various domains of economic and political activity remains a matter of debate (Edwards 2014; Foley and Edwards 1996; Kenny et al. 2017). This lack of clarity over the exact sector or domain of activity included is reflected in the range of labels employed to refer to these organizations and their activities. Among the most common are "non-governmental organizations," "non-profit organizations," "voluntary associations," and "civil society organizations" (Kenny et al. 2017). On the face of it, one can discern that the intent of this set of labels is to emphasize that these organizations are separate from government and the market (and also distinct from the family) and that they ideally foster a sense of civility and a sense of citizenship, a fairly idealistic objective. In this book we employ the label "civil society organizations," or CSOs, in order to emphasize the potential of such organizations to foster civic consciousness and sense of collective agency. The label is also inclusive of many organizations, some of which have fuzzy boundaries when it comes to their relationship to government, unions, political parties, and business.

Before proceeding, it would be useful to further specify characteristics of the types of organizations we are examining. For that purpose, we draw upon the definitional categorization of Lester Salomon and associates that informs the Johns Hopkins Comparative Nonprofit Sector Project (Salamon and Anheier 1996a). For these researchers the entities they include in the category of civil society organizations (1) possess some level of organization, that is they have an institutional structure; (2) are private and are not part of government; (3) are self-governing and control their own activities; (4) do not generate profits either for an individual or stockholders; and (5) are voluntary in that members are not required to participate or contribute. This set of characteristics serves as a useful conceptual starting point to differentiate civil society organizations from political parties, small business, state-sponsored activities, and more, but as we will see, clear distinctions are not always possible or meaningful. In Mexico and elsewhere many civil society organizations receive funding from governments and businesses, as well as support from unions and political parties.

Key Concepts Informing Subsequent Chapters

Active Aging

In addition to civil society, a core theme that informs our presentation relates to the concept of "active aging," which is often referred to using other labels, such as "successful aging," "healthy aging," "productive aging," among others. Regardless of the label, the basic concept is a rejection of traditional disengagement theory or prejudices that view individuals past a certain age as uninterested in and incapable of engaging in community life, and also disinterested in and incapable of learning new skills and understanding complex issues. Active aging has gained great currency in discussions of the actual and ideal situations of older individuals in different social, political, and economic contexts. One widely cited definition of the concept of active aging was offered by the World Health Organization at the Second United Nations World Assembly on Ageing held in Madrid, Spain in April 2002. The definition and discussion of the conditions that encourage active aging are quite long, but the following two paragraphs capture the essence of the idea:

> Active ageing applies to both individuals and population groups. It allows people to realize their potential for physical, social, and mental

wellbeing throughout the life course and to participate in society according to their needs, desires and capacities, while providing them with adequate protection, security and care when they require assistance.

The word "active" refers to continuing participation in social, economic, cultural, spiritual and civic affairs, not just the ability to be physically active or to participate in the labour force. Older people who retire from work and those who are ill or live with disabilities can remain active contributors to their families, peers, communities and nations. Active ageing aims to extend healthy life expectancy and quality of life for all people as they age, including those who are frail, disabled and in need of care.

(World Health Organization 2002, p. 12)

The WHO's description is clearly a normative ideal, that is something that societies should work toward. Unfortunately, the reality for many older individuals falls quite short of this ideal. Many older individuals live in poverty with little family or institutional support. Many are abandoned and lack the basic necessities of a dignified and productive existence, including adequate nutrition, medical care, and education. Many older individuals remain isolated and do not participate in community life. Many are at elevated risk of depression and death.

This reality has given rise to a global consciousness raising movement that promotes the possibilities of active aging, which recognizes the great potential of older individuals to participate in and contribute to family and community life (Kalache 2013). As we illustrate in the following chapters, the image of the older person as physically and cognitively weak and incapable of acting in his or her own behalf or that of others is incorrect and is being challenged by older individuals themselves and by their advocates, who include academics, service providers, legal experts, activists, and more. As we discuss in Chapter four the concept of active or healthy aging has received significant criticism insofar as it reflects the wellness movement that has gained currency in recent years, which states, or strongly implies, that one has nearly complete control over one's own health. From an extreme perspective one need not age. Rather, decline, disability, and disease reflect lifestyle choices that are under one's own control (Lamb 2017; Lamb 2020). Our use of the concept of active aging focuses more on political, economic, and social aspects of aging and less on the attempt to live forever. Our conception is based on the proposition that the physical, emotional, and social well-being of individuals of all ages depends on their structural position and their ability to act in ways that guarantee that they enjoy full human and social rights.

One indicator of the force of the concept of active aging is the WHO Global Age-Friendly Cities initiative that was proposed at the 2005

International Congress of Gerontology and Geriatrics in Rio De Janeiro, Brazil (World Health Organization 2007). This initiative is intended to encourage city planners, administrators, government officials, and others to consider how aspects of urban physical and social environments affect individuals of all ages. Everyone, and certainly the elderly, benefit from safe and clean environments, green spaces in which to enjoy nature and other people, outdoor seating, walkways that are in good repair, safe roads and crosswalks, accessible buildings, essential social services, public toilets, and more. Without these amenities older individuals are at risk of isolation, loneliness, and poor physical health.

Defamilisation

In Chapter two we introduce the concept of "defamilisation," a term which refers to the shift in responsibility for the care of dependent individuals from the family to the State. As we note, this shift is related to the rise of the modern welfare state in which basic education, health care, housing, income supports, and more are provided by various levels of government. While defamilisation refers to a historical process that has affected most middle and high-income countries, its specific forms depend on local historical, political, and cultural factors. Social policies related to the family differ greatly between the Social Democratic states of northern Europe, which maximize the role of the State and reduce that of the family, and the more conservative states of central and southern Europe that maximize the role of the family (Esping-Andersen 1990; Palier 2010). The more conservative systems, among which we place Latin American and Caribbean nations, are based on a traditional male-breadwinner model of family economics. The normative expectation of this approach is that the husband assumes responsibility for income generation, while the wife remains home to care for the household, children, and aging parents (Becker 1981; Esping-Andersen 1990; Horrell and Humphries 1997). Increasingly, even in Latin America that model of family economics is no longer universal. As part of the process of defamilisation, which as we describe is driven by extensive social and demographic changes including lower marriage and fertility rates, higher divorce rates, longer life spans, and the entry of women into the labor force, the State assumes a larger portion of the family's welfare and care functions (Esping-Andersen 1996; Michoń 2008).

We also employ the term "refamilisation" to refer to attempts to reaffirm and reestablish the family's role in the care of old and frail parents. These policies reflect long-standing traditions that are particularly resistant to change even as they are increasingly at odds with social transformations that have reduced the family's ability to provide extensive care and support. Although defamilisation remains far less pronounced in Latin

America and other developing regions than in higher-income nations, even there, non-contributory pensions and other services that we discuss in Chapter two are becoming more important as the family's ability to support and care for aging parents is reduced by the same social changes that have so profoundly affected the developed world. As we illustrate, those changes influence how civil society organizations frame the problems they address and the solutions they propose.

Frame Realignment

We use the term "frame" through the book in reference to the ways in which civil society organizations conceive of and communicate their objectives and attempt to convince a larger audience of the justice of their approaches. In Chapter three we introduce the concept of "frame alignment" to characterize the process of changing the public's perceptions of old age, as well as that of older persons themselves, from that of old age as a period of withdrawal and voluntary or involuntary disengagement from life, to that of old age as a period in which an older individual him or herself, as well as the community, can benefit from a lifetime of experience. One might think of the image of a picture frame that delimits and draws attention to a particular aspect of reality. As we discuss in Chapter three, "frame alignment processes" refer to ways in which social movements or groups attempt to convince a larger audience that their interpretation of some situation is accurate and that their proposed solutions are both just and likely to be effective (Goffman 1974; Snow et al. 1986). As we argue, it is important to understand how specific groups frame the causes of the problems they address in order to understand and evaluate their attempts to alter the status quo.

Objectives of the Book

In the following chapters we will examine the role of civil society organizations in advocating for and providing support and care to older people, many of whom have seriously diminished capacity and require special care. We also examine the extent to which these organizations and the social movements they are part of empower older individuals to act collectively to further their own interests, thereby enhancing active aging and effective citizenship. Latin America has been at the forefront of international efforts to codify the human and social rights of older people through numerous conventions. The extent to which these conventions have done more than simply state general principles and have actually resulted in national, regional, and local level protection of the human and social rights of older persons remains unclear, but what is clear is that a new discourse focused on human and social rights of older individuals and others is an important part of the rise in civil society action.

Historically in Latin America, as elsewhere the family has been the sole or primary guarantor of older parents' well-being. This remains the case in much of the developing world, including Mexico. We often romanticize this aspect of family life and overlook the serious conflicts that often characterize intergenerational family relations. Later we will discuss the problem of children dispossessing their aging parents of their homes, or condemning them to deplorable living conditions. As life expectancy at birth and older ages rises dramatically it is unlikely that we will return to some romanticized past of family solidarity and filial piety. Nor will the state be able to address all of the day-to-day needs of individuals in their communities. This new reality serves as the motivation for what we deal with in this book. If traditional communities are disappearing our human interdependence and our inability to live purely solitary lives makes it imperative that we examine how strangers can assume some of the roles we have traditionally attributed to families.

In our analysis of the growing role of the non-governmental sector we summarize many of the social changes that are altering the roles of the family and the state in the care and support of individuals. Since the end of the 19th Century the state has assumed a growing responsibility for ensuring the welfare of minor children, the disabled, individuals with serious medical conditions, and others. In this book we focus specifically on older individuals, who because of age and the serious functional limitations that often accompany it are at high risk of dependency and the loss of autonomy. Our objective is to examine the institutional arrangements that are available for their care and how those are changing in a middle-income nation. Our unique contribution is to examine the role of the non-profit sector in complementing state efforts or assuming an activist and potentially adversarial role to pressure the state to live up to its obligations to vulnerable citizens.

Our ultimate goal is to illustrate the roles of civil society in furthering the social, as well as political rights of citizens. We focus heavily on the actual and potential role of CSOs in Mexico in dealing with rapidly growing challenges associated with population aging. Mexico, like most other developing and developed nations, is aging at a truly astonishing pace. This demographic transition, which we discuss in detail in Chapter two, is accompanied by numerous social changes that place growing strains on public budgets and that diminish the capacity of the family to fulfil its traditional role of sole provider of material and emotional support to aging parents. Lower fertility and smaller families, migration patterns that separate families on the basis of generation, limited resources, and greatly increased life spans often accompanied by lengthy periods of serious physical and cognitive decline can seriously strain or completely overwhelm the capacity of families to cope.

Although civil society organizations are clearly no substitute for the state, they have become increasingly important players at every level of public and political life in all nations. Although civil society organizations do not exercise direct power, nor serve as democratically elected representatives of the groups they serve, they represent an important aspect of more direct democracy, at least ideally. Of course, not all civil society organizations are progressive in the sense usually attributed to that term, nor are they inclusive of interests other than those of their membership. Indeed, it is not always clear what organizations or political orientations the concept encompasses (Foley and Edwards 1996; Kenny et al. 2017). Nor is the very concept of civil society directly applicable from one society or culture to another (Bebbington, Hickey, and Mitlin 2008; Chambers and Kymlicka 2002; Kenny et al. 2017; Lewis 2002). Yet in an historical period in which disillusionment with political parties, particularly those of the center and left, is growing and in which the populist rejection of democratic institutions and procedures is becoming more common, this domain of collective activity emerges as central to understanding the full range of actors that influence public policy.

Outline of Subsequent Chapters

The following eight chapters cover various themes related to the emerging discourse on human and social rights that has emerged after the return of democracy to the nations of Latin America. Although we deal with human and social rights more generally, we focus specifically on the role of CSOs in addressing the situation of older individuals. We focus specifically on changes in the post-World War II welfare state that are resulting in varying degrees of defamilisation of social care and the shift from an exclusive reliance on the family to a greater reliance on the State. It is in this context that we locate the growing presence of civil society organizations and the social movements of which they are a manifestation.

We address the question as to whether the increase in the number of these organizations represents an increase in direct democracy and the empowerment of those previously marginalized, or the spread of a fragmenting identity politics that reflects the decline of traditional party politics. As we show, neither perspective adequately characterizes what is going on, but it is clear that the growth of particular identities and the spread of identity politics reflects a rejection of traditional hierarchical political and economic arrangements that gave short shrift to gender, racial, ethnic, religious, age, and other differences. We argue that despite the potential limitations in the ability of CSOs to significantly alter the status quo, the limitations that both the State and family increasingly face in providing the support that dependent older individuals need makes understanding the potential role of CSOs vital. These organizations will continue to play an important role in advocacy for and service delivery to older persons, if for no other reason than that there are few other options.

In Chapter two we discuss the defamilisation of social care that has accompanied the rise of the welfare state, by which we mean the growing role of the state in providing financial and material support to individuals in need. Nations differ greatly in the extent to which family policy is based on defamilisation or refamilisation. The social democratic nations of northern Europe manifest high degrees of defamilisation, whereas the more conservative and corporatist nations of central and southern Europe, as well as those of Latin America, have remained highly familistic and cling to policies that look to the family for the care and support of older parents.

In Chapter three we introduce the new Human Rights discourse as it has evolved in Mexico and Latin America and the Caribbean more generally. We introduce the concept of "frame realignment" to summarize attempts to alter public images of older persons, as well as older individuals' own self-image, from that of the old as obsolete, unproductive, and uninvolved recipients of care and charity to that of older individuals as active, productive, and engaged members of the community. A core aspect of this new Human Rights agenda is the affirmation of social rights, which include the right to the material and social means to live a dignified life. In this chapter we summarize the major international conventions concerning the human and social rights of older persons and discuss the extent to which those international conventions have affected national and more local laws and their enforcement related to the rights of the older individuals.

In Chapter four we develop the concepts of active aging and active citizenship. Many CSOs and social movements are involved in fostering active aging, a concept that includes encouraging and supporting social and even political engagement by older citizens. The objective of these organizations is to get older individuals to recognize that they are potentially active contributors to their own support and welfare, and also to that of the community. Active aging from this perspective implies and requires active citizenship. As we illustrate in later chapters, while enhancing the quality of life of older individuals is a central objective of most CSOs, some directly challenge the status quo and take as a core objective raising the consciousness of older individuals themselves so that they can compel the state to recognize and protect their basic rights, as well as those of citizens generally.

In Chapter five we discuss the economic, political, legal, and cultural context in which CSOs operate in Mexico. We review the various federal and state laws that govern formal registration of such organizations. Many non-governmental and community organizations with different degrees of formal organization exist in Mexico and other nations. We focus on those that fit the formal definitions of CSOs by federal and state laws. Unfortunately, there is no complete census of such organizations so our examination is based on a convenience sample of CSOs from various cities in

Mexico in which we have contacts. We present various organizations with different frames of reference ranging from a fairly narrow focus on improving their members' physical and mental quality of life to fairly politicized objectives including insuring pensions for their members and insuring adequate social rights to citizens in general.

In Chapters six through eight we examine specific CSOs with different missions and frames of reference. These missions and frames overlap and many organizations focus on more than one set of objectives, but those we deal with can be usefully classified in terms of their focus on preserving or enhancing the quality of life, assuring older individuals' human and social rights, which include the right to the basic material necessities of a dignified life, and defending their political and human rights more generally. The specific emphasis of any particular organization reflects its history as well as the social and occupational background of its membership.

In Chapter six we examine organizations that consist of retired union members, government employees, teachers, university professors, or other highly-educated professionals. We begin with these groups since they were among the first to engage in active collective conflicts with employers and the state. Many are highly educated, and others have been life-long activists. These individuals have high levels of human and cultural capital and often maintain contacts with their unions and professional organizations to which they belonged in their working years. This higher level of institutional as well as human capital gives them valuable leverage in making demands of the state and protecting their members' human and social rights.

In Chapter seven we examine organizations that focus on participants' quality of life, which includes preserving and enhancing their physical health through exercise and group activities, as well as socialization and community participation to enhance psychological health and avoid isolation. These organizations consist largely of individuals with lower levels of education, few resources, and little formal labor force experience. A large fraction of the memberships of these organizations are women who were housewives, mothers, and caregivers and who have no resources of their own. For them the organizations to which they belong are truly extensions of the family. Their interactions with others, and the organizations' focus on preserving or even improving physical and mental health and avoiding isolation clearly enhances the quality of their lives. Unlike organizations whose members were union activists, government employees, or who have high levels of education these organizations are less political or activist, but even they foster a civic consciousness in their members that reflects a changing sense of the possibilities for mature adulthood.

In Chapter eight we present examples of organizations that go beyond a concern with quality of life to advocate for their members' human and social rights, as well as those of citizens generally. These organizations can be seen as outgrowths of the labor movement and union activism, combined with a concern for enhancing the quality of life. As Mexicans reject traditional clientelist, corporatist, and corrupt political parties, these organizations represent a growing direct democracy that emerges out of earlier union struggles and social movements by various marginalized groups. For these organizations the preservation and extension of social rights is central. Given the fact that fewer than half of older Mexicans have an employment-based pension or receive a formal government pension, most older individuals depend on newly introduced non-contributory pensions. For CSOs, assuring that their participants are aware of and receive the state-sponsored support they are due represents a major objective.

Chapter nine concludes with a summary of the good and the bad aspects of civil society organizations, and what lies ahead as we move deeper into the 21st Century. We reflect on the future of old-age support policies and the role of CSOs in advocacy and support of the older persons given their recent history and growing influence. As we emphasize throughout the book, civil society organizations are no substitute for a beneficent and efficient state. In fact, CSOs find it difficult to function effectively in the face of state opposition or a lack of acceptance of their legitimate role. In such situations, which reflect those in many nations today, and in Latin America during repressive periods, their role remains that of an adversary to the established order. To varying degrees that role remains a core frame for organizations that are committed to improving the lot of marginalized groups, including that of older people. As we point out, without the political power that only an organized party or major social movement can muster, the possibilities for civil society may be limited.

It might be tempting or easy to take an idealized view of civil society organizations as progressive and fundamentally concerned with the welfare of those in need. As we note throughout our discussion, though, civil society organizations are not always progressive or interested in the general welfare. They can be parochial, exclusive, and exclusionary, and they can work to marginalize others. Yet they are an increasingly important and probably inevitable part of modern society. Their influence has clearly been enhanced by modern media and transportation technologies. Yet, as we discuss, rather than leading to a growing cosmopolitanism, social media makes it possible for one to communicate and share ideas only with like-minded individuals. How this new communications technology will affect civil society and governance in general in the future remains to be seen.

References

Adkins, Julie, Laurie Occhipinti, and Tara Heferan (Eds.). 2010. *Not by Faith Alone: Social Services, Social Justice, and Faith-Based Organization in the United States*. New York, NY: Lexington Books.

Aguila, Emma, Nelly Mejia, Francisco Perez-Arce, Edgar Ramirez, and Alfonso Rivera Illingworth. 2016. "Costs of Extending the Noncontributory Pension Program for Elderly: The Mexican Case." *Journal of Aging & Social Policy* 28 (4):325–343.

Albrow, Martin, Helmut Anheier, Marlies Glasius, Monroe Price, and Mary Kaldor (Eds.). 2008. *Global Civil Society 2007/8*. Thousand Oaks, CA: Sage.

Ammerman, Nancy Tatom. 2005. *Pillars of Faith: American Congregations and Their Partners*. Berkeley, CA: University of California Press.

Angel, Jacqueline L., William Vega, and Mariana López-Ortega. 2017. "Aging in Mexico: Population Trends and Emerging Issues." *The Gerontologist* 57 (2):153–162.

Babb, Sarah. 2013. "The Washington Consensus as Transnational Policy Paradigm: Its Origins, Trajectory and Likely Successor." *Review of International Political Economy* 20 (2):268–297.

Babb, Sarah, and Alexander Kentikelenis. 2018. "International Financial Institutions as Agents of Neoliberalism." In *Handbook of Neoliberalism*, edited by Damien Cahill, Melinda Cooper, Martijn Konings, and David Primrose. Thousand Oaks, CA: Sage. Retrieved 8/18/2009 from http://www.kentikelenis.net/up loads/3/1/8/9/31894609/babbkentikelenis2018-international_financial_institu tions_as_agents_of_neoliberalism.pdf.

Bayón, María Cristina (Ed.). 2019. *Las grietas del neoliberalismo: Dimensiones de la desigualdad contemporánea en México*. Coyoacán, México: Universidad Nacional Autónoma de México, Instituto de Investigaciones Sociales.

Bebbington, Anthony J., Samuel Hickey, and Diana C.Mitlin. 2008. *Can NGOs Make a Difference: The Challenge of Development Alternatives*. London, UK: ZED Books.

Becker, Gary S. 1981. *A Treatise on the Family*. Cambridge, MA: Harvard University Press.

Bendaña, Alejandro. 2006. "NGOs and Social Movements: A North/South Divide?" United Nations Research Institute for Social Development, Paper 22. New York, NY: United Nations.

Boli, John, and George M. Thomas. 1997. "World Culture in the World Polity: A Century of International Non-Governmental Organization." *American Sociological Review* 62 (2):171–190.

Boli, John, and George M. Thomas (Eds.). 1999. *Constructing World Culture: International Nongovernmental Organizations Since 1875*. Stanford, CA: Stanford University Press.

Borland, Elizabet. 2006. "The Mature Resistance of Argentina's Madres de Plaza de Mayo." Pp. 115–130 in *Latin American Social Movements: Globalization, Democratization, and Transnational Networks*, edited by Hank Johnston and Paul Almeida. New York, NY: Rowman & Littlefield.

Cameron, Maxwell A. 2009. "Latin America's Left Turns: Beyond Good and Bad." *Third World Quarterly* 30 (2):331–347.

Campbell, John L. 2004. *Institutional Change and Globalization*. Princeton, NJ: Princeton University Press.

Campbell, John L, and Ove K. Pedersen (Eds.). 2001a. *The Rise of Neoliberalism and Institutional Analysis*. Princeton, NJ: Princeton University Press.

Campbell, John L., and Ove K. Pedersen. 2001b. "Introduction: The Rise of Neolibralism and Institutional Analysis." Pp. 1–23 in *The Rise of Neoliberalism and Institutional Analysis*, edited by John L. Campbell and Ove K. Pedersen. Princeton, NJ: Princeton University Press.

Carroll, Thomas. 1992. *Intermediary NGOs: The Supporting Link in Grassroots Development*. West Hartford, CN: Kumarian Press.

CEPAL. 2007. "Demographic Trends in Latin America in Observatorio demográfico N° 3: Proyecretción de población." Retrieved 1/25/2019 from http://www.eclac.cl/publicaciones/xml/0/32650/OD-3-Demographic.pdf.

CEPAL. 2017. "Derechos de las persona mayores: Retos para la interdependencia y autonomía." Retrieved 9/15/2017 from https://www.cepal.org/es/publicaciones/41471-derechos-personas-mayores-retos-la-interdependencia-autonomia.

Chambers, Simone, and Will Kymlicka (Eds.). 2002. *Alternative Conceptions of Civil Society*. Princeton, NJ: Princeton University Press.

CONADEP. 1984. "Report of Conadep (National Commission on the Disappearance of Persons)." Retrieved 8/11/2019 from http://web.archive.org/web/20031013222809/http://nuncamas.org/english/library/nevagain/nevagain_002.htm.

Cotlear, Daniel (Ed.). 2011. *Population Aging: Is Latin America Ready?* Washington, DC: The World Bank.

DeMars, William E., and Dennis Dijkzeul. 2015. *The NGO Challenge for International Relations Theory*. New York, NY: Routledge.

Dillon, Sam. 1998. "Mexico City Journal: Anniversary of '68 Massacre Brings Facts to Light." *New York Times*. Retrieved 8/11/2019 from https://www.nytimes.com/1998/09/14/world/mexico-city-journal-anniversary-of-68-massacre-brings-facts-to-light.html.

Eade, Deborah (Ed.). 2000. *Development, NGOs, and Civil Society: Selected Essays from Development in Practice*. Oxford, UK: Oxfam GB.

Edelman. 2018. "2018 Edelman Trust Barometer Global Report." Retrieved 7/5/2019 from https://www.edelman.com/sites/g/files/aatuss191/files/2018-10/2018_Edelman_Trust_Barometer_Global_Report_FEB.pdf.

Edwards, Michael. 2014. *Civil Society* Cambridge, UK: Polity Press.

Ehrenberg, John. 2017. *Civil Society: The Critical History of an Idea*, Second Edition. New York, NY: New York University Press.

Encarnación, Omar G. 2018. "The Rise and Fall of the Latin American Left: Conservatives Now Control Latin America's Leading Economies, But the Region's Leftists Can Still Look to Uruguay for Direction." *The Nation*. Retrieved 8/19/2019 from https://www.thenation.com/article/the-ebb-and-flow-of-latin-americas-pink-tide/.

Escalante Gonzalbo, Fernando. 2016. *Historia mínima del neoliberalismo*. Mexico City: El Colegio de México, A.C.

Esping-Andersen, Gøsta. 1990. *The Three Worlds of Welfare Capitalism*. Princeton, NJ: Princeton University Press.

Esping-Andersen, Gøsta. 1996. "Welfare States without Work: The Impasse of Labor Shedding and Familialism in Continental European Social Policy." Pp. 66–87 in *Welfare States in Transition: National Adaptations in Global Economics*, edited by Gøsta Esping-Andersen. Thousand Oaks, CA: Sage.

Estes, Carroll. 2001a. *Social Policy and Aging: A Critical Perspective*. Thousand Oaks, CA: Sage.

Estes, Carroll L. 2001b. "Crisis, the Welfare State, and Aging: Ideology and Agency in the Social Security Privatization Debate." Pp. 95–117 in *Social Policy and Aging: A Critical Perspective*, edited by Carroll L. Estes and Associates. Thousand Oaks, CA: Sage.

Estes, Carroll L. 2011. "Crises and Old Age Policy." Pp. 297–320 in *Handbook of Sociology of Aging*, edited by Richard A.SetterstenJr. and Jacqueine L. Angel. New York, NY: Springer.

Fisher, William F. 1997. "Doing Good? The Politics and Antipolitics of NGO Practices." *Annual Review of Anthropology* 26:439–464.

Foley, Michael W., and Bob Edwards. 1996. "The Paradox of Civil Society." *Journal of Democracy* 7:38–52.

Garrard, Virginia. 2017. "Living with Ghosts: Death, Exhumation, and Reburial among the Maya in Guatemala." Pp. 133–144 in *Memory, Truth, and Justice in Contemporary Latin America*, edited by Roberta Villalón. New York, NY: Rowman & Littlefield.

Global Policy Forum. 2010. "*Paper on NGO Participation at the United Nations.*" New York, NY: United Nations.

Goffman, Erving. 1974. *Frame Analysis*. Cambridge, MA: Harvard University Press.

Grzybowski, Candido. 2000. "We NGOs: A Controversial Way of Being and Acting." *Development in Practice* 10 (3–4):436–444.

Hall-Jones, Peter. 2006. "The Rise and Rise of NGOs." Global Policy Forum. Retrieved 12/6/2017 from https://www.globalpolicy.org/component/content/a rticle/176/31937.html.

Hancock, Lanon H. (Ed.). 2016. *Narratives of Identity in Social Movements, Conflicts and Change*. Bingley, UK: Emerald Group Publishing.

Herbert, David. 2003. *Religion and Civil Society: Rethinking Public Religion in the Contemporary World*. Burlington, VT: Ashgate.

Holloway, John. 2002. *Change the World Without Taking Power*. New York, NY: Pluto Press.

Holloway, John. 2010. *Crack Capitalism*. New York, NY: Pluto Press.

Horrell, Sara, and Jane Humphries. 1997. "The Origins and Expansion of the Male Breadwinner Family: The Case of Nineteenth-Century Britain." *International Review of Social History* 42 (S5):25–64.

Huber, Evelyne, and John D. Stephens. 2001. *Development and Crisis of the Welfare State: Parties and Policies in Global Markets*. Chicago, IL: University of Chicago Press.

Huber, Evelyne, and John D. Stephens. 2012. *Democracy and the Left: Social Policy and Inequality in Latin America*. Chicago, IL: University of Chicago Press.

Hudock, Ann C. 1999. *NGOs and Civil Society: Democracy by Proxy?*Cambridge, UK: Polity Press.

Hujo, Katja (Ed.). 2014. *Reforming Pensions in Developing and Transition Countries*, United Nations, UNRISD. Basingstoke, UK: Palgrave Macmillan.

INEGI. 2010. "Censo de Población y Vivienda 2010." Retrieved 8/20/2019 from https://www.inegi.org.mx/app/biblioteca/ficha.html?upc=702825002042.

Issacharoff, Samuel. 2015. *Fragile Democracies: Contested Power in the Era of Constitutional Courts*. New York, NY: Routledge.

Jelin, Elizabeth, and Susana G. Kaufman (Eds.). 2006. *Subjetividad y figuras de la memoria*. Buenos Aires, Argentina: Siglo XXI Editora Iberoamericana S.A.

Kalache, Alexandre. 2013. "*The Longevity Revolution: Creating a Society for All Ages*." Adelaide, Australia: Government of South Australia.

Keck, Margaret, and Kathryn Sikkink. 1998. *Activists Beyond Borders: Advocacy Networks in International Politics*. Ithaca, NY: Cornell University Press.

Kenny, Sue, Marilyn Taylor, Jeny Onyx, and Marjorie Mayo. 2017. *Challenging the Third Sector: Global Prospect for Active Citizenship*. Chicago, IL: Policy Press c/o The University of Chicago Press.

Kinsella, K.G. 1992. "Changes in Life Expectancy 1900–1990." *The American Journal of Clinical Nutrition* 55 (6):1196–1202.

Kochhar, Rakesh. 2014. "10 Projections for the Global Population in 2050." Pew Research Center. Retrieved 11/7/2015 from http://www.pewresearch.org/fact-tank/2014/02/03/10-projections-for-the-global-population-in-2050/.

Korpi, Walter. 2003. "Welfare-State Regress in Western Europe: Politics, Institutions, Globalization, and Europeanization." *Annual Review of Sociology* 29:589–609.

Lamb, Sarah (Ed.). 2017. *Successful Aging as a Contemporary Obsession: Global Perspectives*. New Brunswick, NJ: Rutgers University Press.

Lamb, Sarah. 2020. "'You Don't Have to Act or Feel Old': Successful Aging as a U.S. Cultural Project." Pp. 49–64 in *The Cultural Context of Aging: Worldwide Perspectives*, edited by Jay Sokolovsky. Santa Barbara, CA: Praeger.

Lechner, Norbert, and Pedro Güell. 2006. "Construcción Social de las Memorias en la Transición Chilena." Pp. 17–46 in *Subjetividades y Figuras de la Memoria*, edited by Elizabeth Jelin and Susana Kaufmann. Buenos Aires: Siglo XXI. Retrieved 8/11/2019 from https://www.archivochile.com/Ceme/recup_memoria/cemememo0024.pdf.

Lee, Taedong. 2010. "The Rise of International Nongovernmental Organizations: A Top-Down or Bottom-Up Explanation?" *VOLUNTAS: International Journal of Voluntary and Nonprofit Organizations* 21 (3):393–416.

Lewis, David. 2002. "Civil Society in African Contexts: Reflections on the Usefulness of a Concept." *Development and Change* 33 (4):569–586.

MacDonald, L., and A. Ruckert. 2009a. *Post-Neoliberalism in the Americas*. Basingstoke, UK: Palgrave Macmillan.

MacDonald, Laura, and Arne Ruckert. 2009b. "Post-Neoliberalism in the Americas: An Introduction." Pp. 1–18 in *Post-Neoliberalism in the Americas*, edited by Laura Macdonald and Arne Ruckert. Basingstoke, UK: Palgrave Macmillan.

Márquez, Gabriel García. 1993. *Cien Años de Soledad*. Buenos Aires: Editorial Sudamericana.

Mendelson, Sarah E., and John K. Glenn (Eds.). 2002. *The Power and Limits of NGOs: A Critical Look at Building Democracy in Eastern Europe and Eurasia*. New York, NY: Columbia University Press.

Mesa-Lago, Carmelo. 2008. *Reassembling Social Security: A Survey of Pensions and Health Care Reforms in Latin America*. New York, NY: Oxford University Press.

Meyer, Carrie A. 1999. *The Economics and Politics of NGOs in Latin America*. Westport, CT: Praeger.

Michoń, Piotr. 2008. "Familisation and Defamilisation Policy in 22 European Countries." *Poznań University of Economics Review* 8 (1):34–54.

Monsiváis, Carlos. 1987. *Entrada libre. Crónicas de la sociedad que se organiza.* Mexico City: Ediciones Era, S.A. de C.V.

Montes de Oca Zavala, Verónica. 2013. "La discriminación hacia la vejez en la ciudad de México: contrastes sociolpoliticos y jurídicos a nivel nacional y local." *Revista Perspectivas Sociales/Social Perspectives* 15 (1):47–80.

Montes de Oca Zavala, Verónica, and Paola Carmina Gutiérrez Cuellar. 2018. "La discriminación entre la población mexicana: una revisión para pensar avances y desafíos." Pp. 285–302 in *Por la igualdad somos mucho más que dos. 15 Años de lucha contra la discriminación en México,* edited by Mario Alfredo Hernández Sánchez, Yoloxóchitl Casas Chousal and Marcela Azuela Gómez. Mexico City: CONAPRED and SEGOB.

Mora, Mariana. 2008. "Zapatista Anti-Capitalist Politics and the 'Other Campaign.' Learning from the Struggle for Indigenous Rights and Autonomy." Pp. 151–164 in *Latin American Social Movements in the Twenty-first Century: Resistance, Power, and Democracy,* edited by Richard Stahler-Sholk, Harry E. Vanden, and Glen David Kuecker. New York, NY: Rowman & Littlefield.

Motta, Sara C. 2009. "New Ways of Making and Living Politics: The Movimiento de Trabajadores Desocupados de Solano and the 'Movement of Movements'." *Bulletin of Latin American Research* 28 (1):83–101.

Motta, Sara C. 2014. "Latin America: Reinventing Revolutions, an 'Other' Politics in Practice and Theory." Pp. 21–42 in *Rethinking Latin American Social Movements: Radical Action from Below,* edited by Richard Stahler-Sholk, Harry E. Vanden, and Marc Becler. New York, NY: Rowman & Littlefield.

Nelson, Brian A. 2019. "Hugo Chávez." Encycloaedia Britannica. Retrieved 8/20/2019 from https://www.britannica.com/biography/Hugo-Chavez.

O'Cinneide, Colm. 2014. "Austerity and the Faded Dream of a Social Europe." Pp. 169–201 in *Economic and Social Rights after the Global Financial Crisis,* edited by Aoife Nolan. Cambridge, UK: Cambridge University Press.

Olvera, Alberto J. 2001. *Movimientos Sociales Prodemocráticos, Democratización y Esfera Pública en México: el caso de Alianza Cívica.* Jalapa, Mexico: Universidad Veracruzana, Cuadernos de la Sociedad Civil, no. 6.

Olvera, Alberto J. 2004. "Civil Society in Mexico at Century's End." Pp. 403–439 in *Dilemmas of Political Change in Mexico,* edited by Kevin J. Middlebrook. London, UK: Institute for Latin American Studies.

Olvera, Alberto J. 2010. "The Elusive Democracy: Political Parties, Democratic Institutions, and Civil Society in Mexico." *Latin American Research Review* 45:79–107.

Palier, Bruno (Ed.). 2010. *A Long Goodbye to Bismark? The Politics of Welfare Reform in Continental Europe.* Amsterdam: Amsterdam University Press.

Panizza, Francisco. 2005. "Unarmed Utopia Revisited: The Resurgence of Left-of-Centre Politics in Latin America." *Political Studies* 53 (4):716–734.

Partida-Bush, Virgilio. 2002. "Demographic Transition, Demographic Bonus and Aging in Mexico." Mexico City: CONAPO. Retrieved 5/15/2021 from https://www.un.org/en/development/desa/population/events/pdf/expert/9/partida.pdf: CONAPO.

Pearce, Jenny. 2004. "Collective Action or Public Participation? Complementary or Contradictory Democratisation Strategies in Latin America?" *Bulletin of Latin American Research* 23 (4):483–504.

Pichardo, Nelson A. 1997. "New Social Movements: A Critical Review." *Annual Review of Sociology* 23:411–430.

Poniatowska, Elena. 1980. *Fuerte es el silencio*. Mexico City: Era.

Robinson, M., and R. Riddell. 1995. *Non-Governmental Organizations and Poverty Alleviation*New York, NY: Oxford University Press.

Rodda, John. 1968. "How the Guardian reported Mexico City's Tlatelolco massacre of 1968." *The Guardian*. Retrieved 8/11/2019 from https://www.thegua rdian.com/cities/from-the-archive-blog/2015/nov/12/guardian-mexico-tlatelolco-massacre-1968-john-rodda.

Ruggie, John Gerard. 1998. "What Makes the World Hang Together? Neo-Utilitarianism and the Social Constructivist Challenge." *International Organization* 52 (4):855–885.

Salamon, Lester M. 2003. *The Resilient Sector: The State of Nonprofit America*. Washington, D.C.: Brookings Institution Press.

Salamon, Lester M., and Helmut K. Anheier. 1996a. "The International Classification of Nonprofit Organizations: ICNPO-Revision 1, 1996." Working Papers of the Johns Hopkins Comparative Nonprofit Sector Project, No 19. Baltimore, MD: The Johns Hopkins Institute for Policy Studies.

Salamon, Lester M., and Helmut K. Anheier. 1996b. *The Emerging Sector: An Overview*. Manchester, UK: Manchester University Press.

Salamon, Lester M., and Helmut K. Anheier. 1998. "Social Origins of Civil Society: Explaining the Nonprofit Sector Cross-Nationally." *VOLUNTAS: International Journal of Voluntary and Nonprofit Organizations* 9 (3):213–248.

Salamon, Lester M., Helmut K. Anheier, Regina List, Stefan Toepler, S. Wojciech Sokolowsk, and Associates. 1999. *Global Civil Society: Dimensions of the Nonprofit Sector*. Baltimore, MD: The Johns Hopkins University Press.

Shefner, Jon, George Paskirtz, and Corey Blad. 2006. "Austerity Protests and Immiserating Growth in Mexico and Argentina." Pp. 19–41 in *Latin American Social Movements: Globalization, Democratization, and Transnational Networks*, edited by Hank Johnston and Paul Almeida. New York, NY: Rowman & Littlefield.

Sitrin, Mariana (Ed.). 2006. *Horizontalism: Voices of Popular Power in Argentina*. Oakland, CA: AK Press.

Sitrin, Mariana. 2014. "Argentina: Against and Beyond the State." Pp. 209–232 in *Rethinking Latin American Social Movements: Radical Action from Below*, edited by Richard Stahler-Sholk, Harry E. Vanden, and Marc Becker. New York, NY: Rowman & Littlefield.

Snow, David, Jr., E. Burke Rochford, Steven K. Worden, and Robert D. Benford. 1986. "Frame Alignment Processes, Micromobilization, and Movement Participation." *American Sociological Review* 51:464–481.

Stahler-Sholk, Richard. 2014. "Mexico: Autonomy, Collective Identity, and the Zapatista Social Movement." Pp. 187–207 in *Rethinking Latin American Social Movements: Radical Action from Below*, edited by Richard Stahler-Sholk, Harry E. Vanden, and Marc Becker. New York, NY: Rowman & Littlefield.

Stahler-Sholk, Richard, Harry E. Vanden, and Marc Becker (Eds.). 2014. *Rethinking Latin American Social Movements: Radical Action from Below*. New York, NY: Rowman & Littlefield.

Stahler-Sholk, Richard, Harry E. Vanden, and Glen David Kuecker (Eds.). 2008. *Latin American Social Movements in the Twenty-first Century: Resistance, Power, and Democracy*. New York, NY: Rowman & Littlefield.

Stiglitz, Joseph E. 2008. "Is There a Post-Washington Consensus?" Pp. 41–56 in *The Washington Consensus Reconsidered: Towards a New Global Governance*, edited by Narcís Serra and Joseph E. Stiglitz. New York, NY: Oxford University Press.

Swords, Alicia C.S. 2008. "Neo-Zapatist Network Politics: Transforming Democracy and Development." Pp. 291–305 in *Latin American Social Movements in the Twenty-first Century*, edited by Richard Stahler-Sholk, Harry E. Vanden, and Glen David Kuecker. New York, NY: Rowman & Littlefield.

United States Institute for Peace. 1997. "Truth Commission: Guatemala." Retrieved 8/11/2019 from https://www.usip.org/publications/1997/02/truth-commission-guatemala.

Villalón, Roberta (Ed.). 2017. *Memory, Truth, and Justice in Contemporary Latin America*. New York: Rowman & Littlefield.

Williamson, John. 2004. "The Strange History of the Washington Consensus." *Journal of Post Keynesian Economics* 27 (2):195–206.

Willmore, Larry. 2014. "Old Age Pensions in Mexico: Toward Universal Coverage." Social Science Research Network. Retrieved 9/11/2015 from http://dx.doi.org/10.2139/ssrn.2383768.

World Health Organization. 2002. *Active Aging: A Policy Framework*. Geneva, Switzerland: WHO.

World Health Organization. 2007. *Global Age-friendly Cities: A Guide*. Geneva, Switzerland: WHO.

Wright, Glen W. 2012. "NGOs and Western Hegemony: Causes for Concern and Ideas for Change." *Development in Practice* 22 (1):123–134.

Wuthnow, Robert. 1996. *Christianity and Civil Society*. Valley Forge, PA: Trinity Press International.

Young, Kevin, and Michael Schwartz. 2012. "Can Prefigurative Politics Prevail? The Implications for Movement Strategy in John Holloway's Crack Capitalism." *Journal of Classical Sociology* 12 (2):220–239.

Chapter 2

Defamilisation and the Welfare State

A Life-Long Commitment

On October 11, 2009 Mexican President Felipe Calderon Hinojosa ordered the liquidation of the state-owned electrical company Luz y Fuerza del Centro (Central Light and Power) that provided power to Mexico City, and transferred its functions to the Mexican Federal Electricity Commission (CFE). Forty-four thousand members of the Sindicato de Electricistas de México, SME (the Union of Mexican Electrical Workers), were left without jobs. Retirees and dismissed employees engaged in a struggle for their rights and for reinstatement. Reynaldo Bastida Sáenz, a retired union member, describes what the company and the union have meant to him and other retirees. As Mr. Saenz reveals, retirees remain close to the union.

SÁENZ: Our organization consists of retirees of Central Light and Power and we belong to the Union of Mexican Electrical Workers with a history [going back] one hundred years. It has a marvelous history. Thanks to the union we retired with all the benefits that we fortunately have. We had a more or less [economically secure] life and besides that, they give us the opportunity to participate in the work of the union. Our objectives include preserving democracy for our fellow workers who [wish to return to] work here, and [to make sure they are not hired for] only a few months, but that they get something substantial. For example, we were able to retire after thirty years, but we are at the end of that contract. Right now, the new hires who resisted when [the power company] was liquidated are about to go to work … but they are starting from scratch, they were let go and they must start again … the objective of the union, is to get long-term jobs and get a pension or retirement.

INTERVIEWER: Could you describe the profile of the people who belong to the organization?

SÁENZ: The people who belong to the organization are almost family. That is, since the organization began, they [had] their children join. For example, my dad got me in, I got one of my sons in, and so on. Really, it is a family business, that can be said. And the objective is

DOI: 10.4324/9781003205609-2

like a school, because we begin by grabbing a broom and sweeping, until we reach a managerial post. They give us the opportunity to earn a university degree while we are working ... to improve ourselves intellectually or culturally. In my case, I spent ten years in the operating department ... as a mechanic, I even reached the level of a maintenance mechanic. I finished a training course and I switched to accounting ... and from there I retired [but they still] talk to me all the time; that allows me to be active.

INTERVIEWER: At what age do you retire?

SÁENZ: There are people who retire at 45 years old because they [began at] 14 ... In my case, I [retired after] thirty years as established in the contract. Our style of life as retirees here is not like in other places because [when we] left an operational department we left with a trade as an electrician, as a mechanic, as a bricklayer, as a carpenter, but we left with a trade. Many administrative workers retire as accountants, as editors etc. We have everything here in our company, from laborers to mechanical engineers or dentists all that ... They are given the opportunity here. Many continue to work here [in their own offices]; many others go to look for work elsewhere. But the real benefit that we had was retirement because [we had] all the benefits that no other company provides and we have the opportunity to advise our leaders, another very great prerogative that they do not offer anywhere else. It gives life to us retirees. All this was built by retirees and workers in years past, retirees ... continue to contribute.

INTERVIEWER: Could you describe some of the activities carried out in the organization?

SÁENZ: Retirees and pensioners have political groups, in which we dedicate ourselves to studying issues related to the laws ... in order to [have an informed] opinion; there are like fifteen or twenty groups. We worked for private initiatives and foreign companies for almost twenty years, we had everything ... but the government began to take everything away from us. But they did get us the benefit [as retirees of keeping the same benefits as before].

INTERVIEWER: Are there other cultural activities?

SÁENZ: We have soccer groups for retirees and tournaments ... We have fellow workers who have artistic aptitudes, who offer their services when there are events ... for example, [there are] those who sing rancheros, there are those [with theater experience], those who give Hawaiian dance lessons to the daughters of workers. They keep moving even as retirees.

INTERVIEWER: How often are these activities carried out and who can participate?

SÁENZ: Everyone who likes it, for example the theater, most of them are children of workers. In the ballet it is the girls. Soccer is for children and retirees lead the teams; they are mostly grandparents. Here all events are open to members. For the most part we get together for events for children; we collect toys for children on Kings Day and all that; all retirees contribute.

INTERVIEWER: In the organization have you heard of active aging? Is it encouraged?

SÁENZ: Our retirement is another method of aging, because fortunately we are assured of our daily bread, and workers who participate and who do not participate are dedicated to taking care of their children, they support them. So, aging here is different, here there are people who left work and missed their work, but little by little we helped them to get out of that, we supported them so that they did not fall into depression. Many of us begin to study, we begin to do something else, to give advice, to train. So that one ages in a different way.

INTERVIEWER: From your point of view, what would you understand by active aging?

SÁENZ: I say that active aging is taking advantage of the knowledge that one has ... so as not to lose memory, it is like an exercise. Taking care of yourself physically, doing more sports, also [remaining intellectually active] and being with your family is very important ...

INTERVIEWER: Are the rights of older adults promoted within the organization?

SÁENZ: Yes, we have a good idea of them; when they bring us the INAPAM card (Mexico's discount card for seniors) then fellow workers come to tell us about rights, also about social security. We are aware of everything we are entitled to and we ask about them. They gave us some pamphlets where all our legal and medical rights are explained ... Our union is the only one that still retains democratic rights, people admire that and for that reason they have supported us; we elect our leaders by direct and secret vote. That is something that society admires, even worldwide.

An Extended Family

These excerpts from an interview with a very active and engaged union retiree reveals the close association between retired workers and the electrical workers union. Mexican electrical workers have been very militant and have opposed the government's attempts to privatize the industry. The retirees of the electrical workers union are unique in that they retain a strong identity with the union, rather than forming an entirely separate organization. As Saenz explained, the union and the retiree groups take on aspects of family. As in his case, workers sponsored their family members for jobs, and with the union's support the enterprise became more than just an employer. These workers were clearly unique in the extent of benefits they enjoyed. The close association between the union and retired workers remains a source of belonging and of meaning, as well as a venue for demanding worker and retiree rights. Although not all ex-workers participate, those that do enter a new and active stage in life. As we discuss in later chapters, the missions and objectives of retiree organizations are influenced by the social and cultural capital of their members, as well as the organizational and political environments in which they operate (Angel, Montes-de-Oca Zavala, and Rodríguez 2018). Retiree organizations made up of individuals with union backgrounds, with government service experience, or backgrounds that provide experience in business or social mobilization are very different than those that consist of individuals with less cultural and social capital.

In the following chapters we present different civil society organizations that provide services to or advocate for older people. They are motivated by a wide range of objectives, and different ways of framing the issues they address. We discussed the concept of "framing" in Chapter three. In general, the term refers to how an organization explains a particular situation and the ways in which it might be changed. These objectives range from that of improving the quality of life of the people they serve by enhancing physical and emotional health and encouraging social engagement, to advocacy and political action aimed at forcing agencies of the State to address the needs of citizens and respect their human and social rights. Some organizations engage in a range of activities from support to advocacy. Many address multiple problems and the needs of individuals of different ages, motivated primarily by the grinding need of so much of humanity and a genuine desire to alleviate it. In addition to the cultural and social capital of their participants, the organizations we discuss are also constrained by the economic and political contexts in which they operate, as well as their relation to governmental agencies, unions, political parties, and other organizations.

Before proceeding, though, we review the degree of poverty in Mexico and the changing roles of the family and the State in the economic and social support of older individuals. These determine the range of issues that civil society organizations address, as well as their room for maneuver. Even as its role is changing, the family remains the main source of social and instrumental support in Latin America and the Caribbean, as it does in the highly familistic nations of central and southern Europe (Esping-Andersen 1990; Palier 2010). Nonetheless, even in a context characterized by strong familistic values and a strong sense of filial piety, income support and health care are increasingly provided by the State, which is limited of course by its fiscal capacity to do so.

The Extent of Need: Multidimensional Poverty

The changing role of the family and the State in the support of older citizens in Mexico occurs against the backdrop of serious poverty among all age groups. Let us briefly summarize the extent of poverty among older individuals and compare their situation to that of younger groups. We employ data provided by the Consejo Nacional de Evaluación de la Política de Desarrollo Social, CONEVAL (National Council for the Evaluation of Social Development Policy), an agency of the federal government that provides information on poverty, disability, and other social characteristics among various segments of the total population and that of specific states (CONEVAL 2020). The afflictions of poverty are seriously compounded by mental and physical disability since the disabled are at greatly elevated risk of poverty (SEDESOL 2016) and, of course, the risk of disability increases with age, creating a triple jeopardy for the old, the poor, and the infirm (INEGI 2017a).

In the Unites States poverty is assessed on the basis of a measure that compares an individual's or household's income to officially established poverty thresholds (US Census Bureau 2019). These were originally based on a minimally adequate food basket and have been adjusted over time. Much debate continues over the reasonableness and accuracy of the official measure, but it remains conceptually the same today as when it was introduced. Mexico has gone further and is the first nation to officially adopt a multidimensional operationalization of poverty. This operationalization begins with an estimation of income adequacy based on the cost of food and non-food based baskets of basic necessities, similar to what is done in the U.S., but it also takes account of social rights, that is, access to the basic physical and social necessities of a dignified and healthy life (CONEVAL 2014). These include education, measured negatively in terms of a household's average educational deficit, access to health services, access to social security, size and quality of the living space, adequate nutrition, the degree of social cohesion (a concept that taps various dimensions of social access and participation), and the degree of access to a paved road. This set of measures has been carefully thought out and is highly relevant to Mexico where it reveals a stark reality.

The Mexican government has introduced an important refinement of the measure that differentiates between those living in what we might term moderate poverty and those living in extreme poverty. The first group consists of individuals in households with incomes below the well-being threshold (Línea de Bienestar Económico, LBE), conceptually equivalent to the official poverty thresholds in the U.S., but who also suffer a deficit in at least one of the social dimensions. In 2019 the well-being thresholds for individuals were 2,056.85 pesos, or roughly $110.07 US per month in rural areas, and 3,176.95 pesos, or $170.01 US per month in urban areas.

Extreme poverty is defined on the basis of a lower income, $60.69 US per month in rural areas and $85.54 US per month in urban areas, combined with three or more social deficits. Individuals and households in extreme poverty are clearly in desperate need of assistance.

Such a measure of poverty is clearly not intended to mask the reality of the situation and indeed this measure makes it clear that a large fraction of the Mexican population suffers at least some degree of poverty and deprivation. In fact, in 2018 only 21.9% of Mexicans had adequate incomes and suffered no social service deficits (CONEVAL 2018b). As one would expect, there are significant regional differences with higher rates of poverty in states in the southern part of the country. Chiapas has a poverty rate of 76.4% and an extreme poverty rate of nearly 30%. Over half of the population in Guerrero, Morelos Oaxaca, Puebla, Tabasco, and Veracruz experience moderate or extreme poverty. In the face of such deprivation the fight for basic rights takes on particular significance and calls for effective civil society involvement. As we discuss in the next three chapters the protection and extension of the basic economic and social rights of all persons is a major focus of CSOs.

Despite the magnitude of the need in the population at large, a bit of good news is that the situation of older persons has improved over the last decade, especially in terms of access to medical care and pensions (CONEVAL 2018c). Between 2008 and 2016 the percentage of Mexicans over 65 who lacked adequate health care dropped from 34.1% to 9.5%, and the proportion without pension income dropped from 34.1% to 14.4%. Improvements in health care access clearly reflect the expansion of public medical care through Seguro Popular, the government health program introduced in 2003 for those without other coverage (Gutiérrez Robledo, López Ortega, and Arango Lopera 2012). In 2020 that program was reorganized and renamed el Instituto Nacional de Salud para el Bienestar, INSABI (National Institute of Health for Well-Being). More adequate incomes clearly result from the new non-contributory pension system we discuss below. Even with these improvements, though, a significant fraction of older Mexicans continues to live in poverty, but at rates lower than those of younger groups. In 2016 34.6% of older Mexicans experienced moderate poverty and 6.6% experienced severe poverty. Among children and adolescents under 18, 42.1% lived in moderate poverty and 9.0% lived in extreme poverty (CONEVAL 2018a; CONEVAL 2018c). It is clear that Mexico faces serious challenges in addressing the basic needs of large segments of its population of all ages.

Defamilisation and Refamilisation: Social Policy and Aging

Clearly, then, the level of need among all segments of the Mexican population, including older individuals, is great, as it is in most of Latin America and the Caribbean despite some reduction in extreme poverty in recent years (Fleury 2017). While the family remains the most important source of social support for older people, even in developing countries the welfare state is playing a larger role. It would be useful to provide some general sense of the ways in which various welfare states operate with reference to family policy. Clearly, a core factor that determines the breadth and generosity of any nation's welfare state is its level of economic development. As a convenient starting point we draw upon Esping-Andersen's well-known tripartite classification of welfare states (Esping-Andersen 1990). The typology is based on developed European nations, but raises issues we find useful in a discussion of Latin American welfare states, particularly in terms of the role of the State relative to that of the family in the care of older parents. Although many critics have objected to various aspects of this typology, it continues to serve as a useful starting point for emphasizing major differences in welfare systems.

In his classification Esping-Andersen contrasts "liberal" regimes, characterized by means-tested assistance focused on the most vulnerable, to "conservative" regimes, which look to the family for the support of its members, and "social democratic" regimes which provide comprehensive and universal state-sponsored benefits. The United States represents a quintessential liberal regime. In the U.S. "welfare" is a pejorative term that implies the inability or unwillingness to care for oneself. Federal and state income and support programs are geared to those with the fewest resources. The nations of central and southern Europe represent conservative regimes in which social support policies are geared toward reaffirming the family's role. The Nordic nations, with their universal and comprehensive social support systems, embody the most comprehensive and universal social democratic regimes.

Our focus on Mexico requires modifications and elaboration that we will introduce in the course of our discussion. The major differences between the developed European nations on which this typology is based and those of Latin America and the Caribbean relate to the lower levels of economic development and very different political histories and cultures among the latter. Welfare systems have historically been more extensive and generous in Europe than in Latin America. As we discuss throughout, the relative underdevelopment of Latin American and Caribbean welfare states is an important focus of ongoing debates concerning human and social rights. From our perspective, Mexico, like much of Latin America, combines aspects of the liberal regime, in that the State provides limited support, and income and social service programs are geared to those with the fewest resources. These countries also display aspects of the conservative pattern, in that the family remains the basic source of support and care, and family policy reflects a male-breadwinner model of family economics and welfare, even as the State is playing a greater role in providing support for dependent family members. The limited fiscal capacity of the State, combined with an unwillingness to provide extensive income and material supports associated with neoliberal economic policies, provides clear objectives for civil society organizations.

The term "defamilisation" is commonly used to refer to the shift in responsibility for the care of dependent individuals from the family to the State. The concept and policies informed by defamilisation are theoretically and practically important since they relate to a major shift in the role of the State relative to that of the family in the economic and social support of older persons. Political policies, such as those typical of the social democratic states of northern Europe, that maximize the role of the State and reduce that of the family in the material support of its members contrast profoundly to those of conservative states that maximize the role of the family. Recent policy changes in the United States and elsewhere focused on the devolution of responsibility for individuals from the higher levels of government to local levels and to non-governmental and faith-based groups and organizations reflecta desire to minimize the role of the State and maximize that of local communities and the family.

Nations differ greatly in the extent to which defamilisation is central to family and social policy. In the conservative welfare states of central and southern Europe social policy continues to emphasize the family, whereas in the more social democratic nations of northern Europe, formal state policy assigns many of those tasks to the State (Esping-Andersen 1990; Palier 2010). The more conservative systems, among which we place Latin American and Caribbean nations, are based on a traditional male-bread-winner model of family economics. The normative expectation of this approach is that the husband assumes responsibility for income generation, while the wife remains home to care for the household, children, and aging parents (Becker 1981; Esping-Andersen 1990; Horrell and Humphries 1997). In previous eras this arrangement may have been optimally efficient since it allowed the family to address all of its own social service needs, but circumstances have changed.

In post-traditional societies, which increasingly include even the conservative corporatist nations of central and southern Europe and the nations of Latin America and the Caribbean, that model of family economics is no longer universal. As part of the process of defamilisation, which as we describe is driven by extensive social and demographic changes including lower marriage and fertility rates, higher divorce rates, longer life spans, and the entry of women into the labor force, the State assumes a larger portion of the family's welfare and care functions (Esping-Andersen 1996; Michoń 2008). Although child care and elder care can be purchased on the market, for our purposes we limit the scope of defamilisation to the extent to which the State assumes significant responsibility for directly providing care or subsidizes its purchase.

In contrast to defamilisation, the term "refamilisation" refers to attempts to reaffirm and reestablish the family's role in the care of old and frail parents and other dependent members. These policies reflect long-standing traditions that are particularly resistant to change even as they are increasingly at odds with the social transformations that have reduced the family's ability to provide extensive care and support (Palier 2010). These pervasive transformations include, among other things, a significant and wide-spread decline of the full-employment male-breadwinner family economic model, increased life expectancies accompanied by longer periods of frailty, labor market exclusion and disadvantage, and more (Esping-Andersen 2010; Palier 2010). Although defamilisation remains far less pronounced in Latin America and other developing regions than in higher-income nations, even there, non-contributory pensions and other services that we discuss below are becoming more important as the family's ability to support and care for aging parents is reduced by the same social changes that have so profoundly affected the developed world.

Defamilisation and refamilisation raise issues related to the changing nature of intergenerational solidarity, both at the family level and at the societal level. Recent neoliberal retirement system reforms, as we describe in the next section, have refamilised the economic support of older parents, or rather they have individualized the responsibility for old-age economic security by formally sifting that responsibility from the State or employers to the individual. Rather than older retired workers depending on younger active workers for economic support, they find themselves dependent on themselves. The shortcomings of these privatized systems have forced civil society organizations to demand non-contributory pensions for older individuals, many of whom would otherwise suffer extreme poverty. We discuss this aspect of social solidarity in some detail below and review the role of CSOs in guaranteeing at least a minimum income to older people. The theoretical argument we develop, while focused on Latin America and Mexico, applies more broadly to other middle and even high-income countries.

Financial Security in Old Age

Old-age income security, or at least support, is indisputably one of the major guarantees of the welfare state (Estes 2001; Myles 1989; Quadagno 1988). Although the protections of the welfare state differ greatly among nations and remain more limited in low and middle-income than in high-income countries, in most nations, other than those at the lowest levels of development, these protections have evolved to a point at which citizens increasingly view them as rights. The modern welfare state is commonly traced to Otto Von Bismarck, who as the first Chancellor of Germany from 1871 to 1890 introduced old age pensions, workers compensation, and health insurance, core aspects the modern welfare state in order to blunt the appeal of socialism among the working class (Hennock 2007). In 1935 the United States introduced Social Security and the concept of universal protection was affirmed and codified in England by William Beveridge in his 1942 report *Social Insurance and Allied Services* (Beveridge 1942; Haber and Gratton 1994; Mesa-Lago 2008).

At the end of World War II the principle of the right to social security coverage was asserted by the International Labor organization (ILO), and in 1948 the Universal Declaration of Human Rights affirmed it as a universal right (Mesa-Lago 2008). During the 20th Century Latin American and Caribbean nations introduced social security schemes and other aspects of the modern welfare state. Certain pioneer nations including Argentina, Brazil, Chile, Costa Rica, and Cuba introduced social security systems in the 1920s and 1930s. Mexico is part of a later group that includes Bolivia, Colombia, Ecuador, Panama, Peru, and Venezuela, that introduced social security systems in the 1940s and 1950s. The remainder of Latin American countries introduced their systems in the 1960s and 1970s (Mesa-Lago 2008).

These systems suffered from many problems related to low rates of coverage, low contribution densities, and low replacement rates (Barrientos 1998; CONSAR 2017; Madrid 2003). Perhaps the major weakness of these systems was that they covered only formal sector workers, which continues to be the case. In Mexico approximately 60% of workers are employed in the informal sector, in which they lack formal contracts and do not pay into the social security system (Aguila, López-Ortega, and Gutiérrez Robledo 2018; CONSAR 2017). Many workers move back and forth between formal and informal employment over their working lives and often contribute only for a few years (ILO 2019; Maloney 2004). As a consequence, a large fraction of the population has no or inadequate resources for retirement, forcing many to continue working well into old age (Aguila et al. 2011). Even after fairly drastic reforms, the long-term outlook for pension systems in most of Latin America looks bleak (Alonso, Hoyo, and Tuesta 2015; de la Torre and Rudolph 2018). One of the major objectives of civil society organizations in most nations is to guarantee at least a minimal income to individuals who do not qualify for social security.

In general, then, in Europe and elsewhere problems with conservative family-based social welfare policies are becoming obvious, even as those systems remain particularly resistant to reform. One major criticism of the Bismarckian welfare state model, which is prevalent in central and southern Europe, relates specifically to its familistic basis (Esping-Andersen 1996; Esping-Andersen 2010). Changing marital patterns, female employment and male unemployment, as well as changing social mores means that effective welfare policy can no longer be based on the traditional male-breadwinner model of family security. For many observers the only realistic alternative is a formal policy of defamilisation, but in situations in which the state's capacity to provide adequate support is limited, what alternatives exist? For reasons of history and serious fiscal limitations Mexico continues to look to the family as the main support of citizens, although the family is becoming less able to assume the entire responsibility. Even in a middle-income nation with a long tradition of family support, some degree of defamilisation seems inevitable.

Longer Life: A Mixed Blessing

The major source of the old-age support dilemma that nations face results from greatly increased life spans and decreasing fertility, leading to rapidly aging populations. This demographic transition has particularly profound implications for pension systems. In the early years after such systems are established, most new enrollees are working and will not retire for several years so the ratio of retirees to those who are contributing to the system is favorable. In addition, in previous decades lower life expectancy meant that most retirees receive benefits for only a relatively short period. As these systems mature and as life expectancy increases the number of active workers relative to those who are retired declines. In the United States in 1945, ten years after Social Security was introduced, forty-two active workers supported each retiree. By 2009 that number had dropped to three and continues to decline (Social Security Administration 2013). This dramatic drop in the number of active workers relative to the number of retirees is occurring in both developed and developing nations (United Nations 2017). In addition to this lower ratio of workers to retirees, increases in life spans means that retired individuals will need support for longer periods.

As a consequence, as retirement systems mature, they face serious middle and long-term fiscal shortfalls. The reforms that are needed to address these shortfalls often engender ferocious opposition from those workers who fear they will be forced to work longer or that their benefits will be reduced. Longer life spans clearly increase the number of years a retired worker must be supported financially, but that is only part of the story. Long life can mean many years of illness and the need for expensive medical care. Successes in controlling the ravages of acute and chronic disease represent a clear advance for humanity, but long life introduces a new set of problems for families and for society at large. Ideally, the objective of modern medicine is to compress morbidity, which means to confine it to a short period at the end of the life course. Unfortunately, it appears that substantial compression has not occurred, and may actually not be possible. Longer lives, then, often mean many additional years of illness and disability (Angel and Angel Forthcoming; Angel, Angel and Hill 2015).

This new reality presents developing nations, including Mexico where relatively few individuals have retirement plans, with particularly serious problems (Cotlear 2011; Da Costa et al. 2011; Hujo 2014; Mesa-Lago 2008). Today, as in the past, the family continues to play its traditional roles as the main source of material support and care for frail older parents, even as the number of older individuals who live alone increases (Montes de Oca et al. 2014). Numerous social and demographic changes, then, have contributed to a rapidly changing reality for older individuals (Haber 2006; Quadagno 1982; Thane 2005). Declining fertility is among the most salient. In the United States at the turn of the 20th Century the average American female had nearly four children (Coale and Zelnik 1963; Himes 1989; Tolnay, Graham, and Guest 1982). Traditionally, in most countries, family members, or at least some children, remained close to home and were available to provide daily care to frail parents. Almost no one entered a long-term care facility, other than perhaps a poorhouse or an insane asylum (Grob 1983; Haber 2006; Haber and Gratton 1994; Thane 2005; Wagner 2005). A few rich individuals could pay for their care in monasteries or remain on their estates (Quintanar Olguin 2000). Nursing homes remained a rarity. That remains true today in most parts of the world, although the situation is changing even in countries like India where the number of long-term care facilities is increasing (Liebig 2003).

In Mexico the demographic transition began much later than in today's high-income nations, but it is proceeding at a far more rapid pace (Miles 2017). In the early 1960s Mexican women married early and had an average of seven children (Seiver 1975). Few couples divorced. Beginning in the 1970s, though, marriage rates declined, divorce rates increased, and the number of children born to the average woman decreased dramatically (INEGI 2017b). By 2015 the average number of children born to women had dropped to 2.2, similar to the United States. Other changes that accompanied the demographic transition in Europe and the United States are affecting Mexico. Lower fertility is part of a package that includes higher rates of single-parent households, more female labor force involvement, and higher rates of migration. These trends are not only unlikely to reverse themselves, they are in fact likely to accelerate and do not bode well for the family's ability to care for aging parents who are living longer than ever before.

The problem affects most nations. In western Europe fertility rates have reached historic lows (Sobotka 2006). In many European nations, including Italy and Spain, where up until a generation ago families had many children, fertility rates are below replacement. In 2018 the fertility rate in Italy and Spain was barely 1.3, far below the 2.1 that is necessary for a stable population (The World Bank 2021). In the absence of immigration these countries would shrink in size. South American populations are aging at an astonishing rate as well and will continue to do so well into the 21st Century (Chamie 2005; Palloni, Pinto-Aguirre, and Pelaez 2002). This new demographic and social reality of rapid growth in the proportion of populations in the oldest age ranges, in combination with the other social transformations we have mentioned, requires novel approaches to the care of older adults and the protection of their human and social rights.

Which brings us directly to the question of the potential role of civil society organizations in advocating for and providing services and assistance to growing populations of elders. Given the fact that federal, state, provincial, and municipal governments are limited in what they can provide, the potential complementary role of CSOs could be significant. As of yet, though, we know little of how these organizations frame their missions, who they serve, how they are organized, or the ties they may have with other organizations, government agencies, labor unions, and other potential allies. Nor do we know how successful they are in furthering the interests of their clients. Our objective in this book is to at least begin framing a set of relevant questions.

Pensions as Central to Human Rights

Increasingly, social rights are viewed as a major dimension of human rights as codified in the Universal Declaration of Human Rights and other international treaties and conventions (United Nations 1948). At the most basic level, political rights are clearly central to the exercise of full citizenship. The transformation of peasants and serfs into citizens required guaranteeing their rights to vote, to own property, not to be imprisoned without legally valid cause, and more. The extension of the notion of rights to include positive rights is based on the recognition that basic political rights are of little value without the material means and the cultural capital to exercise them (Marshall 1950). As we discuss in the following chapters, modern concepts of "active citizenship" and "active aging" are based on an affirmation of basic human rights, but also subsume social rights as a core necessity.

Even though the size and extent of the modern welfare state is far greater today than at its beginning, health care and old-age security continue to be the most central and costliest protections that the State guarantees its citizens. Given the rapid aging of the populations of most nations, the fiscal burden on the State of the financial support and health care for older citizens is huge and growing. Responses by governments are shaped by the ways in which the sources of the problems are framed. Christine Lagarde, Managing Director of the International Monetary Fund, and others see the problem as primarily one of demographics and increasing life spans (Hutchens 2016). From this perspective, the dramatic increase in the number of older individuals relative to those of working age creates a dependency burden that is unsustainable.

According to José Piñera a neoliberal economist who was central to the expansion of contributory pensions in developing countries, and who served as Chilean Secretary of Labor and Social Security from 1978 to 1980 under President Augusto Pinochet, the burden of traditional pay-as-you-go retirement plans will inevitably result in resentment among younger workers who will be forced to contribute an ever growing fraction of their earnings to the support of retired workers (Piñera 1995/96). Such arrangements are on the face of it unsustainable. Indeed, it is hard to imagine that there is not a limit to the tax burden one can place on workers. Regardless of one's political position, some solution other than continual increases in payroll taxes must be found. Given the dominance of neoliberal social policies, a radical and extensive redistribution of wealth in any country seems unlikely. So far, most reforms have made rather modest changes to existing systems.

To date, the most radical reforms of pension systems have involved their privatization, a solution that rejects the original solidaristic philosophy on which traditional retirement income schemes were based (Arrizabalo Montoro, del Rosal, and Javier Murillo Arroyo 2019; McCarthy 2017). Nonetheless, in recognition of the obvious fiscal limitations of traditional pay-as-you go defined-benefit arrangements most Latin American and Caribbean nations have adopted various forms of mixed or fully defined-contribution arrangements in which workers are responsible for their own retirement savings (Flores-Castillo 2013; Mesa-Lago 2008). Again, though, since these reforms apply only to workers in the formal labor market, they do little to address problems of informality and limited contributions.

In a defined-benefit plan an individual contributes a specified fraction of his or her salary for a specified number of years after which he or she becomes vested and is entitled to a specified pension, usually some fraction of his or her highest salary or average salary over a number of years, which may be adjusted for inflation, for life. Such plans are usually funded by joint contributions by the employee and the employer. In most schemes of this sort workers' contributions are used to pay the pensions of current retirees and are not placed in an individual savings or investment plan. In a defined-contribution or individually funded retirement scheme, on the other hand, the worker's and employer's contributions are invested in mutual funds, bonds, or stocks. These plans belong to the individual and are managed by an authorized agent, such as an insurance company or a specially licensed investment company. One's income in retirement is based on the amount invested and the return on those investments.

Many developing countries, including most Latin American and Caribbean nations, have adopted some version of this defined-contribution approach (Arza 2019; Madrid 2003; Mesa-Lago 2004; Mesa-Lago 2008), although many have modified their initial plans to deal with a wide range of problems inherent in a defined-contribution scheme, again primarily related to low contribution and savings levels. Argentina abandoned the experiment altogether and returned to a fully defined-benefit arrangement. Despite initial hopes that defined-contribution retirement schemes would increase savings and further economic development, the result was largely disappointing and the schemes were riddled with problems that required fundamental reforms. In most nations high rates of informality meant that only workers in the formal sector or state employees ever receive an adequate pension (Mesa-Lago 2008; Villagómez and Ramírez 2013). Even as late as 2000, only 22% of the Mexican labor force was covered (Willmore 2014).

Non-contributory Pensions: A Survival Income

The shortcomings of both the older defined-benefit and the newer defined-contribution pension schemes have forced many developing nations to provide a minimal guaranteed income to individuals who do not qualify for an employment-based pension. This group is huge and includes individuals who have worked in the informal sector, women who were employed episodically because of child and elder care duties, and others. In many cases, this group represents the majority of workers. Although the fiscal unsustainability of traditional defined-benefit approaches is obvious, many critics of defined-contribution approaches, primarily from the left, continue to see the source of the problem as an unjust and inequitable distribution of wealth. Forcing workers to finance their own retirement security through potentially volatile and risky investments only exacerbates inequities.

Although extreme inequality represents an ongoing problem in Latin America and elsewhere, what is different today than in the fairly recent past is that the problem is not framed in terms of a rhetoric of class struggle, but rather a rhetoric that pits privileged elites against individuals and groups with local identities (Goodhart 2017). In the case of older individuals, such a rhetoric motivates individuals to engage in grass-roots and more organized civil society efforts to address the problem of inadequate incomes. These local efforts reflect a greater involvement of citizens in issues related to governance and the distribution of social benefits. Yet one problem with an excessively local civil society focus arises from the rejection of the hierarchy and discipline typical of political parties, without which activists cannot coordinate their efforts and prevail over the status quo. We discuss this problem more fully in Chapter four.

Whether the term "defamilisation" and the concepts it refers to are useful or not, they emphasize the fact that in high-income countries and increasingly in lower-income countries the financial and social support of older parents is no longer the sole responsibility of the family. Rather than defamilisation, we might refer to this change in the family's responsibility for aging parents as the socialization of support of older individuals. In the United States children do not expect to be the sole or even primary support of their parents, and relatively few would be capable of doing so. Social Security has profoundly changed expectations and practice (Haber and Gratton 1994). As we note in Chapter three where we discuss various Latin American conventions concerning the human rights of older persons, those conventions explicitly affirm the right of older parents to family support. As we document, though, that support role is weakening and, in many cases, aging parents are even the victims of abuse and neglect by their own families.

As the welfare state matured during the latter half of the 20th Century, welfare states faced serious fiscal and political challenges related to far more than just pensions. Many of the challenges are the result of deliberate policies to deal with the social changes that resulted from technological advances, productivity gains that required fewer workers, and increasing unemployment among the working-age population (Védrine 2014). Today France struggles to deal with the consequences of what has become a cultural expectation of early exit from the labor force. That expectation is the result of a deliberate policy of labor shedding and a desire to increase opportunities for younger workers. The expectations that such policies created are extremely difficult to change. Resistance to the government's plans to consolidate pension plans in France is just one example of the importance of a retirement income to older people, and the difficulties governments encounter in attempting to control the continually growing cost of these programs.

Although business groups have been calling for raising the legal retirement age in France to 64 or 65, such a move has long been seen as political suicide for any administration, so at least for the present the legal age of retirement remains 62, although many French workers retire sooner (The Local 2018). In Latin America and the Caribbean seriously incomplete pension coverage results in less resistance to radical change in pension systems, many of which were imposed by totalitarian governments. The pioneering privatized system of Chile, which in 1980 established a defined contribution scheme based on a mandatory contribution of 10% of salary paid only by the employee, was initially considered a major success. Over time, though, high administrative costs and the fact that 10% of a worker's wages are insufficient to guarantee an adequate retirement wage mean that most retirees face serious economic hardship. The huge profits that resulted from mandatory pension investments primarily benefitted the investment managers and the rich (Borzutzky and Hyde 2017).

Although privatized pension plans address the long-term fiscal crises faced by pension systems, they do so at a potentially high social cost. In addition to a loss of whatever bond of solidarity defined-benefit systems fostered, without other reforms defined-contribution plans cannot address problems of incomplete coverage, gender inequity, or episodic contribution. If twenty-five or more years of contribution are required to receive a full pension, workers who spend many years in the informal sector, those who are unemployed for long periods, or women who must raise children or care for aging parents are unlikely to qualify. To address these problems Latin American countries, including Mexico, have introduced various forms of non-contributory pensions or adopted more flexible rules for qualification for state pensions (Barrientos 2012; Rofman, Apella and Vezza 2013). Such non-contributory pensions have become the main source of income security for older individuals in at least forty countries around the world (Newson and Bourne 2012; Willmore 2006).

In Mexico non-contributory pensions have made pension coverage nearly universal (Willmore 2014). Without such pensions most workers would receive no benefits at all. In 2019 only 23% of women and 40% of men had access to a contributory pension (Secretaría de Bienestar 2019). Making matters worse, fully 26% of older adults had neither a pension nor access to public programs. In response to this vulnerability, non-contributory pensions were initially provided by local governments, beginning with Mexico City in 2001. In 2007 the federal government introduced a non-contributory pension program named "Setenta y Mas" (70 and older) for adults 70 years or older living in rural areas with less than 2,500 inhabitants. This program was expanded to all localities with fewer than 20,000 inhabitants in 2008, and to all places with fewer than 30,000 inhabitants in 2009. In 2012 it was extended to all older persons not receiving any other social security benefits or state-level non-contributory pensions (Aguila, López-Ortega, and Gutiérrez Robledo 2018). Currently the program, which is referred to as the Programa Pensión para Adultos Mayores (Pension Program for Older Adults), covers individuals 65 and older who live in indigenous communities and certain individuals registered as special rights holders in the program, and those 68 and older in the rest of the country (Secretaría de Bienestar 2019). In 2019 recipients received 1,275 pesos ($64.87 US) per month paid bimonthly.

Currently, most older adults in Mexico rely on these state or federal non-contributory pensions, which are significantly smaller than social security benefits (Aguila, López-Ortega, and Gutiérrez Robledo 2018). Although these programs have greatly reduced the number of older individuals with no income, the level of support is minimal and a large fraction of Mexican elders live in poverty. Of necessity, many continue to work well past 65 (Aguila et al. 2011). In addition, the reliance on public funding reintroduces the long-term fiscal risks for national economies that older pay-as-you-go pension systems involved (Filgueira and Manzi 2017). Yet in light of the growing number of individuals with little income, few resources, and no retirement plan these basic pensions are an essential lifeline. For that reason, they are a major focus of civil society efforts which work to ensure that older individuals who are entitled to benefits in fact receive them. Like other government support programs once they are introduced, non-contributory pensions take on a life of their own and individuals resist losing them or having their payment levels reduced. Although states must deal with fiscal realities, experiments with neoliberalism and an excessive focus on the market and economic issues alone ignore essential social realities.

Very Real Fiscal Constraints

The welfare state has become such a central part of citizens' lives in middle and high-income nations that attempts to limit its size or even its rate of growth confront serious resistance. Yet as it has matured certain strains have become increasingly obvious. Fully developed, and even less developed welfare states are extremely expensive and require high levels of taxation. Although citizens for the most part accept the necessity of high taxes, ever increasing levels of taxation, often accompanied by reductions in services, eventually elicit serious resistance, especially when accompanied by perceptions of unjust economic and status inequalities. Although few observers advocate the complete elimination of or even major reductions in basic social programs, the need for reform remains widely recognized. The difficulty arises of course in the nature of the reforms proposed by individuals from various segments of society and points on the political spectrum. One's preferred opinions depend on one's views concerning the extent and sources of inequality, as well as one's beliefs concerning equity and justice.

Yet cost is a constant concern, especially in a highly globalized economy in which nations do not have complete control over domestic economic policy. The wave of neoliberal reform that swept the globe in recent decades is in no small part a response to what international financial institutions and others see as unsustainable expenditures for social programs. The defined-contribution pension reforms that we have discussed reflect what many see as perhaps a regrettable, but inevitable abandonment of the intergenerational solidarity that was based on defined-benefit schemes and traditional society more generally (Angel and Angel 2018).

France again offers a telling example of the almost inevitable conflicts that arise when changes are proposed in highly developed welfare states. In 2018 French President Macron's decision to raise taxes on gasoline in order to finance the development of more environmentally friendly alternatives gave rise to the "gilet jeaune" or "yellow vest" movement, a spontaneous uprising involving ordinary citizens who were heavily dependent on their automobiles and who were mobilized by a sense that the tax was unjust. The movement did not reflect the position of one political faction or perspective. Rather, it involved a wide segment of the population. In addition to the increased gasoline tax, the movement was motivated by a sense of broader injustice. The optimism of the early post-war years that the French refer to as the "trente glorieuse" or "the glorious thirty," a phrase that refers to the period from 1945 until approximately 1975 when the country was recovering from World War II and prospering, is long gone. As long as most people's situation was improving the public was generally satisfied with the overall situation. Once the sense that one is benefitting from a general growing prosperity is lost the general faith in the status quo declines. In France as in other nations, even though today's working and middle classes are materially far better off than during the early post-war years their situation is not improving, and in many localities that have been passed over or harmed by globalization, a sense of stagnation and blocked opportunity prevails. Such sentiments contribute to the growing influence of populist anti-elitist, anti-establishment, and anti-immigrant political parties.

Where and How Does Civil Society Fit in?

The phenomenon of defamilisation ultimately relates to a far more general set of changes related to the emergence of post-traditional society (Angel and Angel 2018). These changes are well along in the developed world, but they are transforming basic institutional and social arrangements in lower-income counties as well. In traditional societies all of the institutions that structured one's life, from the social class to which one belonged, to who one married, to the occupation one pursued, were given. One's life was fairly similar to the lives of those who came before. The loss or weakening of tradition opens up new possibilities that are not governed by traditional norms and practices. Post-traditional society is defined by options and the requirement that one choose among different possibilities (Giddens 1991). As a result, one loses much of the security of limited options, but at the same time one gains the possibility of greater personal and group agency.

It is in this context that civil society organizations have expanded and often redefined their missions. What this means for political action and governance at all levels remains uncertain. CSOs and the social movements of which they are frequently a manifestation often reflect a rejection of traditional political parties and a growing desire for more direct democracy. As we argue throughout the following chapters, the rejection of political parties, especially those of the center-left, and a focus on local group interests may increase opportunities for participation by a wider range of individuals, but they do so at the risk of the fragmentation of potential constituencies into conflicting entities, none of which possess the human or material resources to challenge serious inequalities. Critics of identity politics and an excessive focus on parochial group interests fear that such parochial positions could play into the hands of oligarchs and relinquish power to repressive and exclusionary groups.

The demographic, economic, and social changes that gave rise to this changed political environment during the latter part of the 20th and early 21st Centuries are complex and interactive; they have affected all institutions and aspects of life from marriage and reproduction to work and leisure. The new found freedom though comes with greater uncertainty and the increased responsibility of individuals to make difficult decisions and to structure their own lives. In the context of our discussion of pensions and retirement income it comes with a greater responsibility to plan for a long post-retirement period in which one must remain as actively engaged in family, community, and political life as possible. Even in the United States many individuals are ill prepared for the post-work period of life. In Mexico and the rest of Latin America and the Caribbean the situation is far worse, and CSOs are increasingly involved in fighting for the rights of older individuals with limited resources and human capital.

For all of their shortcomings, CSOs are clearly here to stay. In light of increasing disillusionment with government and political parties, what other domain of organized oppositional or self-help effort exists? We suspect there is in reality no substitute for organized political action and some degree of hierarchy and division of labor in order to deal with the institutionalized structures and organizations that perpetuate inequality and disadvantage. In order to significantly affect individuals' lives and secure their human and social rights these organizations will no doubt find that they cannot remain as horizontal and non-hierarchical as they might wish. Our task is to examine the extent to which civil society organizations of various sorts are able to accomplish this goal for specific groups and for society at large.

Debates over the nature, objectives, and effectiveness of civil society organizations will no doubt continue for years, and it is clear that particular organizations differ greatly in all of these aspects. Some effectively further the interests of their membership and benefit non-members, while others are largely ineffective and do little for the community at large. Our objective is not to arrive at some general assessment of this confusing and complex network of organizations with multiple objectives, structures, and outcomes. At most we can document differences in the way they frame their missions and how they involve the individuals whose interests they further in defining that mission. We return to the indisputable fact that the number and range of activities of these organizations is huge and growing. Ignoring their presence leads to a misrepresentation and misunderstanding of a major set of social forces that are defining our modern post-traditional world.

What we argue in this book is that neither the family nor the State are able to provide all of what older individuals, and dependent individuals in general, need. In our modern world smaller families and the migration of children away from their parent's home and community, in conjunction with numerous other economic, political, and social changes mean that the family can no longer provide all of the support and care aging parents need. Who else, then, is in a position to provide that care and support, or who else will advocate for and demand the human and social rights of older persons? Although the State can provide medical and financial support, at least at minimal levels, to elder individuals, it is not well suited to provide the intimate time-consuming involvement that willing families can provide.

In the following chapters we will examine the role of civil society organizations in advocating for and providing support and care to older individuals, many of whom have seriously diminished capacity and require special care. Historically, the family has been the sole or primary guarantor of aging parents' well-being. We often romanticize this aspect of family life and overlook the serious conflicts that often characterize intergenerational family life. In Mexico the abuse of aging parents, including their abandonment, by family members represents a serious problem (INAPAM 2013; Mazatlán Post 2019). As life expectancy at birth and older ages rises dramatically it is unlikely that we will return to some romanticized past of family solidarity and filial piety. Nor will the State be able to address all of the day-to-day needs of individuals in their communities. This new reality serves as the motivation for what we deal with in this book. If traditional communities are disappearing, our human interdependence and our inability to live purely solitary lives makes it imperative that we examine how strangers can assume some of the roles we previously attributed solely to family.

In our analysis of the growing role of the non-governmental sector we summarize many of the social changes that are altering the roles of the family and the State in the care and support of individuals. In the modern world, the State has increasingly assumed major responsibility for ensuring the welfare of minor children, disabled and incapacitated individuals, individuals with serious medical conditions, and others who cannot adequately support or care for themselves. Even with the changes that we document, it is clear that civil society in general or civil society organizations specifically are no substitute for a beneficent, efficient, and powerful State. Yet they are a growing part of a new social reality. In this book we focus specifically on older individuals, who because of age and the serious functional limitations that often accompany it are at high risk of dependency and the loss of autonomy. Our objective is to examine in detail the institutional arrangements that are available for their care and how those are changing. Our unique contribution is to examine the role of the non-profit sector in complementing state efforts or assuming an activist and potentially adversarial role to pressure the State to live up to its obligations to vulnerable citizens. We deal specifically with the implications for the care of older persons and other dependent individuals of the demographic and social changes that have diminished the family's ability to provide all of the care aging parents need.

References

Aguila, Emma, Claudia Díaz, Mary Manqing Fu, Arie Kapteyn, and Ashley Pierson. 2011. *Living Longer in Mexico: Income Security and Health*. Washington, DC: AARP.

Aguila, Emma, Mariana López-Ortega, and Luis Miguel Gutiérrez Robledo. 2018. "Non-contributory Pension Programs and Frailty of Older Adults: Evidence from Mexico." *PLoS ONE* 13 (11):https://doi.org/10.1371/journal.pone. 0206792.

Alonso, Javier, Carmen Hoyo, and David Tuesta. 2015. "A Model for the Pension System in Mexico: Diagnosis and Recommendations." *Journal of Pension Economics and Finance* 14 (1):76–112.

Angel, Ronald J., and Jacqueline L. Angel. 2018. *Family, Intergenerational Solidarity, and Post-Traditional Society*. New York, NY: Routledge.

Angel, Ronald J., and Jacqueline L. Angel. Forthcoming. "Healthy Life Expectancy." in *Wiley Blackwell Encyclopedia of Sociology*, edited by George Ritzer and Chris Rojek. Malden, MA: John Wiley & Sons.

Angel, Ronald J., Jacqueline L. Angel, and Terrence D. Hill. 2015. "Longer Lives, Sicker Lives? Increased Longevity and Extended Disability Among Mexican-Origin Elders." *The Journals of Gerontology Series B: Psychological Sciences and Social Sciences* 70 (4):639–649.

Angel, Ronald J., Verónica Montes-de-Oca Zavala, and Vicente Rodríguez. 2018. "Strengthening Solidarity: A Theoretical Inquiry into the Roles of Civil Society Organizations in the Support of Elderly Citizens in Mexico City." Pp. 159–180 in *Contextualizing Health and Aging in the Americas: Effects of Space, Time, and Place* (Volume 4), edited by William Vega, Jacqueline Angel, Luis Miguel Gutierrez, and Kyriakos Markides. New York, NY: Springer Nature.

Arrizabalo Montoro, Xabier, Mario del Rosal, and F. Javier Murillo Arroyo. 2019. "The Debate on Pension Systems: The Paradigmatic Cases of Chile and Spain." *American Journal of Economics and Sociology* 78 (1):195–223.

Arza, Camila. 2019. "Basic Old-Age Protection in Latin America: Non-contributory Pensions, Coverage Expansion Strategies, and Aging Patterns across Countries." *Population and Development Review* 45 (S1):23–45.

Barrientos, Armando. 1998. *Pension Reform in Latin America*. Aldershot, UK: Ashgate.

Barrientos, Armando. 2012. "Dilemas de las politicas sociales latinoamericanas. ¿Hacia una protección social fragmentada?" *Nueva Sociedad* 239:65–78.

Becker, Gary S. 1981. *A Treatise on the Family*. Cambridge, MA: Harvard University Press.

Beveridge, SirWilliam. 1942. *Social Insurance and Allied Services*. London, UK: H. M. Stationary Office.

Borzutzky, Sylvia, and Mark Hyde. 2017. "The Chilean Welfare State System with Special Reference to Social Security Privatization." Pp. 138–154 in *The Routledge*

International Handbook to Welfare State Systems, edited by Christian Aspalter. New York, NY: Routledge.

Chamie, J. 2005. *World Population Ageing: 1950–2050*. New York, NY: Population Division, Department of Economic and Social Affairs, United Nations Secretariat.

Coale, Ansley Johnson, and Melvin Zelnik. 1963. *New Estimates of Fertility and Population in the United States*. Princeton, NJ: Princeton University Press.

CONEVAL. 2014. "Multidimensional Measurement of Poverty in Mexico: An Economic Well-being and Social Rights Approach." Mexico City: CONEVAL. Retrieved 2/4/2010 from https://www.coneval.org.mx/InformesPublicaciones/FolletosInstitucionales/Documents/Multidimensional-Measurement-of-poverty-in-Mexico.pdf.

CONEVAL. 2018a. "Informe de Evaluación de la politica de Desarollo 2018." Mexico City: CONEVAL. Retrieved 2/5/2020 from https://www.coneval.org.mx/Evaluacion/IEPSM/IEPSM/Documents/IEPDS_2018.pdf.

CONEVAL. 2018b. "Mediación de la Pobreza 2008–2018, Estados Unidos Mexicanos." Mexico City: CONEVAL. Retrieved 2/4/2020 from https://www.coneval.org.mx/Medicion/MP/Paginas/Pobreza-2018.aspx.

CONEVAL. 2018c. "Para La Población Adulta Mayor es Necesario un Sistema de Protección Universal que Sustituya Programas Sociales Inconexos y Dispersos." Mexico City: CONEVAL. Retrieved 2/3/2020 from https://www.coneval.org.mx/SalaPrensa/Comunicadosprensa/Documents/Comunicado-012-Adultos-Mayores-2018.pdf#search=pobreza%20adultos%20mayores.

CONEVAL. 2020. "¿Quiénes Somos?" Mexico City: CONEVAL. Retrieved 2/3/2020 from https://www.coneval.org.mx/quienessomos/Paginas/Quienes-Somos.aspx.

CONSAR. 2017. "Densidades de Cotización en el Sistema de Ahorro para el Retiro en México." Documento de trabajo No. 3. Mexico City: Comisión Nacional del Sistema de Ahorro parael Retiro. Retrieved 8/8/2019 from https://www.gob.mx/cms/uploads/attachment/file/192977/densidad_vf.pdf.

Cotlear, Daniel (Ed.). 2011. *Population Aging: Is Latin America Ready?* Washington, DC: The World Bank.

Da Costa, Rita, Juan Ramón de Laiglesia, Emmanuelle Martínez, and Ángel Melguizo. 2011. "The Economy of the Possible: Pensions and Informality in Latin America." in *Latin American Economic Outlook*. Paris, France: OECD. Retrieved 8/6/2013 from http://www.oecd.org/dev/46937116.pdf.

de la Torre, Augusto, and Heinz P. Rudolph. 2018. "The Troubled State of Pension Systems in Latin America." Brookings Institution. Retrieved 9/1/2019 from https://www.brookings.edu/wp-content/uploads/2018/03/working-paper_torre_rudolph_20182.pdf.

Esping-Andersen, Gøsta. 1990. *The Three Worlds of Welfare Capitalism*. Princeton, NJ: Princeton University Press.

Esping-Andersen, Gøsta. 1996. "Welfare States without Work: the Impasse of Labor Shedding and Familialism in Continental European Social Policy." Pp. 66–87 in *Welfare States in Transition: National Datation in Global Economics*, edited by Gøsta Esping-Andersen. Thousand Oaks, CA: Sage.

Esping-Andersen, Gøsta. 2010. "Prologue: What Does it Mean to Break with Bismarck?" Pp. 13–18 in *A Long Goodbye to Bismarck? The Politics of Welfare Reform in Continental Europe*, edited by Bruno Palier. Amsterdam: Amsterdam University Press.

Estes, Carroll. 2001. *Social Policy and Aging: A Critical Perspective*. Thousand Oaks, CA: Sage.

Filgueira, Fernando, and Pilar Manzi. 2017. "Pension and Income Transfers for Old Age Inter- and Intra-generational Distribution in Comparative Perspective." United Nations (ECLAC). Retrieved 9/14/2017 from http://repositorio.cepal.org/bitstream/handle/11362/42087/1/S1700520_en.pdf.

Fleury, Sonia. 2017. "The Welfare State in Latin America: Reform, Innovation and Fatigue." *Cadernos de Saúde Pública* 33 (2):11–20.

Flores-Castillo, Atenea. 2013. *Transferencias No Contributivas a Personas Mayores. Análisis Comparativo de Dos Programas: 70 y Más y Pensión Alimentaria de la Ciudad de México*. Mexico, DF: United Nations, CEPAL Mexico.

Giddens, Anthony. 1991. *Modernity and Self-Identity: Self and Society in the Late Modern Age*. Stanford, CA: Stanford University Press.

Goodhart, David. 2017. *The Road to Somewhere: The Populist Revolt and the Future of Politics*. London, UK: Hurst & Company.

Grob, Gerald N. 1983. *Mental Illness and American Society*. Princeton, NJ: Princeton University Press.

Gutiérrez Robledo, Luis Miguel, Mariana López Ortega, and Victoria Eugenia Arango Lopera. 2012. "The State of Elder Care in Mexico." *Current Geriatrics Reports* 1 (4):183–189.

Haber, Carole. 2006. "Old Age Through the Lens of Family History." Pp. 59–75 in *Handbook of Aging and the Social Sciences*, edited by Robert H. Binstock and Linda K. George. New York, NY: Academic Press.

Haber, Carole, and Brian Gratton. 1994. *Old Age and the Search for Security: An American Social History*. Bloomington, IN: Indiana University Press.

Hennock, E.P. 2007. *The Origin of the Welfare State in England and Germany, 1850–1914: Social Policies Compared*. Cambridge, UK: Cambridge University Press.

Himes, Michael R. 1989. "Amerian Fertility in Transition: New Estimates of Birth Rates in the United States, 1900–1910." *Demography* 26 (1):137–148.

Horrell, Sara, and Jane Humphries. 1997. "The Origins and Expansion of the Male Breadwinner Family: The Case of Nineteenth-Century Britain." *International Review of Social History* 42 (S5):25–64.

Hujo, Katja (Ed.). 2014. *Reforming Pensions in Developing and Transition Countries*. Basingstoke, UK: Palgrave Macmillan.

Hutchens, Gareth. 2016. "IMF Managing Director Christine Lagarde Warns of Demographic Timebomb." *The Sunday Morning Herald*. Retrieved 1/16/2019 from https://www.smh.com.au/business/the-economy/imf-managing-dir ector-christine-lagarde-warns-of-demographic-timebomb-20160304-gnapv3.html.

ILO. 2019. "Informal Employment (% of Total Non-agricultural Employment)." International Labour Organization, ILOSTAT database. Retrieved 7/16/2019 from https://data.worldbank.org/indicator/SL.ISV.IFRM.ZS?locations=MX.

INAPAM. 2013. "Recomienda INAPAM a las personas adultas mayores buscar ayuda en caso de sufrir maltrato." Instituto Nacional de las Personas Adultas Mayores. Retrieved 1/1/2020 from https://www.gob.mx/inapam/prensa/recom ienda-inapam-a-las-personas-adultas-mayores-buscar-ayuda-en-caso-de-sufrir-maltrato.

INEGI. 2017a. "La discapacidad en México, datos al 2014: Versión 2017." Insti-tuto Nacional de Estadística y Geografía (Mexico). Retrieved 2/5/2020 from http://internet.contenidos.inegi.org.mx/contenidos/Productos/prod_serv/contenidos/espanol/bvinegi/productos/nueva_estruc/702825094409.pdf.

INEGI. 2017b. "Nupcialidad." Retrieved 7/19/2019 from https://www.inegi.org.mx/temas/nupcialidad/.

Liebig, Phoebe S. 2003. "Old-Age Homes and Services: Old and New Approaches to Aged Care." Pp. 159–178 in *An Aging India: Perspectives, Prospects, and Policies*, edited by Phoebe S. Liebig and S. Irudaya Rajan. New York, NY: The Hay-worth Press.

Madrid, Raúl L. 2003. *Retiring the State: The Politics of Pension Privatization in Latin America and Beyond.* Stanford, CA: Stanford University Press.

Maloney, William F. 2004. "Informality Revisited." *World Development* 32 (7):1159–1178.

Marshall, T.H. 1950. *Citizenship and Social Class: And Other Essays.* Cambridge, UK: Cambridge University Press.

Mazatlán Post. 2019. "In Mexico, the Abandonment of Older Adults Is a Real Problem." *The Mazatlán Post.* Retrieved 1/1/2020 from https://themazatlanpost.com/2019/10/15/in-mexico-the-abandonment-of-older-adults-is-a-real-problem/.

McCarthy, Michael A. 2017. *Dismantling Solidarity: Capitalist Politics and American Pensions since the New Deal.* Ithaca, NY: Cornell University Press.

Mesa-Lago, Carmelo. 2004. "An Appraisal of a Quarter-Century of Structural Pension Reforms in Latin America." *CEPAL Review* 84:57–81.

Mesa-Lago, Carmelo. 2008. *Reassembling Social Security: A Survey of Pensions and Health Care Reforms in Latin America.* New York, NY: Oxford University Press.

Michoń, Piotr. 2008. "Familisation and Defamilisation Policy in 22 European Countries." *Poznań University of Economics Review* 8 (1):34–54.

Miles, Richard. 2017. "A Smaller, Wealthier Mexico Is on the Horizon." Center for Strategic and International Studies. Retrieved 9/9/2019 from https://www.csis.org/analysis/smaller-wealthier-mexico-horizon.

Montes de Oca, V., S. Garay, B. Rico, and S.J. García. 2014. "Living Arrange-ments and Aging in Mexico: Changes in Households, Poverty and Regions, 1992–2009." *International Journal of Social Sciences Studies* 2 (4):61–74.

Myles, John. 1989. *Old Age and the Welfare State: The Political Economy of Public Pensions.*Revised edition. Lawrence, KS: University Press of Kansas.

Newson, Lara, and Astrid Walker Bourne. 2012. "Financing Social Pensions in Low- and Middle-Income Countries." in *Pension Watch: Briefings on Social Protec-tion in Older Age.* HelpAge International. Retrieved 5/15/2021 from file:///C:/Users/RON-AD~1/AppData/Local/Temp/24123.pdf.

Palier, Bruno (Ed.). 2010. *A Long Goodbye to Bismarck? The Politics of Welfare Reform in Continental Europe.* Amsterdam: Amsterdam University Press.

Palloni, Alberto, Guido Pinto-Aguirre, and Martha Pelaez. 2002. "Demographic and Health Conditions of Ageing in Latin America and the Caribbean." *Inter-national Journal of Epidemiology* 31 (4):762–771.

Piñera, José. 1995/96. "Empowering Workers: The Privatization of Social Security in Chile." *Cato Journal* 15 (2–3):155–156.

Quadagno, Jill. 1982. *Aging in Early Industrial England.* New York, NY: Academic Press.

Quadagno, Jill. 1988. *TheTransformation of Old Age Security: Class and Politics in the American Welfare State.* Chicago, IL: University of Chicago Press.

Quintanar Olguin, Fernando. 2000. *Atención a los ancianos en asilos y casas hogar de la ciudad de México. Ante el escenario de la Tercera ola.* Mexico City: Plaza y Valdéz, S.A. de C.V.

Rofman, Rafael, Ignacio Apella, and Evelyn Vezza (Eds.). 2013. *Más allá de las Pensiones Contributivas: Catorce Experiencias en América Latina.* Buenos Aires: Banco Mundial.

Secretaría de Bienestar. 2019. "Programa para el Bienestar de las Personas Adultas Mayores." Gobierno de México. Retrieved 9/5/2019 from https://www.gob.mx/bienestar/acciones-y-programas/programa-para-el-bienestar-de-las-personas-adultas-mayores.

SEDESOL. 2016. "Diagnóstico sobre la situación de las personas con discapacidad en México." Mexico City: Secretaría de Desarrollo Social. Retrieved 2/5/2020 from https://backend.aprende.sep.gob.mx/media/uploads/proedit/resources/dia gnostico_sobre_l_8a347852.pdf.

Seiver, Daniel A. 1975. "Recent Fertility in Mexico: Measurement and Interpretation." *Population Studies* 29 (3):341–354.

Sobotka, Tomáš. 2006. "Is Lowest-Low Fertility in Europe Explained by the Postponement of Childbearing?" *Population and Development Review* 30 (2):195–220.

Social Security Administration. 2013. "Ratio of Social Security Covered Workers to Beneficiaries Calendar Years 1940–2013." Washington, DC: Social Security History. Retrieved 12/30/2019 from https://www.ssa.gov/history/ratios.html.

Thane, Pat (Ed.). 2005. *A History of Old Age.* Los Angeles, CA: The J. Paul Getty Museum.

The Local. 2018. "France Unveils Pensions Overhaul but Will Keep Legal Retirement Age at 62." The Local.fr. Retrieved 9/15/2019 from https://www.thelocal.fr/20181011/frances-major-pension-reforms-will-keep-retirement-age-of-62.

The World Bank. 2021. "Fertility Rate, Total (Births Per Woman) – European Union." Washington, DC: The World Bank. Retrieved 1/30/2021 from https://data.worldbank.org/indicator/SP.DYN.TFRT.IN?locations=EU.

Tolnay, Stewert E., Stephen N. Graham, and Avery M. Guest. 1982. "Own-Child Estimates of U.S. White Fertility, 1886–99." *Historical Methods* 15 (8):127–138.

United Nations. 1948. "Universal Declaration of Human Rights." Retrieved 7/22/2019 from https://www.un.org/en/universal-declaration-human-rights/index.html.

United Nations. 2017. "Workers Per Retiree (ages 20–64 per ages 65+)." Retrieved 12/30/2019 from http://www.econdataus.com/workers1565_17.html.

US Census Bureau. 2019. "How the Census Bureau Measures Poverty." Washington, DC. US Census Bureau. Retrieved 2/4/2020 from https://www.census.gov/topics/income-poverty/poverty/guidance/poverty-measures.html.

Védrine, Hubert. 2014. *La France au défi.* Paris, France: Fayard.

Villagómez, F. Alejandro, and Gabriel Darío Ramírez. 2013. "México." Pp. 313–349 in *Más allá de las Pensiones Contributivas: Catorce Experiencias en América Latina,* edited by Rafael Rofman, Ignacio Apella, and Evelyn Vezza. Buenos Aires: Banco Mundial.

Wagner, David. 2005. *The Poorhouse: America's Forgotten Institution.* Lanham, MA: Roman & Littlefield.

Willmore, Larry. 2006. "Universal Age Pensions in Developing Countries: The Example of Mauritius." *International Social Security Review* 59 (4):67–89.

Willmore, Larry. 2014. "Old Age Pensions in Mexico: Toward Universal Coverage." Rochester, NY: Social Science Research Network. Retrieved 9/11/2015 from http://dx.doi.org/10.2139/ssrn.2383768.

Chapter 3

Elder Rights in the Context of the New Human Rights Discourse

Although many cultures supposedly venerate the elderly, that idealized veneration does not necessarily translate into actual respect for and support of their human and social rights. The reality for many older individuals is far from ideal. In most low and middle-income nations older parents are dependent on their children for physical and emotional support. In the absence of a developed welfare state, there are few options. Unfortunately, the ideal of veneration, respect, and support does not apply for everyone, especially for older individuals with few personal resources. In response, in recent decades older individuals and their advocates have engaged in an ongoing struggle to bring the plight of so many older individuals to the public's attention and to demand the legal protection of their rights. These efforts have given rise to a number of international conventions dealing with the human and social rights of older persons. In this chapter we summarize those efforts and also ask whether and how such efforts actually improve the situations of older individuals. Liliana Padilla has been actively involved in the fight for the human and social rights of the elderly for many years. She told of some of her experiences that serve as an introduction to our discussion of the ongoing struggle for the rights of older persons.

LILIANA: My name is Liliana Silva Chávez Padilla. I am 65 years old and I was born in Mexico City. I studied biology, and have a master's degree in psychoanalysis and a master's degree in teacher training. I have worked on issues of feminism, human rights, democracy, and citizenship ... I joined the human rights department of the Director's office for the municipality at the invitation of [name] ... We met [because we were working] on the issue of feminism. We both taught and ... she invited me to join knowing my interests ...

INTERVIEWER: And what are some of the activities you engage in?

LILIANA: It is my duty to respect, promote, enforce, and guarantee people's rights in [city] ... This office did not exist as such. There was a legal department with a human rights section, but when I created the

DOI: 10.4324/9781003205609-3

human rights office, the director ... said to me "... remember that we are to respect and protect the human rights of civil servants." ... I asked him "how?" I don't understand, then. I told him that my obligation was to enforce the rights of citizens, of people, and that is when the differences began. They took everything, they left no information, they scrubbed the computer and left nothing. All they left was a filing cabinet with open cases, they were incomplete; there was no information for the last seven years ... he told me not to worry, you don't have to work much. Offer a few courses and publicize them in the newspaper and that's it. It surprised me ... The only thing they left me was a desk, telephone and a printer. That's it.

INTERVIEWER: Not even a chair.

LILIANA: Nothing, nothing, nothing. We were in the offices of the municipality and they wanted to move us to a building a very long way from here but we came back. I said no we're not staying there, and when we came back there was a confrontation with the union that was thrown out, but I said that I am not leaving, I'm staying in this office. It was a scandal and the union people said "get out!" ... when they saw that we were seven people and I invited several feminists and people to work on human rights protocols that some people were against. They didn't want us, but we stayed. ... I worked for independent bodies, such as the Federal Electoral Institute on federal and local cases. I thought I would not keep the job because they elected a new council and I am grateful that they kept me on.

INTERVIEWER: Yes, I was going to ask you that because I saw that you were a counselor. Are you still doing that?

LILIANA: Yes, because there was a new election ... and I am grateful that it made a difference. Previously I spent seven years in the public defender's office and on the human rights commission for the city ... It was a difficult time because it was after 2006. The reality was that it was very difficult because I was coerced by agents of the State, terribly, because one was unable to open one's mouth ... the truth is that one learns that if one is committed to the idea of human rights and if one believes in the cause and thinks it is possible then one has to defend the rights of everyone. I defended the case of ... the women who were murdered from the radio station that broke the silence, because it was a silencing of the defender's office. I even sent all the information to the inter-American convention. But someone intervened and there was no answer, but nonetheless I have the experience with matters of this type on the commission as a counselor questioning and succeeding ... Well, I carried on ... I have a civil association called [name] and I have worked with resources from SEDESOL (Ministry of Social Development) ... I have worked on issues related to the environment, but with women, women who have the capacity to defend the water because it is a social issue. We form committees made up of men and women and we discuss water and land issues ...

INTERVIEWER: Who is involved?

LILIANA: We have gone out to the edge of the city. The center is very beautiful, but the outlying areas are very poor, marginalized, and in the process of gentrification ... I have been working in [neighborhoods]. But it has been two years since I have been in the municipality and I have not been able to. I have worked with women who produce coffee in order to empower them so they can get ahead. They are the ones who make the tortillas ... they are women who have no right to own land, who cannot get a loan from SAGARPA (Secretariat of Agriculture and Rural Development) because SAGARPA only gives to men, the owners of land, and women stay in the community ...

INTERVIEWER: From the municipal level in the field of rights, could you tell us what else you are doing?

LILIANA: ... I give courses to police and to the authorities ... who are the first ones to violate human rights ... We began to offer courses with the support of the public defender's office and do you know what happened? The police did not come, they were upset by the type of course ... we told them to [be aware that] they are being violent, they harass women ... We couldn't do anything. A police course was scheduled and nothing was done, they did not provide anything, no chairs no tables so I said, OK, today we are offering the course without chairs ... I sent a letter to the municipal president telling him of the shameful conditions ... another thing is that when the media arrive it is when the defender's complaints arrive. They come to me and I have to process them and tell that authority that they have been accused of violating this or that ... and I need a response ... they send me an answer saying that they don't have to answer for anything ...

INTERVIEWER: ... Regarding the rights of older adults, what actions have been taken?

LILIANA: The issue of older adults is something so serious, so painful because [city] is second in the number of older adults in poverty, who have few resources, and it deals with the problem of older adults in poverty and women in the poor neighborhoods in a terrible manner ... The situation isn't just bad, it's terrible.

Rights rather than Charity

Liliana Padilla is clearly a unique individual. She is well educated and highly committed to protecting the human rights of the most vulnerable. She has worked on issues related to feminism, human rights, democracy, and citizenship in various capacities, including that of a municipal official charged with the enforcement of human rights laws. In this position she has had to deal with many individuals and forces that resist change. For that reason, she began a civil society association that focuses on the rights of those with little protection. Liliana Padilla is an example of individuals with high levels of human and cultural capital that they bring to the defense of their own and others' rights. In Chapter six we deal with organizations that are made up of retired union members, retired teachers, retired entrepreneurs, and those with a history of governmental employment that gives them experience in dealing with bureaucracies. These individuals are often keenly aware of the fact that the human rights of many groups and individuals, including older individuals, are restricted or denied. Gaining and protecting those rights represents a central component of the agendas of civil society organizations.

In this chapter we review the various international conventions on the human and social rights of older persons that have been drafted in recent decades, as well as the influence that civil society organizations have had on the drafting of those conventions, focusing largely on Latin America and the Caribbean where they have been particularly important. We begin by asking what exactly human rights consist of and who implements and enforces the guarantees that are enumerated. The conception of human rights that most of us share, which is that they are basic, inviolate, and universal, entered into public discourse only recently. The widespread and serious state-sponsored violations of individual and group rights that has characterized much of human history did not gain widespread public attention until the 1970s (Moyn 2010). Traditional conceptions of rights for the most part saw them as consisting solely of those individual or group prerogatives granted by the State.

Even though widespread public concern for human rights did not draw international attention until the 1970s, the serious violations of human rights and dignity embodied in the Holocaust and the inhumanity of much of the 20th Century demanded attention at the highest levels. In 1948 immediately after World War II the United Nations General Assembly adopted the *Universal Declaration of Human Rights*, the first international statement affirming the existence and universality of such rights (United Nations, 1948). The thirty Articles, or principles, of the Declaration affirm such basic rights as the following:

Article 1: All human beings are born free and equal in dignity and rights. They are endowed with reason and conscience and should act towards one another in a spirit of brotherhood.
Article 2: Everyone is entitled to all the rights and freedoms set forth in this Declaration, without distinction of any kind, such as race, colour, sex, language, religion, political or other opinion, national or social origin, property, birth or other status ...

Article 3: Everyone has the right to life, liberty and security of person.

Article 4: No one shall be held in slavery or servitude; slavery and the slave trade shall be prohibited in all their forms.

Article 5: No one shall be subjected to torture or to cruel, inhuman or degrading treatment or punishment.

Article 9: No one shall be subjected to arbitrary arrest, detention or exile.

Article 14: 1. Everyone has the right to seek and to enjoy in other countries asylum from persecution.

Article 15: 1. Everyone has the right to a nationality.

Article 19: Everyone has the right to freedom of opinion and expression; this right includes freedom to hold opinions without interference and to seek, receive and impart information and ideas through any media and regardless of frontiers.

Article 22: Everyone, as a member of society, has the right to social security and is entitled to realization, through national effort and international co-operation and in accordance with the organization and resources of each State, of the economic, social and cultural rights indispensable for his dignity and the free development of his personality.

Article 25: 1. Everyone has the right to a standard of living adequate for the health and well-being of himself and of his family, including food, clothing, housing and medical care and necessary social services, and the right to security in the event of unemployment, sickness, disability, widowhood, old age or other lack of livelihood in circumstances beyond his control.

The Declaration affirmed both negative rights, which include things that the State or others cannot do to anyone, and positive rights, or what one is entitled to, including food, clothing, and shelter as affirmed in Article 25 listed above. It also listed obligations, as in Article 29 (1), which states that "Everyone has duties to the community in which alone the free and full development of his personality is possible."

This first codification of human rights was an attempt to comprehensively condemn the atrocities of the Nazis and others throughout human history, as well as to affirm personal autonomy and citizenship in terms of democratic participation. At the time it was adopted, many legal scholars and others were sceptical of the declaration's utility given that nation states enjoy absolute sovereignty, meaning that the imposition and enforcement of such principles is largely voluntary for individual nations. Even today many observers are sceptical of the utility and success of international treaties and agreements related to human rights (Hopgood 2013; Posner 2014). Yet during the closing decades of the 20th Century, a general disillusionment with older utopian and grand scale philosophies advocating radical social transformation breathed new life into the more immediate defense of individual human rights (Moyn 2010). Civil society organizations such as Amnesty

International and Americas Watch emerged to address a growing concern with the human and political rights of individuals and victimized groups. Many others, including faith-based organizations, embraced the new agenda.

The concern for human rights includes the rights of women, children, the mentally ill, political prisoners, racial, ethnic, and religious minorities, and others. As a social movement it embodies opposition to capital punishment, genital mutilation, the separation of immigrant children from their parents, and other policies and practices that subject individuals to unjust and cruel treatment. Initially, this new human rights agenda did not specifically mention the rights of older people, but that has changed. Since the 1980s several international conventions have affirmed the human and social rights of older people as a group whose rights have been at particular risk. These conventions are part of an emerging international social movement that rejects traditional views of older people as uninterested, uninvolved, and unproductive. The new discourse embodies a growing affirmation of active aging and active citizenship and the rejection of discredited disengagement theories that proposed that aging individuals voluntarily and inevitably withdraw from active participation in life. The rejection of such notions and the widespread adoption of policies that enable and encourage active aging accompany greatly enhanced life spans and an increase in the proportion of older individuals in the populations of all nations. As life spans increase dramatically, the proportion of very old individuals, those 80 and older, is increasing at an astonishing rate and is expected to quadruple in certain Latin American nations by 2050 (He, Goodkind, and Kowa 2016). Given the new demographic and social reality that accompanies rapidly aging populations, retirement policy, health care systems, social service agencies, legal systems, and more must adapt.

International conventions in general, and those focused on aging in particular, are for the most part only statements of principle. They are not enforceable, nor do they place binding obligations on signatories, other than those that the participating states choose to impose upon themselves. Rather, they are manifestations of changing public perceptions and an evolving discourse related to aging, much as previous conceptions of appropriate gender roles and racial differences have changed in accordance with new discourses that reject sexism and racism. Ultimately, these conventions articulate a changing moral order in which the human, political, and social rights of citizens, including those of older individuals, take on new meanings and importance, as we discuss more fully below.

In what follows we deal with the changing discourse related to the rights of older individuals and their rightful place in the family, the community, and society generally. Our core theme relates to the affirmation of basic human rights that assure one's right not to be interfered with. In the case of older persons these include freedom from violence and intimidation, freedom from economic exploitation, freedom from the fear of abandonment, and more. Basic rights also include the right to vote, the right to lifelong education, the right to health care, and the right to participate fully in family and community life. While such basic rights are central, they are inadequate to insure the effective expression of citizenship. Increasingly, conceptions of human rights include positive social rights, which include the right to the material necessities for a healthy and dignified life. These new human and social rights discourses have important implications not only for older individuals, but for society at large. Unfortunately, as we illustrate in this and later chapters, demands for social rights run headlong into the reality of fiscal limits, especially in low and middle-income countries that face seriously constrained capacities to provide all citizens the material support they need.

Framing the Issue

Before proceeding to a discussion of the various international conventions that deal with the rights of older people, it would be useful to review the various ways in which the role of older people and their rights and duties can be framed. We employ the verb "frame" to refer to the ways in which the situation of older people, including their capacities and appropriate roles, are viewed by older people themselves and by the public at large. In general, frames relate to public perceptions of the appropriate solutions to a particular problem or situation. Although biological aging may be an objective fact, the social situations of older persons, including their rights and obligations, are social constructions (Huerta Benze 2015; Huerta Benze 2016; Estes, 2011). Older people can be viewed as superannuated and unproductive, or they can be seen as autonomous agents who are not only potentially productive and able to care for themselves, but entirely capable of contributing significantly to the commonweal. These different frames clearly have important implications for the ways in which older people are viewed and treated (Estes 1979; Estes 2011).

"Frame analysis" and "frame alignment processes," refer to ways in which social movements or groups attempt to convince a larger audience that their interpretation of some situation is accurate and that their proposed solutions are both just and likely to be effective (Goffman 1974; Snow et al. 1986). In the case of oppressed or marginalized individuals and groups, the basic process involves changing the public's interpretation of their current situation as accidental, unavoidable, or inevitable to the realization that it results from injustice or an intolerable set of imposed circumstances (Turner 1969). In the case of the economic rights of older persons, rather than viewing old-age poverty as the inevitable result of a loss of productive potential, a situation that calls for simple charity, advocates for the social rights of older persons attempt to reframe the problem of poverty as the result of inequitable and unjust social structures and arrangements that operate over the life course to increase the precariousness of certain individuals in old age. These arrangements can and must be altered. Frame analysis complements and adds a new dimension to resource mobilization theory, which focuses on the economic, political, and social resources that a group can bring to bear in furthering its cause. Frame analysis reintroduces cultural and cognitive meaning to extend our focus beyond material, political, and human resources and capacities alone. For groups that lack large reserves of material or political capital, changing hearts and minds takes on ever greater importance.

"Master frames" refer to widely held understandings of the causes of a particular situation, including the ways in which it can be altered. These are more general than specific frames focused on a specific issue. Takeshi Wada presents quantitative data to support the assertion that during the neoliberal period in Mexico earlier claims for social rights took on a new aspect as demands for political rights, which are basic to gaining civil and social rights (Wada 2006). Rita Noonan argues that women were able to protest in Pinochet's Chile in ways that men were not because they could use a master frame of motherhood and femininity to protest human rights abuses since the focus on womanhood was compatible with the regime's own master frame of veneration of the home and family (Noonan 1995). While resource mobilization theory focuses on the material capacity and skills necessary for successful protest, frame analysis adds a focus on individuals' and groups' understandings and the deliberate and strategic actions they take to attempt to change things.

To summarize, then, public perceptions of older people can range from viewing them as the victims of misfortune or unavoidable aging processes to viewing them as potentially active agents who are capable of furthering their own and others' interests. Many variations and combinations of frames are possible, and each has important implications for collective action by older individuals. As a culmination of a long series of international conventions and statements on the rights of older persons, in 2015 the Inter-American Convention for the Protection of the Human Rights of Older Persons issued a major report which affirmed the right of older persons to social participation, as well as political participation and non-discrimination (OAS 2021). The right to participation is held to be central to the protection of other human rights. Theoretically and practically, then, the question that the report leads us to pose is how civil society organizations mobilize citizens and help to create social and political environments in which they can act as effective agents in furthering their own interests and those of others.

Retirement as a Right

In high-income and even middle-income nations retirement has become synonymous with the right to an adequate income after one's working years are over, which given increases in life expectancy can be quite young. Although we may take retirement for granted, leaving the labor force while one is still healthy is a relatively recent practice in human history, even in the developed world (Thane 2005). Prior to the 19th Century most individuals worked until they could no longer do so and then turned to family or the charity of others. That remains the reality in much of the world today. In the past, destitute older individuals with no support often ended up in asylums or workhouses (Grob 1983; Thane 2005). One limiting factor to the social burden that idle individuals might represent was the fact that given relatively short life spans, that period of idleness and dependency was relatively short. Only a few wealthy individuals could afford a life of leisure in old age.

That began to slowly change in the developed world at the end of the 19th Century (Arza and Johnson 2006; Sass 2006). One of the earliest protections offered by the modern welfare state was income security in old age (Myles 1984; Palier 2010; Thane 2006). During the 20th Century private employer and public state pensions became more common in medium and high-income countries (Myles 1984; Thane 2006). Such pensions gave rise to a new phase of the life course in which an individual was freed from the need to work. By the second half of the 20th Century this new life course phase was lengthening rapidly and a growing number of retirees required pension reform, often quite drastic reform, to deal with the growing fiscal burden associated with low fertility and large retired populations. Yet, as we discussed in Chapter two, retirement plans have become a central aspect of advanced industrial societies and have been adopted in most middle-income and even some low-income countries. It is clear they are here to stay, even as they face inevitable limitations.

The Human and Social Rights of Older People: Beyond Demography

The age structure of a population reflects basic demographic processes related to fertility, mortality, and migration. If and when people marry, how many children a woman has, how long people live, and why they decide to migrate, though, reflect many cultural, economic, and political causes that have profound social implications. During the latter half of the 20th Century demographers developed a theory that relates historical changes in fertility and mortality to overall population size (Kirk 1996). Classical demographic transition theory proposed four stages in the transition of human populations from primitive to modern profiles. Stage 1 refers to the period before industrialization and improvements in agricultural production that was characterized by high fertility and high mortality that resulted in a small, but stable population. In Stage 2, as conditions of life improved, mortality rates began to decline while fertility rates remained high, resulting in a rapid increase in population. In Stage 3 as people expected their children to survive, fertility rates began to decline, even as mortality rates continued to drop, resulting in slightly slower population growth. In Stage 4 both fertility and mortality both reach low levels and the population again remains stable, if much larger than at the beginning of this process.

Demographic transition theory is useful in drawing attention to the impact of technological and social changes on population size and composition and also for reminding us that different population age profiles call for different policy and social responses. A young population has different needs for education, health care, economic support, and much more than a population that is much older, and it is likely that in the two cases both levels of economic development and dominant public policies will be quite different. Whether the demographic transition process holds in all of its details for all nations or regions remains disputed (Nielsen 2015; Zaidi and Morgan 2017), but it need not be strictly true in every detail to be useful for our purposes. Whatever the details or exact sequence of events, the aging of the populations of the world is hardly in dispute.

In recent years some observers have proposed a fifth stage to the demographic transition process, again one that implies significant cultural and political adjustments which are relevant to our discussion. This new fifth stage refers to a period when fertility rates drop below mortality rates. Mathematically, such a situation eventually leads to population decline and the sort of rapid population aging we have been discussing. Today, birth rates in Europe are below replacement, as they are in fifteen countries in Latin America (Eurostat 2019; Montes de Oca et al. 2018). In order to replace herself and one male, a woman must bear at least 2.1 children. The fraction is to compensate for some unavoidable loss. Maintaining a stable population requires replenishment from somewhere. Even though Germany's fertility rate is below replacement, it continues to grow as the result of immigration (World Economic Forum 2019). Europe and much of the rest of the developed world are facing serious dilemmas resulting from below-replacement fertility rates and their consequent need for immigrants at a time of growing anti-immigrant sentiment.

As important as the subject of immigration may be, though, it is a bit off topic. The point we wish to make is that the emergence of this fifth stage in the demographic transition brings with it a shift in policy discourse from one focused solely on the needs of younger groups to a greater focus on the welfare and needs of older persons and what they are able to contribute to the commonweal. As we have noted, a major shift in the discourse on human rights is its extension to include social rights as in principle basic and unalienable (Choi, Brownell, and Moldovan 2017; Martin, Rodríguez, and Brown 2015; Montes de Oca et al. 2018; OAS 2021; Rodriguez-Pinzón and Martin 2003). This focus on social rights is rather recent and definitely in a process of evolution. As we have also noted, the extension of social rights is limited by very real fiscal constraints, as well as by institutions that perpetuate injustice and inequality.

The issue of the human and social rights of older persons may at first glance seem uncomplicated. After all, major international conventions, such as the Universal Declaration of Human Rights, and later conventions affirm that all humans are entitled to basic rights (Moyn 2010). Unfortunately, until recently none of these conventions identified older people as a group whose rights require special protection (Rodriguez-Pinzón and Martin 2003). Affirmations of general human rights are useful, but groups with special needs can be overlooked if they are not singled out. More recent conventions, particularly in Latin America, have addressed this omission, at least in principle. The question we are left with is the extent to which this new focus on the rights of older persons is accompanied by real improvements in their political and economic situations.

Are Human Rights Principles Enforceable?

In a recent review of international and regional law related to the rights of older persons Martin, Rodríguez, and Pinzón differentiate between what they term "soft" law and "hard" law related to the rights of older people (Martin, Rodríguez, and Brown 2015). Soft law, which we might really think of as principles rather than law, includes statements such as those expressed in the Universal Declaration of Human Rights, or the United Nations Madrid International Plan of Action on Aging (MIPAA), which sets out general principles related to the rights of older people (United Nations 1948). Such principles are not binding or enforceable in any legal system (Toro Huerta 2006). Hard law, on the other hand, refers to national or more local laws, which are often informed by international conventions and agreements, that are at some level binding. Soft law is couched in terms of general strategies or approaches which may eventually become what the authors term "customary law," which is still not enforceable, but which reflects a greater acceptance of the underlying moral and legal principles espoused. Soft laws or the codification of principles that affirm human rights in principle are useful in changing discourses, but their real success would be reflected in more binding legislation.

An example of how soft law can reify principles to the point that they become customary law, for which there are more mechanisms for monitoring nations' compliance, is the Inter-American Convention of Protecting the Human Rights of Older Persons approved in June 2015 by the Organization of American States (Montes de Oca et al. 2018). States that ratify the convention agree to abide by its principles. In order to monitor implementation and compliance the Convention includes a follow-up mechanism consisting of a Conference of States Parties and a Committee of Experts who are charged with the monitoring task (OAS 2021). Of course, there is no real enforcement mechanism and guaranteeing compliance in effect involves moral suasion, and the fact that signatory nations agree to allow their policies and practices related to the rights of older persons to be made public. Currently five countries, Argentina, Bolivia, Chile, Costa Rica, and Uruguay, have ratified the convention.

In what follows we summarize the major international conventions on the human and social rights of older persons, paying particular attention to the role of civil society organizations in stimulating debates and public pressure that led to their adoption. Latin America has made particularly impressive strides in codifying and affirming the human rights of older persons. The extent to which these conventions have resulted in actual improvements in the situation of older individuals, and especially those with special needs and few resources, remains unclear (Sidorenko and Zaidi 2018). A close examination of the principles reveals that some are little more than affirmations of traditional approaches, such as statements that older people have a right to family support. In what follows we will distinguish between soft principles and hard law, of which there is relatively little related to the human and social rights of older persons in any country.

Are Human Rights Universal?

Since the concept of rights is so central to our discussion, we must briefly examine its meaning and acceptance by different cultural and social groups. Although the term "human rights" may convey the sense of something that is indisputably good, we must point out that it is not a universally accepted or valued concept, nor is it clear that the global struggle for human rights, or at least the Western conception of human rights, is even close to being won. The current rise in populist nationalism in so many parts of the world is frankly disconcerting (Jeppesen 2016; Strangio 2017). More than seventy years after the adoption of the Universal Declaration of Human Rights, many activists, including Amnesty International's Secretary-General, Salil Shetty, have serious concerns regarding real progress in advancing human rights and the possibility that they may be in retreat in many places (Hopgood 2013; Posner 2014; Shetty 2016; Sikkink 2017). The basic problem arises from the fact that legal guarantee of human rights, and especially the enforcement of real protections by local governments, is not guaranteed by any international body. David Kennedy, a human rights activist himself, offers a detailed summary of criticisms of legal conceptions of human rights that have been leveled over the years (Kennedy 2002).

We will not delve into these, except to note that among the most serious criticisms is that traditional human rights claims represent little more than an imposition of Western cultural values on others (García, Klare, and Williams 2015; Hopgood 2013; Kennedy 2002; Moyn 2010; Tharoor 1999/2000). Westerners may privilege the individual and view his or her autonomy and agency as paramount, but other cultures may privilege the will of the group, clan, or tribe over that of the individual. In the absence of a native's understanding of local values and customs, the imposition of ethical concepts, no matter how dearly held by an outsider, could end up doing more harm than good in terms of the well-being of locals. Certain observers have basically given up the hope of extending full human rights to all currently excluded or stigmatized groups. It is important to note, though, that the Human Rights Movement has become far more sensitive to cultural and local differences. Recent efforts at understanding and fostering human rights take cultural differences, gender, and other important distinctions seriously (García, Klare, and Williams 2015).

Kathryn Sikkink defends the utility and basic success of efforts to extend and strengthen human rights (Sikkink 2017). While increases in the number of refugees, and local atrocities, such as those in the Democratic Republic of the Congo or Bosnia, can temper one's optimism, overall Sikkink notes substantial progress in women's rights, the abolition of capital punishment, and more. She offers a plausible explanation for the appearance of a lack of progress when she points out that furthering the agenda entails drawing attention to human rights abuses, a framing tactic that can make it appear that little progress is being made, when in fact the exposure of such abuses affirms the success of the effort. Today, human rights abuses can no longer remain hidden, and governments can no longer violate human rights with impunity as they could just a few years ago (Keck and Sikkink 1998).

For our purposes, an appreciation of cultural differences does not preclude general affirmations of universal basic principles related to the human and social rights of older persons as they are affirmed in the conventions we discuss below. In addition, although progress may be slow, the only alternative to a forceful affirmation and defense of basic rights is despair and acceptance of the status quo, a position that is unacceptable. Additionally, we are less interested in the imposition of external conceptions of human and social rights by specific CSOs. Rather we are more interested in the ways in which local groups define their own agendas and the ways in which they frame the issues they address. Local groups may well be influenced by national and even international social movements and ideas, but those must be implemented at a local level by individuals working in voluntary groups.

The Evolution of an Agenda: From Vienna to Asunción

Although it might not be widely known, debates and advocacy for human and social rights has a long history in Latin America (Montes de Oca et al.

2018; Sikkink 2017). The 1917 Mexican constitution was the first in the world to affirm economic and social rights in addition to civil and political rights. The history of dictatorships and violence in the region might overshadow this reality, but as we discuss below, human and social rights have been a core concern in Latin America and the Caribbean. The history of military and civilian dictatorships in the region clearly have forced the issue onto the public agenda. For present purposes we trace the beginning of the contemporary discourse on the human and social rights of older persons to the Report of the World Assembly on Aging, which met in Vienna, Austria from July 26 to August 6 1982 in the first international convention intended to provide guiding principles that nations could follow in addressing the needs of growing older populations (United Nations 1982).

The Vienna Assembly was preceded by various UN statements on the rights of older persons, but Vienna represented the first modern attempt to comprehensively address the issue. In addition to a long discussion of the demographic and social changes affecting older persons, their families, and communities, the Assembly offered sixty-two recommendations for action to further research, data collection and analysis, training and education of health care providers, and more. The recommendations dealt with health and nutrition, the protection of elderly consumers, housing and environment, family, social welfare, income security and employment, and education (United Nations 1982).

Monitoring and assessing the impact of such general recommendations and principles at the national and more local levels proved difficult and periodic assessments of the situation of older persons in various nations revealed disappointing progress toward the Assembly's goals. Low levels of economic development, political upheavals, recessions, and other factors undermined the implementation of the proposals (Sidorenko and Zaidi 2018). The limited results of the Vienna Assembly led to renewed efforts by the Second World Assembly on Aging (SWAA), which produced the Madrid International Plan of Action on Aging (MIPAA) (Montes de Oca et al. 2018). The Madrid conference framed the situation of aging populations as one that goes beyond issues of demography and population composition to one involving the human and social rights of older persons (United Nations 2002). Point 4 of the introduction of the Assembly's report (p. 5) notes that:

> [p]opulation ageing is poised to become a major issue in developing countries, which are projected to age swiftly in the first half of the twenty-first century. The proportion of older persons is expected to rise from 8 to 19 per cent by 2050, while that of children will fall from 33 to 22 per cent.

The report details unique vulnerabilities associated with gender, rural residence, and more. It calls for "changes in attitudes, policies and practices at all levels in all sectors so that the enormous potential of ageing in the twenty-first century may be fulfilled" (p. 7). Accomplishing this would clearly require an international effort and consciousness raising at all levels of government and society. As with Vienna, implementation at national and local levels remains the challenge.

In the days before SWAA civil society organizations held a forum of their own to affirm the dignity of age and further their agenda related to the basic rights of older people (Montes de Oca et al. 2018). Their efforts included collaborations with academics, government institutions, businesses, and others to begin to build a social movement. These multilateral and civil society initiatives have been carried forward with particular intensity in Latin America and the Caribbean where successive regional and intergovernmental meetings have developed general principles and public policy applicable to the region. These included the regional strategy meetings for implementation of MIPAA in Latin America and the Caribbean. Meetings were held in Santiago de Chile in 2003; Brasilia, Brazil in 2007; San José, Costa Rica in 2012 and Asunción, Paraguay in 2017. Each iteration reaffirmed and refined the basic agenda. In parallel with these meetings, CSOs representing older persons met to produce several declarations. These took place in Santiago in 2003; in Brasilia in 2007; in Tres Ríos, Costa Rica in 2012; and in Ypacaraí, Paraguay in 2017. During this period the Montevideo Consensus on Population and Development (MCPD), drafted in 2013, and the Inter-American Convention for the Protection of the Rights of Older Persons (IACPHROP), drafted by the Organization of American States in 2015, further affirmed the rights agenda. The sequence of these meetings is summarized in Figure 3.1 (Montes de Oca et al. 2018).

These various conferences and meetings of governmental representatives and CSOs were clearly important in furthering the rights dialog related to older persons. We discuss these conventions further in reference to the actions of specific CSOs in Chapter eight. The 2017 Asunción Declaration, with the subtitle "Building Inclusive Societies: Ageing with Dignity and Rights" summarizes the spirit of these efforts. It consists of twenty-two propositions and affirmations and general objectives. The following four serve as examples:

1   Reaffirm the commitment of our Governments to promote, protect and respect the human rights, dignity and fundamental freedoms of all older persons, without discrimination of any kind, and ratify the responsibility of States to ensure ageing with dignity and rights, with the greatest possible quality of life and full enjoyment of the rights of older persons;

2   Reiterate that the San José Charter on the Rights of Older Persons in Latin America and the Caribbean offers a regional framework for public policymaking that States continue to adopt, that complements

	Santiago de Chile Declaration 2003	Civil society Declaration 2007	Tres Rios Declaration 2012		Ypacarai Declaration 2017
Memorandum NGO World Forum on Ageing (Madrid 2002)	Regional CSO Forum on Ageing (Santiago de Chile 2003)	Regional Forum on Ageing (Brasillia 2007)	Regional CSO Forum on Ageing Madrid+10 (San Jose 2012)	**Montevideo Consensus on Population and Development** 2013	Regional CSD Forum on Ageing Madrid+15 (Ypacarai, Paraguay 2017)

2002	2003	2007	2012	2013	2015	2017

Second World Assembly on Ageing (Madrid 2002)	1st Regional Intergovernmental Conference on Ageing (Santiago de Chile 2003)	2nd Regional Intergovernmental Conference on Ageing (Brasilia, 2007)	3rd Regional Intergovernmental Conference on Ageing (San José, 2012)	**Inter-American Convention for the Protection of the Rights of the Older Persons** 2015	4th Regional Intergovernmental Conference on Ageing (Asuncion, 2017)
Madrid International Plan of Action on Ageing (MIPAA 2002)	Regional Strategy of Ageing (Santiage de Chile 2003)	Brasillia Declaration 2007	San José Charter 2012		Declaración de Asunción, 2017

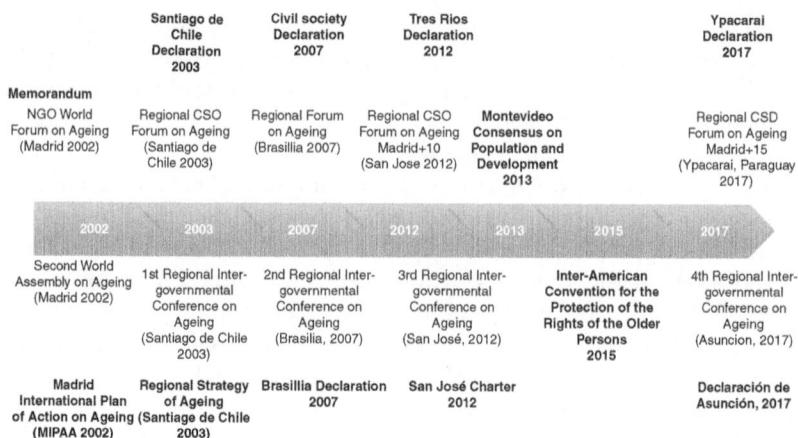

Figure 3.1 International and/or regional meetings and documents relevant to ageing in Latin America and the Caribbean, 2002–2017.
Source: Prepared by Montes de Oca et al. (2018) from United Nations (2002); CEPAL (2013); OEA (2015); CEPAL (2004); CEPAL-UNFPA (2011); CEPAL (2012); CEPAL (2017); Civil Society Declaration, Santiago 2003; Brasilia Declaration 2007; Tres Ríos Declaration, Costa Rica 2012; Ypacaraí Declaration 2017.

the work of other mechanisms at the regional and international levels, and that helps to strengthen protection of the human rights and fundamental freedoms of older persons;

3   Urge the Governments to build the issue of ageing into their development policies, plans and programmes in a cross-cutting manner, and to implement specific policies for older persons that recognize gender inequalities and promote their autonomy and independence, as well as intergenerational solidarity ...

4   Encourage the Governments of the region to consider the situation and interests of older persons, including also the ethnicity, race, gender, disability and generational perspectives, in the design and implementation of national plans and programmes to promote achievement of the 2030 Agenda for Sustainable Development and the Sustainable Development Goals, the Montevideo Consensus on Population and Development, and the Montevideo Strategy for Implementation of the Regional Gender Agenda within the Sustainable Development Framework by 2030.

(ECLAC 2017)

The propositions all begin with terms such as "recommend," "call upon," "urge," and "request," terms which emphasize the principled nature of the propositions. They are soft law in the sense that they do not propose enforceable edicts or specific programs. They serve as policy guidance to individual nations that must take their local and subnational situations into account in applying the general principles. The longer-term questions relate to the responsiveness of governments in adopting policies favorable to the human and social rights of older persons, and the extent to which CSOs have been effective in furthering the adoption of such policies.

From Principle to Practice

As Martin and colleagues note, even though soft laws do not have the force of the courts behind them, they do not lack all effectiveness (Martin, Rodríguez, and Brown 2015). They can lead to changes in public perceptions, redefine acceptable discourse concerning aging and rights, and affect the visibility of various groups. Although several new laws that affirm the rights of older persons have been passed in various nations in Latin America, they have been difficult to put into practice. Laws related to the rights of older persons have been introduced since the early 1990s (Huenchuan 2013) and have been reinforced by institutional commitments and structures (Huenchuan 2016). The specific objectives of these laws differ substantially, and many continue to affirm an assistance perspective which is based on conceptualizations of those over a certain age as unproductive and in need of care and assistance. More recent laws have begun affirming a rights perspective, which includes the right to a dignified life; a dignified death; equality and non-discrimination; physical, psychological, and emotional autonomy; and the right to participate in the social, cultural, and political life of the community (Huenchuan 2013). These principles and rights were fully consolidated in the Inter-American Convention for the Protection of the Human Rights of Older Persons (OAS 2021).

In Mexico, a number of laws dealing with the welfare of older adults have been introduced at the national and subnational levels. These largely reaffirm the family's responsibility for aging parents, while extending and standardizing the provision of diverse services and assistance. Today the family continues to provide most of the care and support that older parents receive (Montes de Oca Zavala 2014). That responsibility is codified in the National Law on the Rights of Older Persons, Article 9 (Cámara De Diputados Del H. Congreso De La Unión (Mexico), 2018, p. 7). Without minimizing the significant advance that this law represents in affirming the rights of older persons, we must note that it does not specifically address the rights of older ethnic group members, nor does it deal directly with economic security or pensions. It reaffirms the right to social assistance and the right to be supported by the family rather than affirming the right to a public pension or support. Despite its shortcomings, though, this reform contributes to the strengthening of subnational laws, and constitutes a substantial move forward in reframing of the justification for social programs and public policies by affirming the proposition that older persons possess basic social rights. It is important to note that these basic principles were again reaffirmed at the Fourth Regional Inter-governmental Conference on Aging and the Rights of Older Persons held in Asunción, Paraguay in 2017 (CEPAL 2017).

Civil Society and the Future of Human and Senior Rights

Despite the shortcomings of human rights initiatives in Latin America and other parts of the world, the context in which the egregious human rights abuses of the fairly recent past occurred has changed. Amnesty International, Americas Watch, and other organizations remain vigilant and active in bringing human rights abuses to the public's attention. Many other smaller and less known groups working in every country, including those that remain highly repressive, carry the human rights agenda forward. As we noted, it is possible to despair of ever arriving at a time when human rights are universally affirmed and respected. The concept of human rights, or at least the highly individualistic way in which the debate over rights is framed in developed Western cultures, is often seen as foreign and rejected by other cultures and nations. Perhaps the problem lies in an insufficiently inclusive conceptualization of human rights that fails to recognize their culturally-based nature that includes obligations to the collectivity, as well as the prerogatives of individuals. It can be rather condescending to imagine that other societies with different values and mores are incapable of respecting the basic rights of individuals and sub-groups. The challenge is to understand different cultural frames of the issue of rights and duties, without abandoning the basic moral values related to life, liberty, and equality.

Against the backdrop of a discussion of human rights generally, we have focused on the human and social rights of older persons and pointed out the fact that the major multilateral conventions that have affirmed their basic rights have been informed by numerous civil society groups that have met before, alongside, or after the formal government-sponsored conventions. These have been instrumental in changing the discourse surrounding aging and the capacities, rights, and duties of older people. A major objective of such efforts is to empower older individuals to act collectively to further their own interests and those of others. This objective involves changing the ways in which society at large, and older individuals themselves view the causes and consequences of their traditionally disadvantaged positions. This change in hearts and minds, or overcoming false consciousness, involves a profound change in individual and public psychology and discourses related to aging. As we noted, resource mobilization theory's traditional focus on the material capacity and skills necessary for successful protest, while valuable, remains incomplete. Frame analysis, or an understanding of how individuals and groups view the causes of and solutions to their current situation, adds an important extension that brings us closer to understanding older individuals as effective actors and advocates. In Chapters six, seven, and eight we will present illustrations of how individuals in civil society organizations focus on a range of objectives, from improving the quality of life of older individuals, to militant actions directed at insuring and extending their basic human and social rights.

References

Arza, C., and P. Johnson. 2006. "The Development of Public Pensions from 1889 to the 1990s." Pp. 52–75 in *The Oxford Handbook of Pensions and Retirement Income*, edited by G.L. Clark, A.H. Munnell, and J.M. Orszag. New York, NY: Oxford University Press.

Cámara De Diputados Del H. Congreso De La Uníon (Mexico). 2018. "Ley de Los Derechos de Las Personas Adultas Mayores." In *Nueva Ley publicada en el Diario Oficial de la Federación el 25 de junio de 2018*, edited by S. G. d. S. Parlamentarios. Retrieved 7/29/2019 from http://www.diputados.gob.mx/LeyesBiblio/pdf/245_120718.pdf.

CEPAL. 2017. *Derechos de las persona mayores: Retos para la interdependencia y autonomía*. Retrieved 9/15/2017 from https://www.cepal.org/es/publicaciones/41471-derechos-personas-mayores-retos-la-interdependencia-autonomia.

Choi, M., P. Brownell, and S.I. Moldovan. 2017. "International Movement to Promote Human Rights of Older Women with a Focus on Violence and Abuse against Older Women." *International Social Work*, 60 (1): 170–181. doi:10.1177/0020872814559562.

ECLAC. 2017. "Asunción Declaration Building Inclusive Societies: Ageing with Dignity and Rights." In ENGLISH ORIGINAL: SPANISH 17–00614, Fourth Regional Intergovernmental Conference on Ageing and the Rights of Older Persons in Latin America and the Caribbean, June 30. Mexico City: Economic Commission for Latin America and the Caribbean. Retrieved 7/25/2019 from https://conferenciaenvejecimiento.cepal.org/4/sites/envejecimiento4/files/c1700614_0.pdf.

Estes, C.L. 1979. *The Aging Enterprise: A Critical Examination of Social Policies and Services for the Aged*. San Francisco, CA: Jossey-Bass.

Estes, C.L. 2011. "Crises and Old Age Policy." Pp. 297–320 in *Handbook of Sociology of Aging*, edited by J. Richard, A. Settersten, and J.L. Angel. New York, NY: Springer.

Eurostat. 2019. "Fertility Statistics." Retrieved 7/24/2019 from https://ec.europa.eu/eurostat/statistics-explained/index.php/Fertility_statistics.

García, H.A., K. Klare, and L.A. Williams (Eds.). 2015. *Social and Economic Rights in Theory and Practice*. New York, NY: Routledge.

Goffman, E. 1974. *Frame Analysis*. Cambridge, MA: Harvard University Press.

Grob, G.N. 1983. *Mental Illness and American Society*. Princeton, NJ: Princeton University Press.

He, W., D. Goodkind, and P. Kowa. 2016. "An Aging World: 2015." International Population Reports (Vol. P95/16–11): National Institute on Aging. Retrieved 1/3/2020 from https://www.census.gov/content/dam/Census/library/publications/2016/demo/p95-16-1.pdf.

Hopgood, S. 2013. *The Endtimes of Human Rights*. Ithaca, NY: Cornell University Press.

Huenchuan, S. 2013. "Los derechos de las personas mayores." Santiago, Chile: CEPAL. Retrieved 12/5/2017 from https://www.cepal.org/celade/noticias/docum entosdetrabajo/8/51618/Derechos_PMayores_M2.pdf.

Huenchuan, S. (Ed.) 2016. *Envejecimiento e institucionalidad pública en América Latina y el Caribe: conceptos, metodologías y casos prácticos*. Santiago, Chile: United Nations, Comisión Económica para América Latina y el Caribe (CEPAL).

Huerta Benze, L.H. 2015. *De la Casa al Aisilo: La Construcción Sociocultural de la Vejez y la Enfermedad en Adultos Mayores en Condición de Internamiento en Los Ramones, Nuevo León*. (Maestra). Mexico City: El Centro de Investigación y Estudios Superiores en Antropología Social (CIESAS).

Huerta Benze, L.H. 2016. "Trayectoria familiar y ocupacional de personas mayores en Monterrey: una mirada antropológica." Pp. 69–97 in *Formas de envejecer: condiciones y necesidades de las personas mayors*, edited by S.G. Villegas. Monterrey, Nuevo León, México: Universidad Autónoma de Nuevo León.

Jeppesen, H. 2016. "Amnesty's Salil Shetty: Human rights 'under attack'." Deutsche Welle (DW). Retrieved 8/12/2019 from https://www.dw.com/en/am nestys-salil-shetty-human-rights-under-attack/a-19068608.

Keck, M., and K. Sikkink. 1998. *Activists beyond Borders: Advocacy Networks in International Politics*. Ithaca, NY: Cornell University Press.

Kennedy, D. 2002. "The International Human Rights Movement: Part of the Problem." *Harvard Human Rights Journal* 15:101–126.

Kirk, D. 1996. "Demographic Transition Theory." *Population Studies*, 50(3):361–387. Retrieved from http://www.jstor.org/stable/2174639.

Martin, C., D. Rodríguez, and P.B. Brown. 2015. *Human Rights of Older People: Universal and Regional Legal Perspectives*. New York, NY: Springer.

Montes de Oca, V., M. Paredes, V. Rodríguez, and S. Garay. 2018. "Older Persons and Human Rights in Latin America and the Caribbean." *International Journal on Ageing in Developing Countries* 2 (2):149–164. Retrieved from https://www.inia. org.mt/wp-content/uploads/2018/09/2.2-8-Montes-de-Oca-edited.pdf.

Montes de Oca Zavala, V. 2014. "Cuidados y servicios sociales frente a la dependencia en el marco del envejecimiento demográfico en México." Pp. 169–181 in *Autonomía y dignidad en la vejez: Teoría y práctica en políticas de derechos de las personas mayores*, edited by S. Huenchuan, and R.I. Rodríguez. Mexico City: CEPAL.

Moyn, S. 2010. *The Last Utopia: Human Rights in History*. Cambridge, MA: Belknap Press.

Myles, J. 1984. *Old Age in the Welfare State: The Political Economy of Public Pensions*. Boston, MA: Little, Brown.

Nielsen, R.W. 2015. "Demographic Transition Theory Contradicted Repeatedly by Data." Retrieved 7/22/2019 from http://arxiv.org/ftp/arxiv/papers/1510/ 1510.00471.pdf.

Noonan, R.K. 1995. "Women against the State: Political Opportunities and Collective Action Frames in Chile's Transition to Democracy." *Sociological Forum* 10 (1):81–111. Retrieved from http://www.jstor.org/stable/684759.

OAS. 2021. "Inter-American Convention on Protecting the Human Rights of Older Persons A-70." Retrieved 5/15/2021 from http://www.oas.org/en/sla/dil/ inter_american_treaties_a-70_human_rights_older_persons.asp.

Palier, B. (Ed.). 2010. *A Long Goodbye to Bismarck? The Politics of Welfare Reform in Continental Europe.* Amsterdam: Amsterdam University Press.

Posner, E.A. 2014. *The Twilight of Human Rights Law.* New York, NY: Oxford University Press.

Rodriguez-Pinzón, D., and C. Martin. 2003. "The International Human Rights Status of Elderly Persons." *American University International Law Review* 18 (4):915–1008.

Sass, S. 2006. "The Development of Employer Retirement Income Plans: From the Nineteenth Century to 1980." Pp. 76–97 in *The Oxford Handbook of Pensions and Retirement Income,* edited by G.L. Clark, A.H. Munnell, and J.M. Orszag. New York, NY: Oxford University Press.

Shetty, S. 2016. "10 Years of the UN Human Rights Council: Remarks by Salil Shetty." Geneva, Switzerland: International Service for Human Rights. Retrieved 3/22/2020 from https://www.ishr.ch/news/10-years-un-human-right s-council-remarks-salil-shetty.

Sidorenko, A., and A. Zaidi. 2018. "International Policy Frameworks on Ageing: Assessing Progress in Reference to the Madrid International Plan of Action on Ageing." *Journal of Social Policy Studies* 16 (1):141–154. doi:10.17323/727-0634-2018-16-1-141-154.

Sikkink, K. 2017. *Evidence for Hope: Making Human Rights Work in the 21st Century.* Princeton, NJ: Princeton University Press.

Snow, D.E., J. Burke Rochford, S.K. Worden, and R.D. Benford. 1986. "Frame Alignment Processes, Micromobilization, and Movement Participation." *American Sociological Review* 51:464–481.

Strangio, S. 2017. "Welcome to the Post-Human Rights World." Foreign Affairs. Retrieved 8/9/2019 from https://foreignpolicy.com/2017/03/07/welcom e-to-the-post-human-rights-world/.

Thane, P. (Ed.) 2005. *A History of Old Age.* Los Angeles, CA: The J. Paul Getty Museum.

Thane, P. 2006. "The History of Retirement." Pp. 32–51 in *The Oxford Handbook of Pensions and Retirement Income,* edited by G.L. Clark, A.H. Munnell, and J.M. Orszag. New York, NY: Oxford University Press.

Tharoor, S. 1999/2000. "Are Human Rights Universal?" *World Policy Journal* 16 (4). Retrieved from http://worldpolicy.org/2009/11/11/tharoor-are-human-right s-universal-world-policy-journal-world-policy-institute/.

Toro Huerta, M.I.d. 2006. "El fenómeno del soft law y las nuevas perspectivas del derecho internacional." *Anuario Mexicano de Derecho Internacional* 6. doi:10.22201/ iij.24487872e.2006.6.160.

Turner, R.H. 1969. "The Theme of Contemporary Social Movements." *British Journal of Sociology* 20:390–405.

United Nations. 1948. "Universal Declaration of Human Rights." Retrieved 7/22/ 2019 from https://www.un.org/en/universal-declaration-human-rights/index.html.

United Nations. 1982. "Report of the World Assembly on Aging." Retrieved 7/26/ 2019 from https://www.un.org/esa/socdev/ageing/documents/Resources/VIPEE-English.pdf.

United Nations. 2002. "Report of the Second World Assembly on Ageing, Madrid, 8–12 April 2002." Retrieved 5/1/2013 from https://documents-dds-ny. un.org/doc/UNDOC/GEN/N02/397/51/PDF/N0239751.pdf?OpenElement.

Wada, T. 2006. "Claim Network Analysis: How are Social Protests Transformed into Political Protests in Mexico?" Pp. 95–111 in *Latin American Social Movements: Globalization, Democratization, and Transnational Networks*, edited by H. Johnston and P. Almeida. New York, NY: Rowman & Littlefield.

World Economic Forum. 2019. "Population, Ageing and Immigration: Germany's Demographic Question." Retrieved 7/24/2019 from https://www.weforum.org/agenda/2017/04/population-ageing-and-immigration-germanys-demographic-question.

Zaidi, B., and S.P. Morgan. 2017. "The Second Demographic Transition Theory: A Review and Appraisal." *Annual Review of Sociology* 43:473–492. doi:10.1146/annurev-soc-060116-053442.

Chapter 4

Active Aging and Citizenship

We introduced the concept of "active aging" in the first chapter and explained that our definition of the term implies far more than a concern for controlling one's health and living as long as possible, although maintaining the highest physical and mental health possible is a clear objective of many of the organizations we studied. Our definition of active aging includes political and activist aspects in that it implies more than a concern for health, but also a willingness to struggle for the social rights that foster health for oneself and others. An important part of assuring optimal health is ensuring access to the basic necessities of a comfortable and dignified life, including good nutrition, safe housing, and medical care. Among the most basic necessities is a minimally adequate income. In Mexico and many other low and middle-income countries a minimally adequate income for older people with few resources and no formal pension comes in the form of a guaranteed non-contributory pension. The struggle for such a pension took years, and assuring the widest possible access is essential. Rosaura Casio Rojo, an inspired and energetic activist from Mérida, Yucatán, described the struggle for guaranteed pensions and other needs of older people.

ROSAURA: My name is Rosaura Magdalena Casio Rojo. I am 59 years old; I have a secondary education. In 2011 we started a movement in support of older adults ... we were a group of artisans ... While investigating we found out that DF (Mexico City) provided an old-age pension and ... we started to fight ... We began to investigate how our members could receive a small pension and we started the fight. There were four of us at first, one unfortunately died, but we grew to more than 10,000 people fighting for that pension.

INTERVIEWER: How were you able to bring together so many leaders of retiree and pensioner organizations?

ROSAURA: We started with a flyer. I have a friend who is an announcer and ... I talked to her about the project and she interviewed me and my colleagues on the radio ... through the radio we began to

DOI: 10.4324/9781003205609-4

mobilize the people and the associations that wanted to support us in this movement ... one interview led to another and we reached municipalities ... and the people ... we had to go to the Congress, the seniors themselves paid for transportation to Mérida. People came from several municipalities in the state.

INTERVIEWER: So, the struggle was for a universal pension? What were the requirements to join your association and to fight for a universal pension?

ROSAURA: ... the fight was for everybody, we fought for retirees of course ... clearly some had a good pension, but even they helped us. They would say "I have a good pension" but the fight is really for my companions. We had managers, teachers, retiree and pensioner organizations with very good pensions. They would say "if it doesn't help me, it doesn't matter. Just so those who have the least receive help."

INTERVIEWER: How many people did you recruit?

ROSAURA: Well, in the demonstrations we reached up to 10,000 ... We needed 4,000 signatures to push the initiative forward. I wondered how we would be able to get that many, but in reality, we ended up with 20,000.

INTERVIEWER: ... What other things were proposed or what other objectives did you begin to develop in order to stay united?

ROSAURA: As a result of walking through the municipalities ... we began to realize the sad reality of older people ... the pension was something important, yes, but they suffer many hardships ... They are abused by their children, dispossessed by their children, by their sons-in-law ... they are even denied medical attention ...

INTERVIEWER: How do you support the association with the expenses that are required to go out into the communities and carry out this work? How is it financed?

ROSAURA: When we started this movement, we all contributed from our own pockets and later on as I witnessed all of the hardships of older people, I began to form other groups in different neighborhoods ... We did a great deal each month and I had to fight for the permits that ... were very difficult to obtain, but from all of that we raised funds. I provided food to the older people each month, they contributed, we cooked, they sold snacks, donated clothing and from there emerged associations for the poor ...

INTERVIEWER: What about donations?

ROSAURA: Nothing, nothing, nothing ... we receive nothing for the association. I make do with my resources because that is what I prefer. I like it and I ... work in the neighborhoods which is not easy because today I have fourteen groups in different neighborhoods.

INTERVIEWER: Have you heard about the term "active aging"? Do you have some idea of how one should achieve it?

ROSAURA: For me active aging is that older people ... have projects ... that they function well, that they can continue to work as much as they can ... enjoy recreation, but often they can't ... They like to dance ... and when I have my fiestas, I play music and they dance and enjoy themselves. I visualize it that way that they have the opportunity to work and if they want to take care of their grand-children, fine, because it brings them pleasure, but it is not an obligation.

INTERVIEWER: Very good. Well, finally tell me about what you think about the issue of the human rights of the older people ... You said that in your speeches you talk about human rights. Do you go for help, do you call upon the Human Rights Commission ... are old people demanding their rights?

ROSAURA: As for human rights, there are none, not for older adults ... here they do not possess them, they do not know about them, they do not exercise them as such ...

INTERVIEWER: ... I understand that the institutions do not do much to protect the rights of older people. What role do the family and the neighborhood play?

ROSAURA: I think that as a result of the movement we started the situa-tion has improved, not as much as we would have liked, but it has improved. As for their children, I can't speak of all of them in general because there are good ones, bad ones, and worse, but there are many who are informed and accompany their parents ... We took on the task of printing some pamphlets to inform them of their rights. At least in the groups I am involved with the majority already know their rights, the right to health, a pension ... and people are becom-ing more interested and I think there is more interest today than when we started eight or nine years ago ... Whatever rights we have to fight for we will do it.

Changing Responsibility for Aging Adults

This interview with a committed and engaged activist reveals an agenda that goes well beyond a focus on the physical and psychological quality of life of older individuals. Rosaura Casio Rojo clearly values health and vitality, but her discourse focuses largely on assuring access to a pension by older individuals with very low incomes and few resources. As she states, her focus on pensions has expanded to address the multiple problems that low-income seniors confront. In addition to being an activist, Rosaura is a community organizer who brings people together, again to do more than simply socialize. Her ultimate objective is to empower older individuals to put pressure on the State to guarantee the material requirements of a dignified life. That is clearly not a job for the timid. Rosaura's struggle for pensions and more general human and social rights is part of what we described in earlier chapters as a global social movement that is bringing the plight of older individuals out of the shadows.

Rosaura's sense of mission is driven by the need she sees, which itself reflects many powerful social changes. As we mentioned in earlier chapters, in Mexico today, as in much of the world, powerful and pervasive demographic and social forces are undermining the family's ability to provide all of the care and support older parents need. At the same time, the State finds itself limited in what it can do. Mexico, like other Latin American and Caribbean nations, and similarly to high-income central and southern European countries, has traditionally relied upon the male-breadwinner family model for the material support of dependent or frail family members. As we discussed in Chapter two, marriage and family patterns are changing rapidly and as the male-breadwinner model of family support is no longer universal, nations are forced to adopt policies of defamilisation that shift responsibility for aging parents from the family to the State. Unfortunately, such policies run headlong into very real fiscal limitations. The combined realities of diminishing family support capacities and limitations in state resources define two major dimensions of the social and economic environment in which CSOs operate. A third dimension relates to the nation's political culture as it is manifested at various levels of governance. Understanding the situation of older persons requires that one address all three. We begin with the role of political institutions and culture, specifically with reference to Mexico, but before proceeding we briefly discuss the concept of active citizenship and the changing political and social roles of older individuals.

Active Citizenship

A major theme that motivates discussions of civil society and the non-governmental sector generally relates to the possibility of fostering active citizenship, which for our purposes basically refers to strengthening individual and group agency, or the ability of vulnerable and powerless groups to act effectively to further their own interests (Gaventa and Tandon 2010; Kenny et al. 2017). Whether and how such objectives can be achieved is the core question. Like most other theoretical positions or conceptualizations, whether the objective is even desirable is contested. The focus on active citizenship, like the concepts of active or successful aging, implies responsibility for oneself, a position that could be seen as compatible with neoliberal objectives of reducing the extent of the welfare state (Estes 2001; Fuller, Kershaw, and Pulkingham 2008; Giddens 1994; Kenny 2002). Our use of the concept of citizenship clearly focuses on responsibility, but not in terms of providing for oneself what the State should provide. Rather, we emphasize the political aspects of active citizenship. Following Kenny and colleagues, we define an action as "activist if it challenges or changes the dominant power relations and structures, regardless of whether it is small scale or large scale in scope" (Kenny et al. 2017, p. 17).

While encouraging self-care and educating people on how best to avoid unnecessary health risks is clearly laudable, exaggerated claims that individuals have complete control over their health and well-being represent what we might call fallacies of misplaced attribution (Lamb 2017; Lamb 2020). Such perspectives attribute health and mortality outcomes that are the result of social, economic, and political forces to individual agency. Taken to the extreme such perspectives privilege the market and private health services, and devalue, or even reject, a more collective public health perspective. A more useful view of active aging is based on a combined human rights and life course perspective (Faber 2015). The combination of a focus on human and social rights and a life course perspective emphasizes the reality that people's work lives, their family and migratory trajectories, and ultimately their health and longevity are shaped by the historical and political contexts in which the life chances of different cohorts are structured (D'Epinay et al. 2011; Elder, Johnson, and Crosnoe 2003; Hareven and de Gruyere 1999). The life course perspective highlights time in all its dimensions, including historical periods, family transitions, and individual growth and aging. Combined with a clear conception of human and social rights it serves as an important corrective to a privatizing functionalist reductionism that ignores the historically determined political, economic, and social forces that constrain an individual's and a group's ability to control the health risks they confront. A life course perspective also draws attention to accumulated inequalities that accompany aging (Ferraro and Shippee 2009) and the need for a clear conception of the defense of human and social rights at all ages.

Clearly, the ability of any non-governmental entity, or any social movement made up of such entities, to challenge or change dominant power relations and structures depends on the social and political contexts in which they operate, in addition to the determination and skill of its leadership and participants (DeMars and Dijkzeul 2015; Mendelson and Glenn 2002). As we have emphasized throughout our discussion, civil society organizations are no substitute for an effective and beneficent state. The ability of social movements and voluntary organizations to bring about significant change in fact depends on a reasonable level of receptivity by the State. Indeed, such organizations are often funded by and even serve as subcontractors to governments (Kenny et al. 2017; Pereira and Angel 2009; Salamon 1995).

Before proceeding we must review important changes related to active citizenship and democracy that have emerged in Latin America, the

Caribbean, and Mexico in recent decades. These changes are closely related to the international adoption of the concept of human rights as possessed inherently and inalienably by each human being, a principle which necessarily implies that they take precedence over state sovereignty (Henkin 1995; Wyatt 2019). The international concern with human rights represents a recent development in international law that has been furthered, if not totally accounted for, by an influential and visible trans-national social movement (Moyn 2010; Sikkink 2017; Stammers 1999). The global reach of this movement and the changing moral discourse it fosters are reflected in the establishment of the International Criminal Court (ICC), created by the Rome Statute of 1998 (ICC 2020). The Court was established to prosecute genocide, crimes against humanity, war crimes, and crimes of aggression largely perpetrated by states against their own people. Since the early 1990s the ICC and other UN tribunals have investigated hundreds of cases of major human rights abuses and have obtained 250 convictions (Kenney and Norris 2018). This broadening of the concept of human rights from prerogatives and protections granted by the State to universal and inviolable basic rights that are possessed by everyone regardless of their nationality or their social position represents a major evolution of the concept of citizenship (Henkin 1995; Kenny et al. 2017; Moyn 2010; Wyatt 2019).

Nonetheless, the basic legal principle, as well as the reality, of state sover-eignty presents human rights law and social movements with serious obsta-cles. Where, and with whom, does the authority to enforce human rights principles lie? The ICC serves as one hopeful example, although it only functions with the consent of the nations that adhere to its basic principles. There is nothing to keep participating nations from reneging, as did Burundi in 2017, and as other nations have threatened. The United States has never ratified the treaty. Without an overarching authority with unquestioned powers of enforcement international human rights agreements are, as we dis-cussed in Chapter three, often little more than paper tigers.

Similar problems arise in the extension of citizenship rights to margin-alized groups within nations. Those without material, political, or social capital have little judicial or legislative recourse for defending their rights and interests. As with the enforcement of human rights principles inter-nationally, national and local social movements and CSOs are often the only options. Human rights, and their extension to include social rights, are part of an ongoing debate over the role of civil society and the various organizations that comprise it in fostering a more direct and effective democracy (Avritzer 2002; Dagnino 2006; Dagnino, Olvera, and Panfichi 2006; Olvera 2004; Olvera 2010; Otero 2004; Teichman 2009). As we mentioned in Chapter three, many observers remain skeptical of the utility or effectiveness of international human rights conventions given the basic reality of state sovereignty (Hopgood 2013; Posner 2014).

The 1980s and 1990s saw the expansion of social movements focused on the democratic inclusion, as well as the human and social rights of excluded sectors of the populations of Latin America and the Caribbean (Olvera 2001; Olvera 2004). These movements were made up of CSOs, unions, leftist parties, indigenous groups, and others (Dagnino 2006; Johnston and Almeida 2006; Stahler-Sholk, Vanden, and Kuecker 2008). As in other nations, they were focused on the rights of racial and ethnic minorities, women, workers, homosexuals, older persons, and others. The specific organizations and actors were motivated by concerns for poverty, the environment, the needs of rural residents, inadequate housing, a lack of health care, low educational levels, violence, and more (Stahler-Sholk, Vanden, and Becker 2014; Stahler-Sholk, Vanden, and Kuecker 2008). An important part of this agenda and the renewed consciousness that surrounded it was a concern with identity and the recognition of cultural and other differences (Dagnino 2006; Kymlicka and Norman 2000).

The extent and nature of this new democratic rights agenda differed depending on the specific situations of individual nations. Those contextual factors included the relative extent of neoliberal market-based state policies and the effectiveness of civil society groups focused on community development (Teichman 2009). In Mexico civil society has historically been weak given the nation's corporatist political structure with power concentrated in the presidency with the legislature and judiciary in subordinate rather than equal positions (Dagnino, Olvera, and Panfichi 2006; Olvera 2010). Clientelism has historically defined the relationship among specific social groups and the Partido Revolucionario Institucional, PRI (Institutional Revolutionary Party) which ruled Mexico uninterruptedly for seventy years from 1930 until its defeat in 2000 (Rodríguez 2000). That history gave rise to a civic culture and political parties that largely reify centralized authoritarian rule centered in the executive branches of national and state governments, a pattern which has not been significantly altered by open and honest elections (Olvera 2004; Olvera 2010).

What Can CSOs Do?

This political reality presents CSOs and democratic social movements generally with serious challenges in changing the basic rules of the game. Lacking extensive political or economic power, their room for maneuver is limited and largely confined to attempting to change hegemonic discourses (Keck and Sikkink 1998). Kenny and colleagues usefully summarize four main features, or what we might think of as ideal characteristics, of civil society organizations that theoretically foster active citizenship. These "cultural frames" include the capacity to foster (1) agency; (2) association; (3) democratic processes; and (4) cosmopolitanism (Kenny et al. 2017, p. 41). Agency refers to the ability of the organization to provide individuals the capacity to define and further their own interests. Association refers to the opportunity to associate with others to address those common ends. Democracy refers to the ability of all to participate on an equal basis. Finally, cosmopolitanism is a complex concept that broadly refers to the organization's ability to foster openness to the larger world among its members. At the extreme it implies the transcendence of local, national, and other parochial affiliations and identities.

As the authors note, these are largely ideal characteristics, which in reality organizations may not possess, or which they may pursue in only a limited fashion. Clearly such a catalog of characteristics can be seen as idealistic, and perhaps even unrealistic, but such a conceptual framework can be of utility in drawing attention to the potential strengths of such organizations, in addition to providing ways of analyzing their short-comings. Many non-governmental organizations do not subscribe to all, or perhaps any of these principles. Organizations and groups can be undemocratic, they can reject outsiders, and they can be parochial and further a narrow range of beliefs and ideas, characteristics which are not likely to foster cosmopolitanism or agency beyond that of their membership.

In addition to theoretical classifications and general characterizations of the functions of CSOs, it is imperative to differentiate between their potential roles with reference to the State. A clear distinction relates to the extent to which such organizations collaborate with or even serve as sub-contractors or agents of the State in providing services to various sub-populations, and the extent to which they assume the role of adversary and advocate to further the agency of those they represent by demanding that their human and social rights be respected. Many organizations that had taken an adversarial stance toward the State during the South American military dictatorships had to redefine their missions and relationship to the State after the restoration of democracy (Meyer 1999; Pereira and Angel 2009). While some organizations, such as those focused on human rights or women's rights, tend inherently to be more adversarial than those focused on such domains as health care or micro-enterprise, it is possible for organizations to engage in both service delivery and advocacy to varying degrees.

Civil Society and the Rise of Identity Politics

The rapid and extensive rise of civil society organizations accompanies an increase in identity politics and a growing awareness of and concern with local identities and interests. This rise in identity politics accompanies a decline in the strength of traditional centrist and leftist political parties globally. As we discussed in the first chapter, post-neoliberalism and the "Pink Tide" that moved many nations to the left at the end of the 20th Century has been followed by a post-post-neoliberal rejection of those leftist sentiments in many nations of the world and in three of the largest Latin American economies, Argentina, Brazil, and Chile (Encarnación 2018). The subsequent return of a Peronist leftist government in Argentina makes it clear that the political situations of many nations are exceedingly fluid. We also noted that many of the post-neoliberal movements and organizations reject hierarchy and espouse a philosophy of horizontalism, which optimizes democracy and participation and rejects the hierarchy of traditional political parties (Motta 2009; Motta 2014; Sitrin 2006).

This philosophy of horizontalism accompanies a growing demand globally by groups defined in terms of race, ethnicity, sexual orientation, religion, region of residence, and more for recognition of their unique identities and cultures (Fukuyama 2018; Kymlicka 1995; Kymlicka 2007; Kymlicka and Norman 2000). These parallel, or even give rise to civil society organizations which, in turn, reinforce local identities and draw attention to real and perceived inequalities and injustices. In Mexico multiple dimensions of disadvantage have drawn increased academic and public attention (Montes de Oca Zavala and Gutiérrez Cuellar 2018). Indigenous women find themselves disadvantaged on the basis of group membership and gender. Destitute older individuals suffer discrimination based on age and poverty. This accumulation of different dimensions of disadvantage and discrimination is often referred to as their "intersection" (Collins and Bilge 2016; Crenshaw 1989). Recognizing this phenomenon contributes to our understanding of the serious discrimination and disadvantage certain groups face and it offers a clear focus for CSO action.

During the last two decades social theorists have begun to address the difficult social issues related to cultural and social group membership, identity, and social rights (Benhabib 2002; Fraser and Honneth 2003; Kymlicka 1995; Kymlicka 2007; Kymlicka and Norman 2000; Taylor 1994). Multiculturalism reflects the demands by previously marginalized groups for recognition of their unique identities in addition to their basic political and social rights. The defense of one's unique identity, though, often includes the rejection of more collective identities, even those associated with nationality. The growing rejection of collective identities and loyalties in favor of more specific group identities strikes some observers as divisive and threatening to the cohesion and sense of common purpose that defines national identities (Fukuyama 2018; Lilla 2016; Schlesinger Jr. 1992). In Federalist Paper #10, James Madison warned of the dangers of factionalism in political life, a warning that one might well apply to an excessive focus on local identities and loyalties (Madison 1787). To organizations such as the International Labor Organization (ILO), a focus on group identities represents the rejection of the sort of class consciousness that is necessary for the exploited of the world to overcome their subjugation (Roman 2004).

One might have imagined that the rapid global diffusion of electronic communication, and especially social media that is proceeding at an accelerating pace would foster greater cosmopolitanism and communication among different groups. Unfortunately, this greater capacity to communicate seems to be accompanied by a growing parochiality and a tendency for individuals to communicate and interact only with those with similar opinions and world views, or those who subscribe to specific ideologies. Increasingly it is difficult to tell fake news from real news, or to recognize what is news at all rather than propaganda. The era of open communication advocated by Jürgen Habermas and other theorists of communicative action does not appear to be upon us (Habermas 1970). A potential down side to the increase in civil society organizations and identity politics, then, is a growing parochiality and polarization between individuals and groups.

David Goodhart, employing mostly British data, characterizes the new political polarization as reflecting a shift from the politics of right vs left to one that pits those individuals who Goodhart labels as from "anywhere" against those from "somewhere," a distinction that emphasizes a cultural divide between the growing group of highly educated, mobile, and cosmopolitan citizens who dominate politics, business, and education and who are comfortable anywhere, and those who are from somewhere and remain in their communities close to where they grew up and identify with the local culture, customs, and people (Goodhart 2017). Recent national and regional elections in many nations show a clear divide between large urban centers and smaller towns and villages that have been left behind by globalization and the shift of manufacturing jobs from the global economic center to the periphery. An emphasis on local initiatives, rights, and grievances again reflects a rejection of older concerns with social class and totalizing political philosophies embodied in Marxist approaches (Therborn 2008).

The force of this greater localism is reflected in various communitarian philosophies whose beliefs vary greatly, but which we might usefully summarize with reference to the Catholic principle of subsidiarity, which holds that human needs should be addressed at the lowest possible level. Communitarians reject extreme individualism, as well as big government, and privilege "community" as the basis of social organization. From this perspective families, neighbors, and local communities embody mutual responsibility and are the principle socializing agents of citizens, as well as their basic sources of support (Bellah 1985; Etzioni 1995; MacIntyre 1984; Putnam 2000). Much of modern communitarian thinking reflects Alexis de Tocqueville's 1840 observation that America is a nation of joiners who participate in any number of local and community organizations, including churches, clubs, associations, and so on (Tocqueville 2000 (1835,1840). These, for de Tocqueville serve as a buttress against excessive individualism at one level and state domination at another. Local associations, in conjunction with philanthropy and mutual assistance, reinforce communal identities.

Robert Putnam identifies what he sees as the collapse of such associational activity as resulting in the weakening of civic culture in the United States (Putnam 1995; Putnum 2000). Putnam's claims have been vigorously criticized because of inadequate data and a potential misrepresentation of the ways in which the nature of association has changed in the modern world in which communication media and much else have changed (Skocpol 1996). Indeed, de Tocqueville's earlier observations have been criticized for an excessive focus on voluntarism and an inadequate understanding of the institutional factors that have encouraged Americans to associate since colonial times (Skocpol 1996). Although membership in certain organizations may have declined in recent years, assuming that this represents a decline in civic consciousness may not be justified. Change occurs, but one may unjustified in viewing change negatively.

These are just a few examples of perspectives that are compatible with and even encourage CSO approaches to social problems. The growing presence of CSOs in countries like Mexico raises intellectual and practical questions concerning the potential of civil society generally to bring about significant change. While local collective efforts represent potentially useful forms of direct democratic engagement, it is hard to imagine that significant structural change can be achieved without power of the sort that only effective political parties can exert. The hope for civil society action derives in part from the fact that revolutionary movements have been largely unsuccessful in bringing about radical reform (Holloway 2019). Unfortunately, the reality is that local community efforts, or even uncoordinated larger-scale efforts, cannot almost by definition, dismantle established structural sources of the sorts of extreme inequality that are typical of Latin America and the Caribbean. One serious criticism of horizontal social movements, and center left and far left parties more generally, is that although they mount serious critiques of neoliberal economics and politics, they offer no viable alternatives to eliminate serious social inequities and underdevelopment (Panizza 2005). This reality requires a reassessment of the extent of change that civil society organizations or the social movements of which they are a part can bring about. The reality may be far more limited than the ideal.

The Power of Beliefs and Ideas

In an insightful critique of theories of civil society Foley and Edwards point out that such theories emphasize either the inherent capacity of voluntary organizations to foster civility and social cohesion or the potential of such organizations to serve as venues for political enlightenment and effective political agency (Foley and Edwards 1996). Indeed, a major question that emerges in discussions of civil society relates to the extent to which voluntary organizations go beyond attending to the needs and interests of their members to an effective ability to influence politics. Antonio Gramsci, the Italian communist who was imprisoned by Mussolini for many years, is perhaps the best known modern theorist to use the term "civil society" (Gramsci 1971). His work influenced the Latin American left in the 1980s and 1990s to reevaluate the role of civil society as a counterpoint to political parties and an opportunity for more local engagement in bringing about change (Allen and Ouviña 2017; Bruhn 1999; Pearce 1996; Pearce 2004). Gramsci's theory reflects Marxist concerns with subordination and false consciousness. In his conceptualization he differentiated between "political society," which relates to the realm of power and control, and "civil society," which consists of the sorts of lower-order organizations and collectivities we have mentioned, in which civic consciousness and individual's conceptions of how society is and should be organized are formed and reinforced. For Gramsci, political and civil society are clearly related in that popular conceptions of the just or acceptable political order are buttressed by the beliefs and conceptions promulgated through civil society (Buttigieg 1995). Any particular social order is maintained by the fact that the ideologies of the dominant classes become "hegemonic," meaning that subordinate groups accept them as legitimate.

For Gramsci, then, oppression is largely cultural and related to prevailing ideas. For him, changing the social order entails replacing hegemonic ideas and beliefs with "counter-hegemonic" ideas and ideologies that reverse and reject previous notions of how society should be organized. Gramsci criticized claims that social revolution must precede changes in class consciousness. Social change, and certainly radical social change, begins with a change in culture and the world views of subordinate groups. This change in culture occurs at the level of civil society. For Gramsci, change begins with altered consciousness and world views and proceeds from the bottom up, rather than from higher levels of organization, such as political parties, to lower levels. In the context of our discussion, the relevance of Gramsci's conceptualizations arises from the focus on local organizations and institutions. In light of the general failure of revolutionary movements to strengthen democracy or improve the lot of the poor in Latin America, the appeal of Gramsci's proposal to pursue civil society options is understandable. Indeed, many subsequent theorists have built upon the potential of civil society in various domains. The horizontal philosophy that we discussed in Chapter one shares many of the same objectives as Gramscian civil society, to the point that some observers imagine that movements like the Zapatistas were directly influenced by Gramsci, although Subcomandante Marcos, the leader of and spokesman for the Zapatistas, may not reflect such a direct influence even if his communiques share a similar philosophy (Henck 2013).

Old People in Post-traditional Society

The situations in both Mexico and the United States reflect the new reality of post-traditional societies in which the traditional family support systems upon which older parents relied can no longer bear the entire burden (Angel 2011). Yet as we have noted, the State faces serious limitations in what it can provide in terms of material and social support. One clear advantage of local voluntary efforts arises from the fact that many of the needs of frail older individuals are routine and personal and require the sort of close and frequent contact that the family has traditionally provided. Organized and concerted non-governmental efforts to assist individuals who would otherwise suffer severe isolation and perhaps worse represent a potentially effective addition to formal state programs. In this capacity these organizations act as allies of or even subcontractors to the State. Such a role does not preclude the more adversarial role we have mentioned in which these organizations place pressure on the State to live up to its obligations to citizens, especially the most vulnerable.

The challenge for all nations, then, is to determine how best to combine the efforts of non-governmental actors and organizations with those of official agencies. The challenge for individual organizations and even groups of organizations is to define their roles as allies or adversaries of the State. What seems clear is that the role of non-governmental organizations is potentially great, especially in areas that are hard to reach or among populations with unique needs, cultures, languages, or beliefs (Pereira and Angel 2009). To the extent that secular non-governmental and faith-based organizations foster or directly provide social support and integration, they could potentially greatly enhance the quality of life of older individuals and their families. Encouraging such caregiving and interaction is a logical and natural extension of basic community ties. Such informal social support is provided by community members to one another every day.

Elder Rights as a Social Movement

Although non-governmental organizations exist and operate in repressive and totalitarian societies, for the most part their ability to influence policy in those contexts are seriously constrained. We confine our discussion to fairly open democratic societies in which civil society organizations have at least some ability to function and even challenge authority. This does not mean that civil society organizations in such societies are not repressed or interfered with. Rather, it means that they have at least a basic ability not only to provide services to the individuals they wish to help, but also to advocate for those individuals and groups and engage in what is basically political activity. The organizations of civil society, though, are in fact defined by the welfare state, which motivates their agendas, defines their legal status, and determines their ability to act on the behalf of those they serve.

In Latin America and the Caribbean the limited success of previous social welfare reforms and the continuing problem of serious inequities in access to social services gave rise to the promotion of active citizenship that we discussed above. The serious inequality that continued even after the initial neoliberal reforms of health and pension systems convinced even supporters of those reforms of the need to involve citizens in governance and fiscal decision making in order to assure the legitimacy and sustainability of reform efforts (Chiara and Virgilio 2005; Peruzzotti and Smulovitz 2002; Tussie, Mendiburu, and Vázques 1997). Although the need for citizen involvement is widely recognized, how exactly that objective might be accomplished remains unclear.

One obvious possibility is to mobilize older citizens themselves to engage in collective action and participate in civic life. A number of studies find that Mexicans, including older adults, provide a significant amount of voluntary unpaid aid and support to family and community members (Burcher 2008; HSBC 2015). The National Survey on Health and Aging in Mexico found that 15.8% of those 55 and over (13.8% of men and 17.2% of women) participate in voluntary unpaid work at least once a week (Enasem 2013). CSOs could clearly play a major role in mobilizing older people to aid one another and to work together to achieve joint objectives. There are simply few alternative collective actors. This possibility leads us again to raise an important theoretical and practical question as to whether increasing CSO activity related to the rights and welfare of older people reflects the emergence of a new transnational social movement, much like the women's movement, the human rights movement, or the environmental movement (Keck and Sikkink 1998).

CSOs and Older People Internationally

Although our focus is on CSOs and their role in advocacy and service delivery to older Mexicans, let us briefly mention other CSOs in other nations to illustrate that they address similar issues. The domains in which civil society organizations operate differ greatly along many dimensions. Within each domain the cultural, political, and social contexts in which they operate constrain these organizations' options. CSOs that deal with environmental issues and those dealing with human rights, women's rights, and the rights of native peoples differ in mission and structure from those that provide medical, educational, and support services in emergency situations. Understanding the potential utility of such organizations requires not only a focus on their structure and organization, but also an understanding of the needs of the populations they serve, and the contexts within which they operate. Clearly, those needs are different in highly developed and affluent welfare states than in lower-income countries with limited old-age supports.

Different cultural, social, and political environments place varying demands on CSOs in terms of service provision and advocacy. Immediate needs for assistance must be addressed at the same time that actions aimed at addressing structural inequalities and barriers though legislation, public awareness campaigns, and other activities must be pursued. Organizations like Amnesty International that focus on human rights or organizations like Greenpeace that oppose the exploitation of animal species engage primarily in advocacy. Other organizations like Habitat for Humanity, Doctors without Borders, Oxfam, and the Red Cross focus more on service delivery and the needs of individuals in distress. Many CSOs engage in both activities to one degree or another, providing services while they engage in advocacy and political action aimed at changing laws and practices to encourage democracy, safeguard civil rights, or develop local capacities to deal with longer-term needs.

One of the reasons for the renewed interest in CSOs as service providers is that they often enjoy certain advantages in dealing with the more routine and manageable needs of specific populations (Pereira and Angel 2009; Pereira, Angel, and Angel 2007). For example, although complex and expensive high-tech medicine can only be paid for or provided by the State, routine and relatively inexpensive services, such as basic primary care, assistance with activities of daily living, and companionship can often be more effectively provided by CSOs and other local groups. As we have emphasized, CSOs are clearly no substitute for an efficient and beneficent State, but ideally such groups can complement the State in supporting older individuals in the community and enhancing the quality of their lives. Because of their more detailed knowledge of the legal, transportation, nutritional, and other needs of older people they could potentially act as both service providers and advocates. Although a comprehensive catalog of such organizations is beyond the scope of this book, some examples of organizations that deal with issues related to older individuals would be useful.

Service to Older Individuals

CSOs not only provide valuable assistance with basic activities of daily living to older individuals, they also encourage pro-social activities, ultimately strengthening communities (Etzioni 1993; Etzioni 1995). Clearly they provide much needed companionship and care to older people (Idler 2006). Faith-based international CSOs such as *CARITAS, Catholic Charities*, and *Lutheran Social Services* provide assistance to older people, as well as others in need. The Red Cross, and numerous international and local relief agencies identify older people as uniquely vulnerable in crisis situations. A quick perusal of CSO directories on the Web yields hundreds of organizations with some focus on older people as a vulnerable population in every country.

In addition to CSOs that offer assistance to older persons with special needs or in times of crisis, many other international, national, and local organizations of differing sizes and reach provide care to older individuals. Again, their number is too large for even a partial enumeration but some examples help illustrate the point that eldercare and issues related to older people are drawing greater attention. In the United States the *Meals on Wheels Association of America* (http://www.mowaa.org) is the oldest and best known non-governmental nutrition program for older individuals in the country. Founded during World War II the organization is dedicated to ending hunger among older people. In addition to providing nutritious meals, volunteers provide important human contact to older persons. The less well-known *Little Brothers – Friends of the Elderly (LBFE)* (https://littlebrothers.org/), a volunteer-based organization with branches in the U.S., provides companionship to older people to reduce isolation and loneliness. It is a member of a larger international network of non-profit organizations, the Fédération Internationale des petits frères des Pauvres (International Federation of Little Brothers of the Poor, http://www.petitsfreres.org). Another international organization is the *Fédération Internationale des Associations de Personnes Agées* (International Federation of Associations of Older Persons, FIAPA: https://ec.europa.eu/justice/grants/results/daphne-toolkit/content/fiapa-international-federation-associations-elderly-people_en) headquartered in Paris, which also takes as a core mission the prevention of isolation and the improvement of older individuals' quality of life.

Three examples illustrate the potential of CSOs in eldercare in less developed countries. India, like most of the rest of the world, is facing a serious problem related to the care of a growing older population. Even as developing nations with high fertility rates remain comparatively young, their older populations are growing in absolute and relative size. In India CSOs are important advocates for and service providers to older people (Sawhney 2003). *Dignity Foundation* (http://www.dignityfoundation.com), a member of the American Association of Retired Persons (AARP) Global Network, provides housing, companionship, recreation, and other services to older individuals in several Indian cities. *HelpAge India* (http://www.helpageindia.org) has a similar service mission. This CSO provides financial, medical, and emotional support to poor older Indians. HelpAge operates in many other nations, including Mexico. HelpAge India has introduced new programs and is extending its services to previously underserved areas. One example highlighted on the organization's website is a Mobile Medicare Unit (MMU) program that provides basic health care. The organization is introducing new initiatives such as disability aids, shelter assistance, yoga, specialized home visits, and psychological therapy.

The cases of Dignity Foundation and HelpAge India are examples of eldercare CSOs moving into resource starved areas in which formal supports are rare. Another example in a more developed nation is *Hogar de Cristo* (Christ's Home: http://www.hogardecristo.cl) in Chile (Pereira, Angel, and Angel 2007). Hogar de Cristo is a Catholic organization in a highly Catholic country, a fact that no doubt has contributed to its success. Begun in 1944 by a Catholic priest named Alberto Hurtado, from its founding the organization has focused on the needs of poor Chileans. Given the specific vulnerabilities of older persons, especially in light of the seriously curtailed social services that were part of the neoliberal reforms introduced by the Pinochet dictatorship, Hogar's mission has expanded to provide the full range of services to poor older individuals. These services include day care, nutritional programs, and even housing. In the absence of an adequate old-age welfare state Hogar de Cristo fills a void that is created by limited government commitments or capacities to address serious social problems.

In the United States a similar comprehensive care approach named *On Lok*, a Cantonese term which means "peaceful, happy abode," was begun in the early 1970s in San Francisco to provide services to frail Asian older individuals in certain Bay area communities in order to allow them to remain in their own homes (http://www.onlok.org) (Bodenheimer 1999). The success of this program led to its formal adoption by Congress as a model for the *PACE* program (Program of All-inclusive Care for the Elderly), which provides comprehensive services paid for primarily by Medicare and Medicaid to high-need frail older individuals (Gross et al. 2004). The On Lok experience serves as an example of how private non-governmental initiatives can serve as laboratories in which best practices related to the care of older persons can be tried and eventually inform state initiatives. Currently, seventy PACE programs employ interdisciplinary teams of care providers who develop care plans for each individual and monitor their progress with the objective of allowing them to enjoy the highest possible quality of life. In addition to primary care, the programs offer specialty care, home health aides, transportation, recreation, and companionship (Gross et al. 2004).

Hundreds of examples similar to these can be found in all nations of the world and it would be impossible to summarize the activities of even a few. As the PACE example shows, there is often a blurring of the distinction between governmental and non-governmental support activities. PACE programs rely heavily on Medicaid and Medicare for financing their operations. The category of non-governmental, therefore, includes many different degrees of government/civil society cooperation. As we mentioned in Chapter one, of the literally tens of thousands of CSOs identifiable on the Web and elsewhere, relatively few define their core missions with reference to older people, yet a closer examination reveals that many of these organizations include assistance to older individuals as part of their missions. As the older population of the globe grows at an ever-increasing pace, defamilisation will continue and the State and CSOs will increasingly take on aspects of family.

Advocacy for Social and Economic Rights

As important as services are for vulnerable older individuals especially in developing nations, basic assistance does not change the fundamental vulnerabilities that undermine their well-being. While basic assistance with food, medical care, and housing might alleviate some of the most immediate problems that older individuals face they are no substitutes for more comprehensive and continuous social security programs (HelpAge International 2009; Willmore 2006). Adequate pensions and other legal guarantees require changing laws, and that objective requires different approaches and organization than short-term crisis interventions.

In addition to service delivery, then, a major role of CSOs is advocacy for older people. In the United States the *American Association of Retired Persons* (AARP) is undoubtedly the most well-known and effective advocate for its membership (Binstock 2004). Other advocacy organizations include the national *Committee to Preserve Social Security and Medicare* (NCPSSM: http://www.ncpssm.org/), the *Alliance for Retired Americans* (ARA: http://www.retiredamericans.org), and the *National Hispanic Council on Aging* (NHCOA: http://www.nhcoa.org/).

According to its Web page NHCOA's mission includes advocacy, the support of research, the funding of community-based projects, as well as the creation of support networks, capacity-building in Hispanic communities, and the support and strengthening of Hispanic community-based organizations. The organization's core objective is to "empower Hispanic community organizations and agencies, as well as Hispanic older adults and their families."

The organization offers educational programs focused on the major health risks to Hispanics like diabetes, and it has developed an e-course on cultural competence that educates health care professionals about their culture their patients' cultures (http://edu.nhcoa.org).

Smaller local organizations, such as Family Eldercare of Austin, Texas (http://www.familyeldercare.org), one of the author's home town, provide important legal services and perform what are basically case-management services in coordinating a wide range of services that the organization's poor and largely minority clientele needs in terms of housing, legal advice, instrumental support, and more. The organization participates in a summer fan drive that collects fans and money to purchase more for older individuals without air conditioning in a part of the country in which the heat of summer can be life threatening. These activities are replicated in various forms by any number of non-governmental organizations all over the world.

The Future of Active Citizenship

The international focus on human rights is fairly recent. United Nations tribunals and the International Criminal Court began only in the 1990s, even with the precedent of the Nuremburg trials after World War II. Rather rapidly, though, an organized social movement driven largely by civil society efforts has drawn attention to major violations of basic human rights. The International Criminal Court represents a noble attempt to bring teeth to international law focused on human rights. The reality of state sovereignty and the lack of any viable policing possibilities limits the effectiveness of international efforts, including the peace keeping missions of the United Nations, to truly guarantee human rights. That stark reality, though, does not deter advocates, nor does it diminish their attempts to improve things, even in the face of inevitable setbacks.

This international affirmation of human rights, especially when extended to include social rights, accompanies a greater concern for the rights of specific groups defined in terms of gender, race, ethnicity, religious affiliation, and more. Among the new foci are the rights of older individuals for whom the objective is fostering active citizenship as part of active aging. Often age intersects with other identities to give rise to specific demands by particular groups of older persons. The core objective of this new agenda involves changing older citizens' self-image and the public's stereotype of them as superannuated and disengaged people who are no longer productive to the realization that humans remain active and engaged well into old age. This clearly involves challenging older hegemonic images of older individuals and the aging process. As important as this change of frames and self-consciousness among the older population might be, a major objective of civil society organizations is protecting their social rights, a task that requires the mobilization of marginalized groups to engage in political action. This objective clearly involves not only changing individuals' and groups' self-image, but getting them to realize that not only can one do something collectively to protect their rights, they have a duty to do so.

As we mentioned in the first chapter when we introduced the concept of active aging, our use of the term and concept differs significantly from that of the wellness movement as criticized by Sarah Lamb and others for stating or implying that one has nearly complete control over one's health and the aging process (Lamb 2017; Lamb 2020). Clearly many residents of Planet Earth have little control over any aspect of their lives, including their health. Clearly, rich individuals in high-income countries have far more control over their lives than poor individuals in impoverished countries or than marginalized groups in developed nations (Angel and Angel Forthcoming). Active citizenship is very clearly more than a reflection of individual initiative; it is constrained by the material, political, and social context in which it is expressed.

Another aspect of an active citizenship and active aging agenda that calls for caution is the possibility that these concepts serve as a smokescreen for neoliberal efforts to dismantle important aspects of the old-age welfare state, or in the case of Latin America and the Caribbean to fail to attend to the desperate needs of older individuals with few resources (Estes, Mahakian and Weitz 2001). Active aging and active citizenship clearly involve engagement with and contribution to the general welfare. Older individuals have much to contribute to their families and communities. Part of that contribution is furthering the rights of children, workers, women, indigenous peoples, and others. The concept of active aging and citizenship should not imply a radical reduction in support for health care, housing, nutrition, entertainment, and the rest of what is required for a safe and productive life. In the next chapter we delve more deeply into the legal, political, and social context in which CSOs operate in Mexico. Then in Chapters six, seven, and eight we present case studies of organizations with varying missions.

References

Allen, Nicolas, and Hernán Ouviña. 2017. "Reading Gramsci in Latin America." New York, NY: The North American Congress on Latin America. Retrieved 8/25/2020 from https://nacla.org/news/2017/05/28/reading-gramsci-latin-america.

Angel, Ronald J. 2011. "Civil Society and Eldercare in Post-Traditional Society." Pp. 549–581 in *Handbook of Sociology of Aging*, edited by Richard A. Settersten and Jacqueline L. Angel. New York, NY: Springer.

Angel, Ronald J., and Jacqueline L. Angel. Forthcoming. "Healthy Life Expectancy." In *Wiley Blackwell Encyclopedia of Sociology*, edited by George Ritzer and Chris Rojek. Malden, MA: John Wiley & Sons.

Avritzer, Leonardo. 2002. *Democracy and the Public Sphere in Latin America*. Princeton, NJ: Princeton University Press.

Bellah, Robert N. 1985. *Habits of the Heart*. Berkeley and Los Angeles, CA: University of California Press.

Benhabib, Seyla. 2002. *The Claims of Culture: Equality and Diversity in the Global Era*. Princeton, NJ: Princeton University Press.

Binstock, Robert H. 2004. "Advocacy in an Era of Neoconservatism: Responses of National Aging Organizations." *Generations* 28 (1):49–54.

Bodenheimer, Thomas. 1999. "Long-Term Care for Frail Elderly People – The On Lok Model." *The New England Journal of Medicine* 341 (17):1324–1328.

Bruhn, Kathleen. 1999. "Antonio Gramsci and the Palabra Verdadera: The Political Discourse of Mexico's Guerrilla Forces." *Journal of Interamerican Studies and World Affairs* 41 (2):29–55.

Burcher, Jacqueline (Ed.). 2008. *México solidario: Participación ciudadana y voluntaiado*. Mexico, DF: Limusa.

Buttigieg, Joseph A. 1995. "Gramsci on Civil Society." *boundary 2* 22(3):1–32.

Chiara, Magdalena, and Mercedes di Virgilio. 2005. *Gestión Social y Municipios. De los escritorios del Banco Mundial a los barrios del Gran Buenos Aires*. Buenos Aires: Prometeo Libros-UNGS.

Collins, Patricia Hill, and Sirma Bilge. 2016. *Intersectionality*. Malden, MA: Polity Press.

Crenshaw, Kimberle. 1989. "Demarginalizing the Intersection of Race and Sex: A Black Feminist Critique of Antidiscrimination Doctrine, Feminist Theory and Antiracist Politics." University of Chicago Legal Forum 1989 (1), Article 8. Retrieved 9/10/2019 from https://chicagounbound.uchicago.edu/cgi/viewcontent.cgi?referer=&httpsredir=1&article=1052&context=uclf.

Dagnino, Evelina. 2006. "Meanings of Citizenship in Latin America." *Canadian Journal of Latin American and Caribbean Studies / Revue canadienne des études latino-américaines et caraïbes* 31 (62):15–51.

Dagnino, Evelina, Alberto Olvera, and Aldo Panfichi (Eds.). 2006. *La Disputa por la Constución Democrática en América Latina*. Mexico City: Centro de Investigaciones y Estudios Superiores en Antropología Social (CIESAS) and Instituto de Investigaciones Histórico-Sociales, Universidad Veracruzana.

DeMars, William E., and Dennis Dijkzeul. 2015. *The NGO Challenge for International Relations Theory*. New York, NY: Routledge.

D'Epinay, Christian Lalive, Jean-François Bickel, Stefano Cavalli, and Dario Spini. 2011. "El curso de la vida, emergencia de un paradigma interdisciplinario." Pp. 11–30 in *La vejez en el curso de la vida*, edited by José Alberto Yuni. Catamarca, Argentina: Encuentro Grupo Editor.

Elder, Glen H., Monica Kirkpatrick Johnson, and Robert Crosnoe. 2003. "The Emergence and Development of Life Course Theory." Pp. 3–19 in *Handbook of the Life Course*, edited by Jeylan T. Mortimer and Michael J. Shanahan. Boston, MA: Springer US.

ENASEM. 2013. "Encuesta Nacional sobre Salud y Envejecimiento en México." Retrieved 12/5/2017 from http://www.mhasweb.org/index_Esp.aspx.

Encarnación, Omar G. 2018. "The Rise and Fall of the Latin American Left: Conservatives Now Control Latin America's Leading Economies, but the Region's Leftists Can Still Look to Uruguay for Direction." *The Nation*. Retrieved 8/19/2019 from https://www.thenation.com/article/the-ebb-and-flow-of-latin-americas-pink-tide/.

Estes, Carroll. 2001. *Social Policy and Aging: A Critical Perspective*. Thousand Oaks, CA: Sage.

Estes, Carroll L., Jane L. Mahakian, and Tracy A. Weitz. 2001. "A Political Economy of 'Productive Aging'." Pp. 187–199 in *Social Policy & Aging: A Critical Perspective*, edited by Carroll L. Estes. Thousand Oaks, CA: Sage.

Etzioni, Amitai. 1993. *The Spirit of Community: Rights, Responsibilities, and the Communitarian Agenda*. New York, NY: Crown Publishers.

Etzioni, Amitai (Ed.). 1995. *New Communitarian Thinking: Persons, Virtues, Institutions, and Communities*. Charlottesville, VA: The University Press of Virginia.

Faber, Paul. 2015. *Envejecimiento Activo: Un marco político ante la revolución de la longevidad*. Río de Janeiro, Brazil: International Longevity Centre Brazil (ILC-Brazil).

Ferraro, K.F., and T.P. Shippee. 2009. "Aging and Cumulative Inequality: How Does Inequality Get under the Skin?" *Gerontologist* 49 (3):333–343.

Foley, Michael W., and Bob Edwards. 1996. "The Paradox of Civil Society." *Journal of Democracy* 7:38–52.

Fraser, Nancy, and Alex Honneth. 2003. *Redistribution or Recognition? A Political-Philosophical Exchange*. New York, NY: Verso.

Fukuyama, Francis. 2018. *Identity: The Demand for Dignity and the Politics of Resentment*. New York, NY: Farrar, Straus and Giroux.

Fuller, Sylvia, Paul Kershaw, and Jane Pulkingham. 2008. "Constructing 'Active Citizenship': Single Mothers, Welfare, and the Logics of Voluntarism." *Citizenship Studies* 12 (2):157–176.

Gaventa, John, and Rajesh Tandon (Eds.). 2010. *Globalizing Citizens*. London, UK: Zed Books.

Giddens, Anthony. 1994. *Beyond Left and Right: The Future of Radical Politics*. Oxford, UK: Polity Press.

Goodhart, David. 2017. *The Road to Somewhere: The Populist Revolt and the Future of Politics*. London, UK: Hurst & Company.

Gramsci, Antonio. 1971. *Selections from the Prison Notebooks of Antonio Gramsci*, edited by Quintin Hoare and Geoffrey Nowell Smith. New York, NY: International Publishers.

Gross, Diane L., Helena Temkin-Greener, Stephen Kunitz, and Dana B. Mukamel. 2004. "The Growing Pains of Integrated Health Care for the Elderly: Lessons from the Expansion of PACE." *The Milbank Quarterly* 82 (2):257–282.

Habermas, Jürgen. 1970. "Towards a Theory of Communicative Competence." *Inquiry* 13(1–4):360–375.

Hareven, Tamara K., and Aldine de Gruyere. 1999. "La generación de enmedio: Comparación de cohortes de ayuda a padres de edad avanzada dentro de una comunidad estadounidense." *Desacatos* 2:50–72.

HelpAge International. 2009. *Working for Life: Making Decent Work and Pensions a Reality for Older People*. London, UK: HelpAge International.

Henck, Nick. 2013. "The Subcommander and the Sardinian: Marcos and Gramsci." *Mexican Studies/Estudios Mexicanos* 29 (2):428–458.

Henkin, Louis. 1995. "Human Rights and State Sovereignty." *Georgia Journal of International and Comparative Law* 25(1 & 2):31–46.

Holloway, John. 2019. *Change the World Without Taking Power*. New York, NY: Pluto Press.

Hopgood, Stephen. 2013. *The Endtimes of Human Rights*. Ithaca, NY: Cornell University Press.

HSBC. 2015. "El futuro del retiro. Decisiones para la tercera edad. Informe de México." Retrieved 12/6/2017 from https://www.hsbc.com.mx/1/PA_esf-ca-app-content/content/inicio/ofertas/retiro/estudio_futuro_retiro.pdf.

ICC. 2020. "International Criminal Court." Retrieved 1/17/2020 from https://www.icc-cpi.int/Pages/Main.aspx.

Idler, Ellen. 2006. "Religion and Aging." Pp. 277–300 in *Handbook of Aging and the Social Sciences*, edited by Robert H. Binstock and Linda K. George. New York, NY: Academic Press.

Johnston, Hank, and Paul Almeida (Eds.). 2006. *Latin American Social Movements: Globalization, Democratization, and Transnational Networks.* New York, NY: Rowman & Littlefield.

Keck, Margaret, and Kathryn Sikkink. 1998. *Activists Beyond Borders: Advocacy Networks in International Politics.* Ithaca, NY: Cornell University Press.

Kenney, Carolyn, and John Norris. 2018. "International Justice on Trial? Taking Stock of International Justice Over the Past Quarter Century." Center for American Progress. Retrieved 1/20/2020 from https://www.americanprogress. org/issues/security/reports/2018/03/28/448415/international-justice-trial/.

Kenny, Sue. 2002. "Tensions and Dilemmas in Community Development: New Discourses, New Trojans?" *Community Development Journal* 37 (4):284–299.

Kenny, Sue, Marilyn Taylor, Jenny Onyx, and Marjorie Mayo. 2017. *Challenging the Third Sector: Global Prospect for Active Citizenship.* Chicago, IL: Policy Press c/o The University of Chicago Press.

Kymlicka, Will. 1995. *Multicultural Citizenship: A Liberal Theory of Minority Rights.* New York, NY: Oxford University Press.

Kymlicka, Will. 2007. *Multicultural Odysseys: Navigating the New International Politics of Diversity.* Oxford, UK: Oxford University Press.

Kymlicka, Will, and Wayne Norman (Eds.). 2000. *Citizenship in Diverse Societies.* Oxford and New York, NY: Oxford University Press.

Lamb, Sarah (Ed.). 2017. *Successful Aging as a Contemporary Obsession: Global Perspectives.* New Brunswick, NJ: Rutgers University Press.

Lamb, Sarah (Ed.). 2020. "'You Don't Have to Act or Feel Old': Successful Aging as a U.S. Cultural Project." Pp. 49–64 in *The Cultural Context of Aging: Worldwide Perspectives,* edited by Jay Sokolovsky. Santa Barbara, CA: Praeger.

Lilla, Marc. 2016. "The End of Identity Liberalism." P. SR1, November 19, in *New York Times,* Opinion Piece. Retrieved 6/12/2019 from https://www.nytim es.com/2016/11/20/opinion/sunday/the-end-of-identity-liberalism.html.

MacIntyre, Alasdair C. 1984. *After Virtue.* Notre Dame, IN: University of Notre Dame Press.

Madison, James. 1787. "Federalist No. 10." University of Texas College of Liberal Arts Archive. Retrieved 11/16/2019 from https://liberalarts.utexas.edu/cor etexts/_files/resources/texts/c/1787%20Federalist%20No%2010.pdf.

Mendelson, Sarah E., and John K. Glenn (Eds.). 2002. *The Power and Limits of NGOs: A Critical Look at Building Democracy in Eastern Europe and Eurasia.* New York, NY: Columbia University Press.

Meyer, Carrie A. 1999. *The Economics and Politics of NGOs in Latin America.* Westport, CT: Praeger Publishers.

Montes-de-Oca Zavala, Veronica, and Paola Carmina Gutiérrez Cuellar. 2018. "La discriminación entre la población mexicana: una revisión para pensar avances y desafíos." Pp. 285–302 in *Por la igualdad somos mucho más que dos. 15 Años de lucha contra la discriminación en México,* edited by Mario Alfredo Hernández Sánchez, Yoloxóchitl Casas Chousal and Marcela Azuela Gómez. Mexico City: CONAPRED and SEGOB.

Motta, Sara C. 2009. "New Ways of Making and Living Politics: The Movimiento de Trabajadores Desocupados de Solano and the 'Movement of Movements'." *Bulletin of Latin American Research* 28 (1):83–101.

Motta, Sara C. 2014. "Latin America: Reinventing Revolutions, an 'Other' Politics in Practice and Theory." Pp. 21–42 in *Rethinking Latin American Social Movements: Radical Action from Below*, edited by Richard Stahler-Sholk, Harry E. Vanden, and Marc Becler. New York, NY: Rowman & Littlefield.

Moyn, Samuel. 2010. *The Last Utopia: Human Rights in History*. Cambridge, MA: Belknap Press.

Olvera, Alberto J. 2001. *Movimientos Sociales Prodemocráticos, Democratización y Esfera Pública en México: el caso de Alianza Cívica*. Jalapa, Mexico: Universidad Veracruzana, Cuadernos de la Sociedad Civil, no. 6.

Olvera, Alberto J. 2004. "Civil Society in Mexico at Century's End." Pp. 403–439 in *Dilemmas of Political Change in Mexico*, edited by Kevin J. Middlebrook. London, UK: Institute for Latin American Studies.

Olvera, Alberto J. 2010. "The Elusive Democracy: Political Parties, Democratic Institutions, and Civil Society in Mexico." *Latin American Research Review* 45:79–107.

Otero, Gerardo. 2004. "Global Economy, Local Politics: Indigenous Struggles, Civil Society and Democracy." *Canadian Journal of Political Science* 37 (2):325–346.

Panizza, Francisco. 2005. "Unarmed Utopia Revisited: The Resurgence of Left-of-Centre Politics in Latin America." *Political Studies* 53 (4):716–734.

Pearce, Jenny. 1996. "Between Co-option and Irrelevance? Latin American NGOs in the 1990s." Pp. 257–274 in *NGOs, States and Donors: Too Close for Comfort?*, edited by David Hulme and Michael Edwards. New York, NY: Palgrave Macmillan.

Pearce, Jenny. 2004. "Collective Action or Public Participation? Complementary or Contradictory Democratisation Strategies in Latin America?" *Bulletin of Latin American Research* 23 (4):483–504.

Pereira, Javier, and Ronald Angel. 2009. "From Adversary to Ally: The Evolution of Non-Governmental Organizations in the Context of Health Reform in Santiago and Montevideo." Pp. 97–111 in *Social Inequality and Public Health*, edited by Salvatore Babones. Bristol, UK: Polity Press.

Pereira, Javier, Ronald J. Angel, and Jacqueline L. Angel. 2007. "A Case Study of the Elder Care Functions of a Chilean Non-Governmental Organization." *Social Science and Medicine* 64:2096–2106.

Peruzzotti, Enrique, and Catalina Smulovitz (Eds.). 2002. *Controlando la Politica: Ciudadanos y Medios en las nuevas democracias Latinoamericanas*. Buenos Aires, Argentina: Temas Grupo Editorial SRL.

Posner, Eric A. 2014. *The Twilight of Human Rights Law*. New York, NY: Oxford University Press.

Putnam, Robert D. 1995. "Bowling Alone: America's Declining Social Capital." *Journal of Democracy* 6 (1):65–78.

Putnum, Robert D. 2000. *Bowling Alone: The Collapse and Revival of American Community*. New York, NY: Simon & Schuster.

Rodríguez, Rogelio Hernández. 2000. "La historia moderna del PRI. Entre la autonomía y el sometimiento." *Foro Internacional* 40 2 (160):278–306.

Roman, Joseph. 2004. "The Trade Union Solution or the NGO Problem? The Fight for Global Labour Rights." *Development in Practice* 14(1 & 2):100–109.

Salamon, Lester M. 1995. *Partners in Public Service: Government–Nonprofit Relations in the Modern Welfare State*. Baltimore, MD: The Johns Hopkins University Press.

Sawhney, Maneeta. 2003. "The Role of Non-Governmental Organizations for the Welfare of the Elderly: The Case of HelpAge India." *Journal of Aging & Social Policy* 15 (2/3):179–191.

Schlesinger Jr., Arthur. 1992. *The Disuniting of America*. New York, NY: Norton.

Sikkink, Kathryn. 2017. *Evidence for Hope: Making Human Rights Work in the 21st Century*. Princeton, NJ: Princeton University Press.

Sitrin, Mariana (Ed.). 2006. *Horizontalism: Voices of Popular Power in Argentina*. Oakland, CA: AK Press.

Skocpol, Theda. 1996. "Unravelling From Above." *The American Prospect* 25 (March–April):20–25.

Stahler-Sholk, Richard, Harry E. Vanden, and Marc Becker (Eds.). 2014. *Rethinking Latin American Social Movements: Radical Action from Below*. New York, NY: Rowman & Littlefield.

Stahler-Sholk, Richard, Harry E. Vanden, and Glen David Kuecker (Eds.). 2008. *Latin American Social Movements in the Twenty-first Century: Resistance, Power, and Democracy*. New York, NY: Rowman & Littlefield.

Stammers, Neil. 1999. "Social Movements and the Social Construction of Human Rights." *Human Rights Quarterly* 21:980–1008.

Taylor, Charles. 1994. "The Politics of Recognition." Pp. 25–73 in *Multiculturalism: Examining the Politics of Recognition*, edited by Amy Gutman. Princeton, NJ: Princeton University Press.

Teichman, Judith A. 2009. "Competing Visions of Democracy and Development in the Era of Neoliberalism in Mexico and Chile." *International Political Science Review* 30 (1):67–87.

Therborn, Göran. 2008. *From Marxism to Post-Marxism?* New York, NY: Verso.

Tocqueville, AlexisDe. 2000 (1835,1840). *Democracy in America*. Translated and edited by Harvey G. Mansfield and Delba Winthrop. Chicago, IL: University of Chicago Press.

Tussie, Diana, Marcos Mendiburu, and Patricia Vázques. 1997. "Los nuevos mandatos de los Bancos Multilaterales de Desarrollo: su aplicación al caso de Argentina." Pp. 63–105 in *El BID, el Banco Mundial y la sociedad civil sus nuevas modalidades de financiamiento internacional*, edited by Oficina de Publicaciones del CBC/FLACSO-Argentina. Buenos Aires, Argentina: FLACSO.

Willmore, Larry. 2006. "Universal Age Pensions in Developing Countries: The Example of Mauritius." *International Social Security Review* 59 (4):67–89.

Wyatt, Samuel James. 2019. "The Responsibility to Protect and Cosmopolitan Human Protection." Pp. 97–126 in *The Responsibility to Protect and a Cosmopolitan Approach to Human Protection*. Cham, Switzerland: Springer International Publishing.

Chapter 5

The Political and Legal Contexts of Eldercare in Mexico

Civil society organizations operate in complex social and legal environments that can often be difficult to navigate. As in the United States, Mexico has a range of laws and federal and state agencies that regulate the operation of officially registered CSOs and specify their fiduciary obligations and the activities they can pursue. Different CSOs emphasize different objectives, from addressing the need of older persons for social interaction and participation to more activist attempts to bring about political and legal changes. These different objectives largely reflect the education, occupational backgrounds, and social activist experience of their members. In this chapter we discuss the different ways in which CSOs with different membership profiles frame their missions. We pay particular attention to the Mexican labor movement, as well as a more recent history of social movements, two venues in which individuals gained experience in dealing with bureaucracies and fighting for their rights. Although labor unions have been traditionally weak in Mexico, they provided the first large-scale venue in which the struggle for rights could begin. Ivonne Arlette Jagüey Camarena, the founder and Director of the Fundación Ofeleia, illustrates the dedication, tenacity, and persistence that is often required to establish an independent CSO as she offers an account of the process of starting the foundation on her Facebook page:

> Today is an important day in my life. The Ofeleia Foundation A.C. is 5 years old. This adventure began on September 8, 2015, although the desire to do so dates back many years ...
>
> It is a non-profit organization which I have been thinking of since 1997 when the idea of being a volunteer in an old-age home occurred to me, but as a requirement for the position they asked me to take religious vows, a condition that I did not accept ... years later in the spring of 2003 I made a request to serve as a volunteer in a nursing home run by nuns where I was rejected by the Mother Superior for not having a medical background, nor from her perspective having a useful profession for working with the Seniors. At that time I was

DOI: 10.4324/9781003205609-5

studying Sociology at the UNAM, however, as I walked around the neighborhoods I was faced with the pain of the elderly ...

In that same year, as a response to the pain I felt ... and with the conviction of dealing with it more profoundly, I began to make myself known to a place close by consisting of older women who lived in Casa Betti ... one day I knocked on the door and expressed my interest in being a volunteer, but they rejected me over and over again. I tried again one to two days a week for an entire year ... I was about to give up ... finally on April 19, 2004 I was accepted as a volunteer to assist with social work support ... I contributed my time and volunteer work for 4 years, there, without realizing it at the time the project to do something for the elderly who, due to various circumstances, are in a situation of vulnerability and social abandonment was born ... The Ofeleia AC Foundation began to take shape.

Foundation Ofeleia A.C. was born on September 8, 2015, having as assets a computer, my brain full of ideas, and my desire. Its name serves as testimony and tribute to María Ofelia Camarena Quiroz, the founder's grandmother, who in her life was generous enough to share her granddaughter with other grandmothers and older women, whose work she always encouraged and supported. Ofeleia is of Greek origin and means: "the one who helps ... the one who provides aid ...".

Foundation Ofeleia A.C. is a non-profit civil organization whose main objective is the well-being of the elderly understood as an old age that is vital, participatory, generative and linked to the younger generations ... but above all [an organization] whose efforts are aimed at helping seniors enjoy their lives, their bonds, and discover their inherent potential.

Foundation Ofeleia A.C. has created its own model called *Therapeutic Environments*, under which it has developed various projects with older people, among which we can mention:

- **Cheer up, get active**: Occupation and recreation for seniors.
- **Club Casino (I almost never get sick ...)**: Playroom for the promotion of healthy habits and lifestyles with the elderly.
- **Club I must take care of myself**: Promotion of healthy habits and lifestyles to prevent and control high blood pressure and diabetes among older persons.
- **GYM, Large Movement**: *Strengthening ourselves outside and inside*. Resilience and Seniors.

Through initiatives and actions such as these, we wish to contribute to the physical, mental and social well-being of the elderly by combining their knowledge, experience, participation and commitment to arrive at this objective. We have also developed a series of *Self-Care Guides for Seniors (10 installments)* with various topics, as a way to disseminate affordable and accessible information to the general population. And in 2017 we produced an internet television program called *Anímate, Activate: Sport for Everyone*.

In addition, Foundation Ofeleia A.C. provides conferences, talks, workshops and courses to various audiences: seniors, families, primary caregivers, youth, professionals who work with seniors and the general public on issues related to aging and the elderly.

The activities we carry out are not for profit and those of us who participate in the different actions are volunteers, we are moved by the commitment to the cause of Seniors and the older people that we will become.

The importance of our work lies in giving life to the years left, favoring the well-being of Seniors, and promoting awareness of the value of this population as an invaluable asset for the younger generations and society as a whole.

(https://www.facebook.com/ofeleialeia/)

I Must Do Something

Ivonne Arlette Jagüey Camarena is clearly a dedicated individual with a serious desire to do something to improve the lives of older individuals with few resources. Her account of how Foundation Ofeleia came into existence underscores the difficulty that individuals often face in their attempts to engage in civic and volunteer activity. Camarena's initial attempts to volunteer were rebuffed for various reasons, many of which we are unaware of, but in the end, her motivation and persistence allowed her to begin her own successful CSO, which is currently providing support and services to older persons in need.

Camarena's account illustrates both the potential obstacles to starting a CSO and also the fact that establishing such entities requires the total commitment of one or a few dedicated individuals with a particular mission in mind. Camarena's story is incomplete in that we do not know about the funding sources of the organization, nor the process she engaged in to become an Asociación Civil, A.C. (Civil Association), the legal designation granted by the government that allows the organization to receive tax-exempt donations. The fact that she acquired the designation and is celebrating the foundation's fifth anniversary indicates that she has been successful. Although Foundation Ofeleia was not one of the organizations we studied, it is typical of many organizations that have come into existence since the 1970s.

In this chapter we deal with the political and legal environment in which civil society organizations operate in Mexico. Although Mexico has its own federal and state laws governing the incorporation and funding of civil society organizations, the basic legal constraints that such organizations confront are similar to those in other nations. We also develop a theoretical classification of civil society organizations based on the cultural and human capital of their members. Cultural and human capital includes higher levels of education, prior union membership, influential business experience, a social activist background, and more. These sources of cultural and human capital can be translated into political and social capital for the purposes of furthering a group's agenda, and they influence the ways in which an organization frames its objectives. These frames have important implications for the sort of collective actions in which organizations that deal with issues related to the welfare and rights of older individuals engage.

Few Formal Alternatives

As we have mentioned, CSOs take on particular importance in the care of older persons in Mexico largely because there are few formal alternatives. Federal or state-sponsored residential or community care is rare and families have few options in caring for their infirm older members (Gutiérrez-Robledo et al. 1996; OECD 2011). As we discuss further in later chapters, non-institutional community-based options could be particularly important in a nation like Mexico in which publicly-funded nursing home care is rare and privately purchased care remains prohibitively expensive for all but the most affluent. Yet, as potentially beneficial as it might be, government-funded or sponsored day care is rare. The federal *Instituto Nacional de las Personas Adultos Mayores*, INAPAM (The National Institute for Older Adults), a federal agency begun in 1979 to provide services and assistance to older individuals, operates seven day care centers, six in Mexico city and one in Zacatecas (INAPAM 2016a; INAPAM 2016b). The federal *Instituto de Seguridad y Servicios Sociales de los Trabajadores del Estado*, ISSSTE (Federal Institute of Social Security and Services for State Workers) operates twenty-one centers, two in Mexico City and the others in the rest of the country (ISSSTE 2020). Other organizations sponsor day care centers, but without hard data on their actual number and the extent of unmet need that exists, it is impossible to know how many older individuals suffer isolation and loneliness. Suffice it to say, that number is likely great.

Publicly funded residential long-term care facilities are particularly scarce in Mexico. Most of those that exist are part of two programs that operate at the federal and state levels, by INAPAM and *El Sistema National para el Desarollo Integral de la Familia*, DIF (the National System for Integral Family Development) (DIF Nacional 2010). These agencies address a wide range of needs among individuals of all ages. Although, they provide useful services, what they offer falls far short of what is needed. INAPAM has a small number of residences that provide comprehensive care to older individuals who have no family support or financial resources. DIF provides care for older people in shelter homes and related nursing homes. In 2010, DIF operated four homes for older people, each housing approximately 470 individuals (Gutiérrez Robledo, López Ortega, and Arango Lopera 2012; OECD 2011).

In addition to limited access to long-term care, basic economic survival remains a serious challenge for older Mexicans. Which brings us back to the role of civil society organizations in advocating for and defending the social rights of older Mexicans. In recent years a growing number of secular and faith-based CSOs have begun to focus on topics related to the needs of the aging population (Gutiérrez-Robledo et al. 1996; Montes-de-Oca 2000; OECD 2011). Unfortunately, we do not have a complete census of these organizations, but some examples of the sorts of services available from government-sponsored and private sources is useful to reiterate the objectives and challenges of long-term care in a limited-resource environment. First, though, we should provide some basic information concerning the legal status of civil society organizations in Mexico.

The Legal Status of CSOs in Mexico

Civil society organizations in Mexico, as elsewhere, come in every form and size. At the most informal level, individuals join together in social groups or in groups with some particular objective, like opposing a new waste treatment facility or demanding services or infrastructure improvements. These groups often have no formal structure or organization, nor are they registered with or regulated by the State. As a consequence, we do not include them in this discussion of the legal status of CSOs. Although CSOs have some universal characteristics, primarily the fact that they are not part of government, since each nation and even states and provinces have their own laws related to incorporation and tax-exemption, it is impossible to characterize the category of CSO internationally.

The rapid growth in the number of CSOs since the 1970s and 1980s in Mexico reflects not only a growing recognition of the potential role of such organizations by citizens and advocates of various sorts, but also significant changes in the legal framework in which these organizations operate. In 2004 the *Ley de Fomento a las Actividades Realizadas por las Organizaciones de la Sociedad Civil* (Federal Law for the Promotion of the Activities of Organized Civil Society) was passed. The objective of this new law was to make it easier to establish such organizations and to clarify the legal environment in which they operate. This law and ongoing advocacy by civil society representatives have clearly resulted in a more favorable environment for CSO activity. Yet legal, administrative, and tax impediments stand in the way of a full development of civil society in Mexico (Díaz Aldret, Titova, and Arellano Gault 2020; Huerta, Ablanedo, and Vázquez del Mercado ND; Magaña Hernández and Figueroa Díaz 2018). It is clear that in order to further the possibilities for significant civil society contributions to the nation's overall welfare clear operational rules, transparency in funding and management, and greater integration of federal and state regulations are necessary (Díaz Aldret, Titova, and Arellano Gault 2020; Huerta, Ablanedo, and Vázquez del Mercado ND).

In the U.S. and Europe CSOs are fairly easily established and are subject to relatively little governmental oversight (Advocates for International Development 2017; Organization for Security and Co-operation in Europe 2004; U.S. Department of State 2017). Those that apply for tax exemption and receive charitable donations are usually required to document what they receive and how it is used on a regular basis. Of course, not all governments welcome CSOs or any other outside influence, and in many countries CSO activities are closely monitored or even banned. Russia, for example, has banned two of George Soros' charities, the Open Society Foundations (OSF) and the Open Society Institute (OSI), for activities that the State sees as hostile (CNBC 2015). Needless to say, the more critical an organization is of a host government's policies or actions the more likely this is to happen.

In the U.S., most of us are familiar with the 501(c)(3) designation for tax-exempt charitable organizations. In Mexico, the basic logic related to the registration of such organizations is similar. In order to receive tax exempt donations civil society organizations must register with the relevant federal or state agencies and receive "authorized donee status," which allows them to issue tax-deductible receipts to donors. These organizations can engage in many recognized socially beneficial activities, as long as those are not primarily for profit (Council on Foundations 2018). The category of authorized donee status includes three types of organizations that are established and governed in accordance to Mexican state laws. These include the *Asociación Civil*, AC (Civil Associations), the *Institución de Asistencia Privada*, IAP (Private Assistance Institutions), and the *Sociedad Civil*, SC (Civil Society). These organizations provide financial aid, medical and psychological care, educational and employment training, legal and funeral assistance, assistance to migrants, and much more. They work with disaster victims, refugees, and many others. They are major players in the fight for gender equality and human rights. Similar organizations operate in many nations of the world. Despite local differences, most promote active citizenship and active aging through civic engagement (Wanderley 2009).

A fourth type of charitable initiative in Mexico includes *fideicomisos* (Trusts), that are formed by individuals who donate money or property for a particular socially beneficial purpose. These are governed by federal law (*Ley General de Títulos y Operaciones de Crédito*, LGTOC (General Law of Titles and Credit Operations)). As elsewhere, the specifics of Mexican state and federal laws governing civil society organizations are complex and specify rules of organization, governance, dissolution, and more. We will not summarize those in any detail. Our objective is only to emphasize the fact that civil society organizations are rapidly becoming an important part of civic action and even governance.

A Typology of CSOs that Deal with Older Persons in Mexico

Mexico, like most other nations of the world, has numerous civil society entities. As we explained earlier, our focus is on organizations with a sufficient level of organization and structure to give them some identity and longer-term presence. We are not interested in groups that reflect the informal efforts of one or a few individuals. Such entities simply lack the capacity to do much beyond offering some minor material support or emotional succor to those involved. On the other hand, as we have discussed, relatively unorganized groups are often active participants in social movements. We present an example of land invasion by a relatively small and disorganized group in Chapter eight. The serious shortage of housing available for migrants to large cities from the countryside spawned many land invasions and the development of squatter settlements on vacant land in many parts of Mexico. These movements provided experience in collective actions, and in some cases, they resulted in ongoing community and neighborhood associations. Our analysis, though, focuses on organizations that have some recognized legal status as defined by state or federal statutes, laws, and regulations. This is clearly not a rigorous definition, but it serves as a general guideline to our investigation of what is inherently a highly varied range of civil society organizations.

In order to characterize the objectives of the organizations we deal with we adapt a general classification of frames of reference proposed by Alfama et al. (2013) that summarizes the basic objectives of various public policies and programs related to active aging. Frames of reference, as we discussed in Chapter three, refer to the ways in which particular states of affairs are portrayed, and the various solutions that are offered to address them. The classification includes three general frames based on a review of international conventions, as well as local municipal policies in Spain, but it can be adapted to deal with more specific framing issues and other countries.

The classification's utility lies in drawing attention to the new concern with human rights, as well as the health and welfare of older citizens. It also draws attention to issues of the economic sustainability of the old-age welfare state. The classification identifies three general policy emphases. The first focuses on the quality of life and self-development of older people; the second on rights; and the third on economics and system sustainability. These frames are not mutually exclusive; they represent ideal types that for our purposes serve as useful analytic or heuristic categorizations. The emerging focus on active aging from which this categorization arises draws attention to the causes and consequences of the inequality and injustice that undermines the welfare and well-being of older individuals. It emphasizes the right to the basic material requirements of a dignified life, as well as the right to autonomy and participation. Let us briefly explain what each frame focuses upon and how we apply each in our analysis. We deal with elaborations and extensions of each of these frames in Chapters six, seven, and eight in which we examine how different organizations combine elements of each.

The first frame of reference emphasizes the quality of life and self-development of older persons. It reflects the new reality of population aging and the need for individuals to remain healthy and engaged for many more years than was common, or even possible, in previous eras. In order for individuals to remain active and engaged they need the material and social resources to make that possible. This includes high-quality health care, a safe environment, education, opportunities for social engagement, and the rest of what is required to allow an individual to remain physically and emotionally sound and productive throughout the life course. Furthering this objective implies changes in policies related to education, health care, the labor force, cultural activities, and more. Given high levels of poverty in the older population all three frames explicitly or implicitly focus on the need for adequate retirement income, which in a situation in which the majority of workers spend much or all of their working years in the informal sector, means fighting for pension reform and non-contributory pensions.

The second frame of reference focuses on rights, with the objective of eliminating discrimination based on age, increasing employment opportunities for older persons, and furthering the recognition of their autonomy and productivity. A core objective of this frame is to change the stereotype of older people as superannuated or obsolete and in need of assistance to the realization that they can be actively engaged citizens who are capable of controlling their own lives and contributing to the community. This objective requires the elimination of all forms of abuse and neglect, an equitable intergenerational distribution of resources, and a recognition of the many contributions that older individuals can and do make.

The third frame focuses on economics and system sustainability. It addresses the problem facing most nations that results from rapid population aging. This problem relates to rapidly increasing old age dependency ratios, which refers to the number of individuals 60 and older relative to those 15 to 59. As fertility declines and life expectancy increases the dependency ratio grows, meaning that the number of workers available to support the retired population shrinks. At some point the burden on the working-age population becomes prohibitive and the system cannot be sustained. This new reality calls for fairly radical policy innovations, again including providing opportunities for older individuals to work longer if they are able and wish to. Given the new demographic reality, the consequences of labor force policies, including those that allow or even encourage early retirement, must be reassessed. Older individuals who have no employment-based income or savings and who are incapable of continuing to work need direct state support. Many low and middle-income nations, including Mexico, have introduced non-contributory pensions to provide a minimal floor of support.

Many other reforms are also necessary. In order for older individuals to participate and remain productive for longer investments in health and human capital over the life course are necessary. Since the State, and particularly the governments of low and middle-income countries, cannot provide all of the material or instrumental assistance older people need, enhancing the capacity of informal caregivers, who are primarily family members, to provide assistance to older individuals is necessary, even as defamilisation proceeds apace. It is clear that CSOs have a major role to play in filling the gaps left by the State and the family.

The affirmation of human rights in general, and of older persons in particular, is clearly a core part of a larger political agenda. A focus on rights and a civil society approach to rights, though, includes more than political activity or the simple affirmation of rights in statutes and legal rulings. Rather, it involves consciousness raising among older persons, with the objective of getting them to realize that they can and should live free from abuse and neglect, and that they do not have to tolerate marginalization and exclusion. It also involves changes in public perceptions. The focus on rights, then, refers to consciousness raising at a personal level, in addition to a change at the level of formal political discourse. This view of rights relates to Gramsci's argument that we discussed in Chapter four, in which he proposes that the process of overcoming oppression begins with a change of consciousness among the oppressed. What civil society organizations do in this context is help older people recognize what they might already know at some level, but have not yet articulated in a manner that allows them to demand justice. This recognition and exercise of rights, then, is not confined to political mobilization on a large scale, although that might be an ultimate objective, but includes more local and smaller group action. The concept of rights that informs our investigation, then, is that of a wide range of activities that vary from the daily affirmation of the most basic human and social rights to the organized and often militant action of unions and political parties.

This classification of frames of reference hardly exhausts the possible classification of approaches to the problems older people face, nor of the possible responses to them, but it serves as a useful beginning in attempting to understand the objectives of civil society organizations and how they frame their missions. This classification, modified as necessary, guides our description of various CSOs in Mexico in terms of their objectives and the focus of their organizational efforts. As we will see, the frames they employ, and the way in which particular organizations define a problem area and potential solutions, are clearly influenced by the human and cultural capital, as well as the employment and social activist history, of their memberships. Certain groups are inexperienced in the workings of government agencies and have few political contacts. These groups have relatively little success in leveraging benefits for their memberships. Others, primarily those consisting of retired government workers, ex-union members, and retired educators, bring much more experience to bear in dealing with State bureaucracies. Their continuing contacts with political parties, unions, and agencies place them in a far more powerful position in terms of leveraging benefits and advantages for their constituents, although even then their ability to bring about major change is often limited.

Our adaptation of the Alfama et al. (2013) categorization of organizational frames follows the historical emergence of efforts to further the rights of different groups, beginning with workers in the formal sector, followed by demands by peasants, ethnic minorities, women, and others who were traditionally outside of the formal sector, for recognition of their identities, as well as their basic rights. The discussion culminates with greater focus of contemporary civil society organizations on human and social rights more generally. This focus on rights goes well beyond those of older persons, and espouses a new and invigorated civil society that empowers individuals of all ages and backgrounds to act as agents in their own behalf. We summarize our approach briefly here and then examine each category of organizations in the following chapters in greater detail.

The Beginning: The Mexican Labor Movement

Our examination of the role of civil society organizations in furthering the basic rights of older individuals begins with an examination of the role of unions and the Mexican labor movement in furthering the rights of workers. Although the labor movement has never been strong in Mexico, it served as perhaps the earliest proponent of rights, in terms of worker rights. As we discuss in Chapter six, labor disputes and job actions began in the 19th Century, but never gave rise to an effective and widespread worker's movement (Huber and Stephens 2012). Official government policy, international competition, and the desire of factory owners to increase profits resulted in serious repression or cooptation of unions and the suppression of wages and workers' ability to improve working conditions. The fact that even today over half of the Mexican labor force works in the informal sector was also a major impediment to widespread unionization.

Yet unions were important in providing their members experience in organizing, striking, and demanding their rights. Many independent unions were quite active and often leftist, and in many cases their members inculcated a militant attitude and a sense of earned rights, and the realization that those rights had to be fought for. Unfortunately, most unions have not been independent, rather they were established by management who appointed their leaders and dictated their policies for the benefit of the enterprise rather than that of workers. Despite these union weaknesses, though, retirees with union backgrounds, those who worked in the government sector, as well as retired teachers and university professors who have high levels of human and cultural capital tend to assume an activist role and frame their objectives in terms of worker rights, including an adequate income, high-quality health care, political rights, and more. For these groups active aging implies more of a collective confrontational stance than is the case for those organizations whose membership does not have these backgrounds and that are focused primarily on individual quality of life.

The labor movement, then, structures an important frame of reference for civil society organizations. But Mexico, much as the rest of Latin America and the Caribbean, has a long history of social movements in addition to labor unions (Escobar and Alvarez 1992; Foweraker and Craig 1990; Johnston and Almeida 2006; Stahler-Sholk, Vanden, and Becker 2014; Stahler-Sholk, Vanden, and Kuecker 2008). Like the older labor movement, these social movements not only reflect increasing demands by the poor and the middle classes for more honest and effective governance, they provide venues in which individuals inculcate more activist perspectives, even as many have adopted more horizontal and non-hierarchical or authoritative organizational and political philosophies (Sitrin 2006; Stahler-Sholk, Vanden, and Becker 2014). These perspectives influenced the frames of the organizations we discuss in Chapters seven and eight. The period of the 1960s and 1970s saw a particularly high level of protest by various groups who were demanding recognition (Escobar and Alvarez 1992; Johnston and Almeida 2006; Stahler-Sholk, Vanden, and Becker 2014; Stahler-Sholk, Vanden, and Kuecker 2008).

As in other Latin American countries, this unrest is fueled by massive social inequalities, widespread poverty, and completely inadequate state policies to address major social problems. As numerous observers have noted, neoliberal policies that gave rise to many of these problems lost legitimacy (Motta 2013; Stahler-Sholk, Vanden, and Becker 2014; Webber and Carr 2012). The serious debt crises that shook Latin America and that resulted in the Mexican default in 1982, in addition to the government's inept response to a major earthquake in Mexico City in 1985, marked the beginning of the decline of the PRI (Hartlyn and Morley 1986; Martínez 2015; Monsiváis 1987). Discontent was widespread and reactions were often violent.

In addition to widespread protests, the period saw the emergence of numerous guerrilla movements (Mendoza García 2011). Protests and strikes were carried out by teachers, railroad workers, doctors, copper miners, peasants, and university students. Most of these movements were aggressively repressed (Minetti 2017). The official state response focused on the elimination of opposition to the ruling party, the PRI, through violently repressive actions that became known as the "dirty war," in which thousands of individuals were killed (Calderon and Cedillo 2012; Mendoza García 2011). The 1968 student protests in the Plaza de las Tres Culturas in Tlatelolco that we mentioned at the beginning of Chapter one ended in the massacre of hundreds of students.

These social movements were part of a growing concern with basic social rights accompanied by a growing rejection of the old corporatist politics. In the newer discourse that we discussed in Chapter three this demand for social rights gave rise to a more generalized identity politics and demands by specific groups, including older individuals and their supporters, for recognition and respect of their basic human as well as social rights. As part of this frame realignment, organizations focus on the quality of life of older individuals. Respect for human rights clearly involves providing not only the basic material necessities of a productive and satisfying life, but a recognition of the basic human need for respect, for participation in family and community life, life-long education, and freedom from fear. These objectives are clearly implicit in all of the other frames, but for certain groups the focus on quality of life was central. Many of these groups, as we explain in Chapter seven include members who do not have union experience or even formal labor force experience, who do not have high levels of education, and who are not veterans of social movements. The majority of the members of these organizations are women.

This declining dominance of the PRI, open and honest elections, growing middle-class and student discontent with the old regime resulted in more general demands for the respect of human rights and for greater economic justice. Latin America and the Caribbean, including Mexico, is characterized by massive income and wealth inequality, which translates directly into massive differentials in power and the inability of many individuals and groups to control their own lives. In recent years, transnational social movements, as well as more local movements, have fostered demands by various groups for recognition. These have included demands by older individuals and their representatives. These are part of a more general concern for human rights that has been instrumental in the passage of the many international conventions that affirm the dignity and rights of older citizens that we summarized in Chapter three. We present more detailed descriptions of these sorts of organizations and their frames in Chapter eight. Here, though, we provide some brief examples of CSOs

in Mexico that frame their missions and objectives in terms of variations
on the issue frames we have summarized.

Union Affiliations and Activism

The labor movement clearly represents a core aspect of civil society. Strong
labor unions can serve as a catalyst for significant social change. One
might expect that after they retire union members retain the confrontational perspective into which they were socialized in the union. This could
conceivably lead to more active, and perhaps more effective, social
engagement by union retirees. As we discuss further in Chapter six,
though, in Mexico unions have had mixed success in furthering their
members' interests or in bringing about political change more generally.
The labor movement in Mexico has been largely coopted by the ruling
party and many unions were simply fronts for State and company interests.
Yet it is clear that the experiences, as well as the human and cultural
capital, of a group's membership structures its framing of issues and its
actions. Our interviews revealed important differences among organizations of retirees depending on their work histories and union membership.

The organizations that stand out in this category include those whose
members have experience in government or unions and have knowledge of
bureaucracies and the ways in which the system works. Examples include
pensioners of the *Instituto de Seguridad y Servicios Sociales de los Trabajadores
del Estado*, ISSSTE (Institute of Security and Social Services of State
Workers), retirees of the *Instituto Mexicano del Seguro Social*, IMSS (Mexican
Institute of Social Security), retired members of the *Sindicato Mexicano de
Electricistas*, SME (Mexican Union of Electricians), the *Coordinadora Nacional de Trabajadores de la Educación*, CNTE (National Coordinating Committee of Education Workers), and retired faculty of the Autonomous
University of Mexico (UNAM), *Pioneros de Creatividad En Libertad*,
PICRELI (Pioneers in Creativity in Freedom). These groups are characterized by strong political organization and memberships with medium to
high levels of education, a characteristic that enhances their collective
effectiveness. Except for those groups consisting of educators, members of
these organizations are predominantly male, although more women are
participating as they enter the labor force in increasing numbers.

These organizations do not frame their missions in terms of active aging
or quality of life, as do other organizations we describe below and in
Chapter seven. For the most part, they retain a discourse focused on labor
rights, which is part of the union culture. One ex-union member
explained that a union consciousness is shared among retirees and workers.
He explained that "we cooperate with the union, they call us to advise the
boys, that helps us to be active, to participate and to live with our companions; we learn to live with young people too." Because most spent their

working years in the formal economy in which they received good salaries, many retired early and receive adequate pensions. Many government workers and workers in strategic sectors of the economy enjoyed defined-benefit retirement plans through patronage arrangements. They are in a completely different class than those workers who spent all or a large fraction of their working lives in the informal sector.

Today, many find the gains they won or were granted threatened by various reforms to the retirement system. In 1997 IMSS, and in 2010 ISSSTE replaced their traditional defined-benefit pension plans with defined-contribution plans. The earlier plans were funded on a pay-as-you-go basis and guaranteed a set income for life; the latter require that the worker fund his or her own retirement, potentially resulting in a very low retirement income if a worker's savings are insufficient, or in losses if economic conditions deteriorate. The privatization of the electric sector and planned reforms in the education sector have also mobilized those workers. Although these organizations retain a confrontational rhetoric and agenda focused on their members' rights, they also pursue a broader agenda focused on economic security and demands for the rights of ex-workers in general. A major focus is adequate medical care to which retired workers are entitled and which represents a major benefit. This larger focus leads to some limited attempts to forge bonds with other unions or groups of older people.

Militant Electricians and Teachers

Retirees of the electrical workers union, the Sindicato Mexicano de Electricistas (SME), present an interesting case of militancy. The union has had a long history of leftist activism and has had confrontations with the State. In addition to seeking protection of their own benefits as ex-workers in a strategic sector that was privatized during the Felipe Calderón administration, retired electrical workers have expanded their mission to combat the adoption of undemocratic practices that affect the country's workers. Participation in the union is framed as an exercise of democratic rights and participation in decision-making related to important social issues. Because of the experience of its members and its politicized discourse, this group and groups like it represent important actors in the political culture of the country. However, the neoliberal policies we discussed earlier have weakened Mexican labor unions, which were never that powerful to begin with. Whatever potential exists for the labor movement to influence government policy, that possibility could be seriously diminished if the union culture is further weakened.

Retired teachers illustrate another aspect of this frame. Given their educations, retired teachers possess a high level of human and cultural capital. The union of retired teachers, the Coordinadora Nacional de Trabajadores de la Educación, CNTE (National Coordinator of Education

Workers) is highly democratic in its internal governance. This organization fosters a social justice discourse advocating active engagement by educators. In terms of aging, their discourse reflects a concern for optimal physical functioning, but even more so for social integration and active engagement. These frames reflect the traditional trade union struggle, and a concern for solidarity with younger generations. Yet, given the historical State and industry opposition to their organizing efforts, they have had to be realistic about the possibilities. As one informant told us, "above all, we must think of goals and still be able to realize them. Fortunately, they can be realized, but we also have to be realistic, to know what we can still do, what influence we have."

A Focus on the Quality of Life and Self-Development

The labor movement, governmental employment, high levels of education, and other experiences with social movements provide experiences and knowledge that can enhance the willingness and ability of other retiree groups to express their agency. Not all groups, though, include individuals with those backgrounds or experiences. Our second organizational category includes groups that focus primarily on maintaining or improving the quality of life of those they serve. *Amanecer Veracruzana* is located in the Iztapalapa alcaldía (borough) of Mexico City, a marginal district whose residents have low incomes and little social capital. We have no exact number, but our informal observations suggest that many such organizations exist. Although the organization's members may be aware of the new human rights discourse, the organization's formal discourse does not focus on rights per se. Rather it emphasizes individual well-being and optimal functioning. The organization's participants consist primarily of women 75 and over, most of whom are widows and in poor health. The vast majority suffer from diabetes and hypertension. Most have very little education and spent their lives as homemakers. Yet one would describe their lives as active. Their activities, which are centered in the neighborhood and focused on recreation, are intended to maintain optimal physical functioning despite chronic disease and mobility problems.

Participation clearly improves the quality of life of these women. It allows them to avoid isolation and remain as physically functional and socially active as possible. Two participants describe their experience in the following way: "It helps me not to think about things I should not, it helps my health because we spend a nice time because … we are rehearsing, or we are exercising." Another said, "they keep us active and we keep the body in motion so that we will not become crippled." Yet because of the members' low levels of human and social capital, and the fact that the local government has not offered support to these sorts of organizations, Amanecer has not been able to obtain significant support from municipal or State authorities. Given the organization's focus on the old and infirm, younger generations are not involved, perhaps contributing to the organization's inability to obtain governmental support. To a large extent, the organization's inability to significantly affect the material and social situations of its membership reflects the particularly disadvantaged position of the older population itself, but also the high degree of marginalization of many of the districts and neighborhoods in which it and similar organizations operate. It also reflects a general lack of governmental programs targeted to older people.

In addition to engaging in physical activity, participants also engage in art projects. A major objective of these group activities is to prevent isolation. As part of its frame realignment efforts one of the group's major objectives is to transform the participants' self-image and the public's image of older people from one that focuses on disease and functional decline to one that portrays older individuals as active agents in control of their lives. Although the organization's activities clearly reflect frame realignment, they do not include a discourse on rights, nor do they involve direct political action.

Rights as a Core Objective

Other groups engage in a newer discourse based on frames with the protection and extension of rights as a core objective. One such organization is the *Renueva Group* located in the Gustavo A. Madero alcaldía in Mexico City. Although the borough is relatively poor, it is slightly less marginalized than the Iztapalapa neighborhood where Amanecer Veracruzana is located. As with Amanecer, the organization's philosophy clearly emphasizes active aging based on the principle that the maintenance of autonomy and independence is central to a high quality of life. A basic focus on physical and mental health is part of the frames of most of the organizations we studied. Speaking about her experiences at Renueva one respondent noted that participation benefits her:

> in the best way possible, being aware of ... what we have to do, without straining ... to grow old in a better way with enthusiasm because that also helps us a lot because it opens our understanding of ourselves and also others ... That's what I mean by active aging, being aware of oneself and taking care of yourself, because then there are people who [feel] abandoned and they get mad at everything because they are cooped up and have no other vision, they do not leave their house, because they do not want to get involved or maybe they can't because they already have a disability ... But this aging is a process that slowly ... It is slow and we accept it and how better than with that spirit.

Another respondent revealed her main reason for participation when she told us that:

> [t]he fact that people feel more cheerful is something that one notices immediately. Participation, also health and the improvement of everyone's health because I have been touched to see people who arrive almost unable to walk because they are fat. Others are not fat but their bones and their muscles hurt. It is simply that there is someone who one approaches, with whom one can talk about different things that are happening, feel support, feel that there is under-standing and that comforts the soul. The spirit feels good, one does not feel that everything has to be kept in and I am getting sicker because I do not have ... I feel cornered, or I feel alone ... one finds that warmth, that shelter where one is supported.

In addition to autonomy and independence, the organization fosters perso-nal mobility as part of its focus on intellectual and physical development. The active aging approach is clearly informed by an awareness of the aging process, but it emphasizes the individual's responsibility for controlling that process to the greatest extent possible. The organization has been successful in its appeals to governmental authorities to obtain locations and resources to support its activities. Through its own revenue generation efforts and with resources it obtains from the authorities the organization sponsors workshops, lectures, recreational activities, conferences, a cinema club, and much more.

What distinguishes Renueva from organizations like Amanecer is the fact that in addition to its focus on mental and physical functioning, Renueva's frame of reference goes beyond the quality of life frame to explicitly add a rights dimension. This focus reflects the affirmation of the rights of older citizens codified in the various international conventions we discussed in Chapter three. One woman who is active in Renueva explained to us that the members' understanding of their rights and their ability to exercise those rights is enhanced by their participation. As she told us that the members:

> are aware of their rights because of the work we do here ... The organization offers us a course on the rights of the elderly ... because human rights and adult rights are completely different, they are dif-ferent and they [the members] are exercising them. From the moment of deciding what I am going to do, it is my right to decide, ... they can no longer tell me, they can no longer deprive me of my right to decide so easily, because the rights of the elderly forbid dispossession and mistreatment ... they [the members] needed only to know what they could do, what they are entitled to and what their obligation is.

As I tell them "we have learned our rights, now what is my obligation?" It remains to exercise your rights ... and they do exercise their rights.

Renueva's membership is predominantly female with higher levels of education than is the case for Amanecer, and they often have work experience. Although many of these women have some employment history, not all enjoy economic security in old age. Most are married. Many continue their education through informal courses, and participants have organized a Center for Social and Cultural Development. This organization clearly benefits its membership and provides convincing evidence that older individuals with few personal resources can act collectively to significantly improve their quality of life and engage in collective activity to protect and extend their basic social rights.

The Combination of Quality of Life, Economic Sustainability, and Rights

Certain groups of retirees combine many aspects of each of the three major frames we have outlined, largely because of the unique characteristics of their members. One such group consists of retirees and pensioners of the Autonomous University of Mexico (UNAM), *Pioneros de Creatividad en Libertad*, PICRELI (Pioneers in Creativity in Freedom). This group is characterized by loose social organization but a high level of participation among those who join. The organization's discourse is not narrowly focused on a defined objective, but rather focuses on multiple ways of exercising members' rights and enhancing the quality of their lives. Clearly, their high levels of education facilitate the defense of members' rights. The majority of members are women with doctorate degrees and a substantial work history. The organization's objectives are to maintain the organization and to communicate with other groups, but above all to remain informed about important policies that affect members and society at large. Four participants of a focus group we conducted with PICRELLI members explained their objectives. They clearly feel a sense of generativity and a desire to maintain some connection to the University. As they explained:

> we try to help the new retirees so that it does not cost them as much work as it cost us ... it cost us from the formalities in the ISSSTE that leave you sitting hours, they bring you back again and again eeeeh ... At least for me it was a disaster ... at UNAM, we realize that ... our office has disappeared, our job ... has been given to another person, we can no longer park because our credentials disappeared, they took them away, then we no longer have a place to come to park, or to come and visit, to see, and we feel that our time has been wasted

because we have more than 30 years of experience ... Ah ... everyone is worth it, right? And when we could counsel, we could give tips, we could advise ... give some seminar, give some talk, give some workshop ... most of us have a lucid mind ... there are some others that already have begun to have mental problems, but most of us have a clear mind ... are struggling to be given a place ...

... to propose to the University that it benefits from our experience ... we have proposed many things that we could do but also that the University, as I understand it, has a place for us ... since we have worked at UNAM for a long time ...

Active aging has a lot to do with transmitting all the experience one has acquired throughout one's life ...

I think it's also an attitude of not simply to wait for death or to wait for visits from children or grandchildren ... I have a good relationship with my son and my granddaughters ... but that can't be everything. One needs economic independence, intellectual independence, the ability to make decisions, to own one's own life.

Caring for Those Who Cannot Care for Themselves

Although our focus is on groups that consist of individuals who are able to potentially engage in activities to improve their quality of life or even engage in collective action to further their own and others' welfare, it is clear that eventually the reality of declining health and cognitive capacity can seriously diminish one's autonomy, perhaps completely. *Un Granito de Arena* A.C., (A Grain of Sand) operates a residential facility for older people with serious cognitive impairments and little personal mobility. This organization serves both men and women who can no longer live alone, although more women than men use its services. This organization differs from the previous organizations we mentioned in the fact that those it serves are so seriously impaired cognitively and functionally that they are unable to care for themselves at all. They have simply lost their autonomy and are unable to act individually or collectively on their own behalf. Active aging, as we have characterized it, is no longer possible.

As is the case for minors or individuals with diminished capacity, others must care for them and act as their proxies. That role is assumed by a dedicated staff who assure that the residents have adequate health care and enjoy as much freedom and autonomy as possible. Granito and other organizations like it address an increasing need for attention to a segment of the population that lives alone, but with seriously compromised autonomy. As Mexico ages rapidly this segment will grow. Although the ideal is to allow people to remain in the community and in their own homes, at some point that may become impossible. As we noted earlier in the chapter, government-sponsored residential care is seriously limited in

Mexico. Caring for elders with serious physical and cognitive impairments poses massive challenges. It is likely that in the future more secular and faith-based non-governmental organizations will move in to at least partially fill the gap.

Residential long-term care poses challenges not only for the State and for care givers, but for the older person him or herself. Having to leave one's familiar environment and the disruption of long-standing routines that it entails is difficult for an older person. As one informant who was forced to make the move told us:

> I suffered a lot because I did not plan to come here. Who would have thought that I was going to end up here? ... that made me very sad and I cried a lot but ... because my daughter ... supports me I could not help her in any way other than by coming here. I have a pension but very little.

She explained that her health meant that she could no longer live alone. As she said:

> I was defenseless. I lost weight. I vomited up everything because I had a terrible gastritis, and everything I ate came back ... I had esophagus damaged from vomiting and not being able to eat. They injected me in the veins, they gave me serum and I spent fifteen days in the hospital, but while I was in the hospital my sister met someone from here who told her about this place.

Defamilisation and Active Aging

Although Mexico is experiencing some degree of defamilisation of the care of older parents, especially in terms of economic support with the introduction of non-contributory pensions, financial and political realities limit the degree to which greater responsibility for older persons could be shifted to the State. In many cases that means that older parents receive limited or inferior care. While we might romanticize the family and imagine that all families are motivated by deeply felt norms of filial piety, the fact is that in the absence of adequate defamilisation in the form of sufficient state supports, the quality of many older parents' lives is compromised. Although we lack reliable information on the extent of the problem, elder abuse occurs and is likely to become a more serious problem as Mexico ages (Giraldo-Rodríguez, Rosas-Carrasco and Mino-León 2015; Giraldo Rodríguez and Agudelo Botero 2020).

Given the limited availability of non-family sources of old-age support, family care arrangements dominate research on the material welfare of older Mexicans and Mexican-origin individuals in the U.S. (Angel and

Angel 2009; Garay Villegas, Montes de Oca Zavala and Guillén 2014; Montes de Oca et al. 2014). While this literature provides extensive descriptions of the family status of older persons, little research has examined the larger institutional contexts that structure the economic and social situations of older persons and the possibilities they have for social and political engagement. Again, this lack of focus on extra-familial contacts largely reflects the fact that traditionally few extra-familial sources of interaction and participation, other than perhaps the Church, were available. Today, as new possibilities emerge, new theoretical paradigms such as those focused on *active aging* and *active citizenship* that we discussed in Chapter four, emphasize the importance of social interaction and engagement with the larger community (Martínez-Maldonado, Correa-Muñoz and Mendoza-Núñez 2007; Gutiérrez Cuéllar 2019; Kenny et al. 2017; Mendoza-Ruvalcaba and Fernández-Ballesteros 2016; WHO 2002).

The practical objective of initiatives motivated by such paradigms, which are promoted aggressively by CSOs, is to create environments that encourage and empower people at different life course stages to defend and exercise their human and social rights at the individual and collective levels. Theoretically and practically, then, social participation represents a core aspect of active aging. One of the major objectives of international and local CSOs is to prevent isolation by encouraging active social engagement by older individuals. Broadly construed, active aging involves not only interactions among individuals, but active engagement with institutions that are vital to fostering and sustaining individual and collective well-being. Communication, dialogue, and face-to-face interactions are necessary preconditions for such effective social participation (Madariaga 2005).

The Future of Long-Term Care in Mexico

The formal long-term care situation in Mexico lags, then, far behind what is needed now, and certainly far behind what will be needed in the relatively near future. It remains unclear whether and how the long-term care industry will develop in Mexico. Even with an abundance of low-cost labor, the cost of institutional long-term care is likely to remain prohibitively high for most older Mexicans and their families. Few have the resources to purchase nursing home care, and unlike the United States in which older individuals can qualify for Medicaid when their personal resources are depleted, Mexico has no state-sponsored long-term care financing program.

In the future, greatly extended life spans with longer periods of disability may increase nursing home use, but given capital and fiscal barriers dramatic increases in publicly-funded long-term institutional care seems unlikely. Of course, publicly-funded formal institutions are not the only option. Many unlicensed and unregulated private nursing homes operate in Mexico. Unfortunately, it is basically impossible to find out anything about the nature and quality of care this sector provides. For the foreseeable future, then, it seems clear that for older Mexicans the family is likely to remain the major source of long-term care, even as its capacity to provide all of the care aging parents need becomes increasingly strained.

Ironically, future growth of the long-term care industry in Mexico may result more from demand by North Americans rather than Mexicans. A brief search on the web reveals numerous sites aimed at U.S. and Canadian residents that extol the benefits of assisted living in Mexico. On a rather modest retirement income a North American retiree can enjoy a much higher quality of life in Mexico or other Latin American and Caribbean countries than would be possible in a facility at home. In the U.S. many individuals find that when they need nursing home care, their resources are quickly depleted. Given the low labor costs in Mexico, and the excellent medical care available in major cities, retirement communities that cater to North Americans might define the future, especially if it were possible for expatriates to use Medicare in Mexico. Although this is an intriguing possibility, it is a bit off our point.

Our review of long-term care options in Mexico clearly illustrates the vacuum of care that CSOs are beginning to address. As we have mentioned before, there are simply few alternatives to civil society initiatives and involvement. Civil society organizations represent a broad range of interests, from those of international organizations to those of local self-help initiatives organized by citizens themselves. In this and earlier chapters we have provided a general overview of the relationship among civil society organizations, government agencies, and other organizations dealing with elder advocacy and eldercare. In the next three chapters we examine the role of organizations with different missions and objectives, from those focused on improving the quality of life of older individuals, to those whose mission involves insuring social rights to those that are more political and focused on more general political, as well as social, changes.

References

Advocates for International Development. 2017. "EU Registration Options for NGOs – Preparing UK-based NGOs for Brexit: A Guide to Establishing NOGs in Europe." Retrieved 7/20/2019 from https://nuso.org/media/articles/downloads/3847_1.pdf.

Alfama, E., R. Canal, and M. Cruells. 2013. "Las políticas de envejecimiento activo en el Estado español (2002–2012): ¿promoviendo la ciudadanía y la participación de las personas mayores?" Universitat Autònoma de Barcelona, Spain. Retrieved 5/10/2021 from https://ddd.uab.cat/record/190632.

Angel, Ronald J., and Jacqueline L. Angel. 2009. *Hispanic Families at Risk: The New Economy, Work, and the Welfare State.* New York, NY: Springer.

Calderon, Fernando Herrera, and Adela Cedillo. 2012. *Challenging Authoritarianism in Mexico: Revolutionary Struggles and the Dirty War, 1964–1982.* New York, NY: Routledge.

CNBC. 2015. "Russia Bans George Soros Charity as 'Security Threat'." Retrieved 7/20/2019 from https://www.cnbc.com/2015/11/30/russia-bans-george-soros-charity-as-security-threat.html.

Council on Foundations. 2018. "Mexico." Retrieved 7/26/2019 from https://www.cof.org/country-notes/nonprofit-law-mexico.

Díaz Aldret, Ana, Elena Titova, and David Arellano Gault. 2020. "Legitimidad y transparencia de las organizaciones de lasociedad civil en México: ¿Actores neutrales o interesados?" *Revista mexicana de ciencias políticas y sociales* 65 (239):25–60.

DIF Nacional. 2010. "Aultos Mayores." Mexico City: Directorio Nacional de Instituciones de Asistencia Social – DNIAS. Retrieved 2/7/2020 from http://dnias.dif.gob.mx/informacion-para-todos/adultos-mayores/.

Escobar, Arturo, and Sonia E. Alvarez (Eds.). 1992. *The Making of Social Movements in Latin America.* Boulder, CO: Westview Press.

Foweraker, Joe, and Ann L. Craig (Eds.). 1990. *Popular Movements and Political Change in Mexico.* Boulder, CO: Lynne Rienner Publishers.

Garay Villegas, Sagrario, Verónica Montes-de-Oca Zavala, and Jennifer C. Guillén. 2014. "Social Support and Social Networks among the Elderly in Mexico." *Journal of Population Ageing* 7 (2):143–159.

Giraldo Rodríguez, Liliana, and Marcela Agudelo Botero. 2020. "Elder Abuse in Mexico." Pp. 73–88 in *International Handbook of Elder Abuse and Mistreatment*, edited by Mala Kapur Shankardass. Singapore: Springer Singapore.

Giraldo-Rodríguez, Liliana, Oscar Rosas-Carrasco, and Dolores Mino-León. 2015. "Abuse in Mexican Older Adults with Long-Term Disability: National Prevalence and Associated Factors." *Journal of the American Geriatrics Society* 63 (8):1594–1600.

Gutiérrez Cuéllar, Paola Carmina. 2019. "¿Qué envejecimiento? El problema público de la vejez en la Ciudad de México." *Iztapalapa. Revista de Ciencias Sociales y Humanidades* 87 (40):143–174.

Gutiérrez Robledo, Luis Miguel, Mariana López Ortega, and Victoria Eugenia Arango Lopera. 2012. "The State of Elder Care in Mexico." *Current Geriatrics Reports* 1 (4):183–189.

Gutiérrez-Robledo, L.M., G. Reyes-Ortega, F. Rocabado-Quevedo, and J. López-Franchini. 1996. "Evaluation of Long Term Care Institutions for the Aged in the Federal District. A Critical Viewpoint." *Salud publica de Mexico* 38 (6):487–500.

Hartlyn, Jonathan, and Samuel A. Morley (Eds.). 1986. *Latin American Political Economy: Financial Crisis and Political Change.* Boulder, CO: Westview Press.

Huber, Evelyne, and John D. Stephens. 2012. *Democracy and the Left: Social Policy and Inequality in Latin America.* Chicago, IL: University of Chicago Press.

Huerta, María, Ireri Ablanedo, and Mariana Vázquez del Mercado. ND. "The Legal Environment for Civil Society Organizations in Mexico. Analysis and Recommendations." Washington, DC: United States Agency for International Development. Retrieved 10/22/2020 from https://socialimpact.com/wp-content/uploads/2017/01/USAID-Civil-Society-Activity_The-Legal-Environment-for-CSOs-in-Mexico.pdf.

INAPAM. 2016a. "Albergues y Residencias de día INAPAM ." Retrieved 2/7/ 2020 from https://www.gob.mx/inapam/acciones-y-programas/albergues-y-r esidencias-diurnas-inapam.

INAPAM. 2016b. "Inapam, 37 años al servicio de los adultos mayores de México." Retrieved 2/7/2020 from https://www.gob.mx/inapam/articulos/inapam-37-a nos-al-servicio-de-los-adultos-mayores-de-mexico?idiom=es.

ISSSTE. 2020. "Directorio de Casas de Día." Retrieved 2/7/2020 from https:// www.gob.mx/issste/es/articulos/directorio-de-casas-de-dia?idiom=es.

Johnston, Hank, and Paul Almeida (Eds.). 2006. *Latin American Social Movements: Globalization, Democratization, and Transnational Networks.* New York, NY: Rowman & Littlefield.

Kenny, Sue, Marilyn Taylor, Jenny Onyx, and Marjorie Mayo. 2017. *Challenging the Third Sector: Global Prospects for Active Citizenship.* Chicago, IL: Policy Press c/o The University of Chicago Press.

Madariaga, Alberto Viveros. 2005. "Lecciones sobre Envejecimiento y Participación Social." La Federación Iberoamericana de Asociaciones de Personas Adultas Mayores (FIAPAM). Retrieved 12/7/2017 from http://fiapam.org/wp-content/up loads/2013/11/Lecciones.pdf.

Magaña Hernández, DianaMargarita, and Luis Figueroa Díaz. 2018. "Análisis de las Organizaciones No Gubernamentales y Organizaciones de la Sociedad Civil en México." *Administración y Organizaciones* 16 (31):131–149.

Martínez, Alejandra Leal. 2015. "El despertar de la sociedad civil: sismo del 85 y neoliberalismo: Los 30 años del sismo del 85 también marcan el aniversario de la aparición de un nuevo concepto en la esfera pública mexicana: la 'sociedad civil'." Mexico City: Horizontal. Retrieved 6/22/2020 from https://horizontal. mx/el-despertar-de-la-sociedad-civil-sismo-del-85-y-neoliberalismo/.

Martínez-Maldonado, María, Elsa Correa-Muñoz, and Víctor Manuel Mendoza-Núñez. 2007. "Program of Active Aging in a Rural Mexican Community: A Qualitative Approach." *BMC Public Health* 7 (1):276.

Mendoza García, Jorge. 2011. "La tortura en el marco de la guerra sucia en México: un ejercicio de memoria colectiva." *POLIS* 7 (2):139–179.

Mendoza-Ruvalcaba, Neyda Ma, and Rocío Fernández-Ballesteros. 2016. "Effectiveness of the Vital Aging Program to Promote Active Aging in Mexican Older Adults." *Clinical Interventions in Aging* 11:1631–1644.

Minetti, Mariana Mas. 2017. "A Victory for the Truth about Mexico's 'Dirty War'." Washington, DC: Open Society Justice Initiative. Retrieved 6/16/2020 from https:// www.justiceinitiative.org/voices/victory-truth-about-mexico-s-dirty-war.

Monsiváis, Carlos. 1987. *Entrada libre. Crónicas de la sociedad que se organiza.* Mexico City: Ediciones Era, S.A. de C.V.

Montes-de-Oca, Verónica. 2000. "Experiencia institucional y situacíon social de los ancianos en la ciudad de México." Pp. 419–456 in *Las políticas sociales en México al fin del milenio. Descentralizaíon, diseñño y gestión,* edited by Rolando Cordera and Alicia Ziccardi. Mexico City: Coordinación de Humanidades/Facultad de Economia/Miguel Angel Porrúa.

Montes-de-Oca, V., S. Garay, B. Rico, and S.J. García. 2014. "Living Arrangements and Aging in Mexico: Changes in Households, Poverty and Regions, 1992–2009." *International Journal of Social Sciences Studies* 2 (4):61–74.

Motta, Sara C. 2013. "Introduction: Reinventing the Lefts in Latin America: Critical Perspectives from Below." *Latin American Perspectives* 40 (4):5–18.

OECD. 2011. "Mexico: Long-Term Care." Retrieved 9/23/2019 from https://www.oecd.org/mexico/47877877.pdf.

Organization for Security and Co-operation in Europe. 2004. "Fundamental Principles on the Status of Non-governmental Organisations in Europe." Retrieved 7/20/2019 from https://www.osce.org/odihr/37858.

Sitrin, Mariana (Ed.). 2006. *Horizontalism: Voices of Popular Power in Argentina.* Oakland, CA: AK Press.

Stahler-Sholk, Richard, Harry E. Vanden, and Marc Becker (Eds.). 2014. *Rethinking Latin American Social Movements: Radical Action from Below.* New York, NY: Rowman & Littlefield.

Stahler-Sholk, Richard, Harry E. Vanden, and Glen David Kuecker (Eds.). 2008. *Latin American Social Movements in the Twenty-first Century: Resistance, Power, and Democracy.* New York, NY: Rowman & Littlefield.

U.S. Department of State. 2017. "Non-Governmental Organizations (NGOs) in the United States." Retrieved 7/20/2019 from https://www.state.gov/non-governmental-organizations-ngos-in-the-united-states/.

Wanderley, F. 2009. "Prácticas estatales y el ejercicio de la ciudadanía: encuentros de la población con la burocracia en Bolivia." *Iconos* 34:67–79.

Webber, Jeffrey R., and Barry Carr (Eds.). 2012. *The New Latin American Left: Cracks in the Empire.* Lanham, MD: Rowman & Littlefield.

WHO. 2002. "Active Ageing. A Policy Framework." Retrieved 12/5/2017 from http://apps.who.int/iris/bitstream/10665/67215/1/WHO_NMH_NPH_02.8.pdf.

Chapter 6

Labor Unions and the Struggle for Political Power

At both the international and national levels the labor movement has been a driving force in the complex evolution of the welfare state. Labor's struggle for better working conditions, higher wages, health care, and dignity have motivated generations of workers and others to fight for their collective and individual rights. These efforts are part of a growing social movement, the objective of which is to guarantee the social rights of workers and citizens more generally (Briggs 1961). Although the labor movement in Mexico has been hampered by a highly centralized and clientelistic State, it has been one of the fundamental venues in which workers collectively sought to further their collective interests. Strikes and other labor actions have forced entrepreneurs, government officials, and even presidents to attend to workers' demands, often with violent repression. The industrial labor movement in Mexico has been closely associated with other social movements by doctors, teachers, agricultural workers, miners, transportation workers, and other activists who are engaged in an ongoing struggle for human and social rights. One important union was the Retirees and Pensioners of Sindicato Mexicano de Electricistas (JPSME), the Mexican electrical workers union. It was the oldest democratic union in the country and was nearly destroyed by the Calderon administration in 2009 for its opposition to privatization. The workers did not all disband and many continued their struggle and are making a comeback today. Javier Leyba, a retired member of the SME who lives in Mexico City, told us of what the union meant to him.

LEYBA: My name is Javier Leyba and I am 58 years old. I am married and have one child. I have been retired for six years. I worked for twenty-nine years. I am from the Federal District ... I studied until high school. Right now, in the union I was elected as a representative for the 2016–2018 period. I am a representative of retirees of the Mexican union of electricians ...

INTERVIEWER: What are the objectives of your organization?

LEYBA: First, is to safeguard the rights that we have already acquired as retirees ... because as you know neoliberal policies at the international

DOI: 10.4324/9781003205609-6

level are constantly trying to undermine those rights that we have, so the main thing is to protect our rights, and also attend the needs of retirees of the Mexican electricians union, their health, socially, morally, and psychologically. When we discover that a partner has a problem we try to help.

INTERVIEWER: What is the gender and age profile of the union?

LEYBA: Well, most of them are men, although many retired women also participate. They are between 55 to 80 years old ... There are professionals ... but I believe that there is a predominance of middle school, high school level or so.

INTERVIEWER: What activities do they generally engage in?

LEYBA: Well, right now we have a forum consisting of the national confederation of retirees of the Federal District, where there are speakers who explain how governments try to modify the laws. They address such questions as, what is their plan? In what ways do they want to change them? We try to keep the retirees well informed. Currently we also have marches and rallies, sometimes sit-ins in the different government agencies, but yes, we engage in all of the political activity possible. The union also sponsors recreational and sports centers where there are soccer tournaments. They also have workshops where retirees can go to paint if they want ... These are places for retirees, but sometimes retirees bring a guest or family member ...

INTERVIEWER: In general, what are the retired pensioners most concerned with?

LEYBA: The political question because in reality it is the one that always affects us directly. If you see that there is a change in policy, we have to keep up with the changes, including the claims that the government makes, because as you know, unfortunately the policies are dictated by the World Bank, the International Monetary Fund, and the rest, the great powers that come to invest their money here.

INTERVIEWER: What motivates individuals to participate in political, as well as physical and recreational activities?

LEYBA: The union has been in existence for more than 100 years, and it has been a constant struggle not only for those of us who are currently active, but also those who came before. So, we have inherited the fight that we must carry on because we know that the enemy, for generations of humanity, has been stalking us. I believe that this is what drives us to remain vigilant in the fight, for the inheritance that our ancestors left us ... It is the continuation of the struggle.

The Ongoing Struggle

Javier Leyba may not fit our usual notion of a retiree. A few individuals who work in strategic sectors of the formal economy in Mexico are able to retire early, but they are relatively rare, which makes Javier's situation somewhat unusual. He is 58 and has been retired for six years. Which means he retired at 52 and is still a relatively young man. Javier represents the retirees of the Sindicato Mexicano de Electricistas (JPSME) (the Mexican electrical workers union), historically a highly political and activist union with leftist leanings. Given the dangerous nature of the work many electrical union members retire early and remain highly protective of the rights they have earned. As the interview with him reveals, Javier is very much involved with issues related to retirement, but from a highly politicized perspective, one that has been structured by his union experience. Unlike other unions, the SME was not coopted and was never an instrument of the government or power industry. The union's 44,000 members were fired in 2009 during the neoliberal period during which the government attempted to privatize the electrical power sector, and only recently has the union experienced some recovery (Bacon 2019; Comas 2018).

Retired electrical workers remain closely tied to the union and do not belong to a completely separate group or retiree organization. Their experience in union struggles for worker rights and benefits, and their continuing ties to the union places them in a very different position relative to the State compared to the groups we will describe in the next chapter whose members have less political and activist experience. The relatively young age of many retired electrical workers and the group's history of union activism mean that these retirees have the experience and capacity to engage in collective efforts, and they have extensive experience in fighting for benefits. Like other unions, the Mexican electrical workers union has had a complex relationship with the PRI, the party that governed unopposed for seventy years.

In previous chapters we dealt with issues related to the role of civil society in general, and in Mexico more specifically. Although social movements and union actions have been common since the 19th Century, it was not until the 1960s that large-scale movements by students, doctors, workers, and the middle class began to confront the corporatism, clientelism, and corruption of the old regime. One major example of the growing demands by the middle classes was the widespread doctors' strike of 1964 and 1965 (Casas-Patiño, Reséndiz-Rivera, and Casas 2009). The movement, which was led by doctors, but included other health professionals, was a reaction against the ruling party's attempts to control all employee organizations, and the medical workers' demands for higher wages and better working conditions. Several work stoppages and hospital shutdowns resulted in serious State repression (Casas-Patiño, Reséndiz-Rivera, and Casas 2009). Another example was the student movement of 1968, one of the movements with which we began Chapter one, which was ended by brutal State repression resulting in the death of hundreds of students in the Tlatelolco Square in Mexico City.

In this and the next two chapters we investigate the roles of specific civil society organizations that deal with issues related to the situation of older persons and describe how they frame issues of power, rights, and active aging from different perspectives. We investigate how issues related to aging and the well-being and welfare of older people are framed for the purpose of mobilization of older people themselves, and for the purpose of attempting to change public perceptions of the roles and rights of older people in the community. We begin with those organizations whose origins and identities lie close to the labor movement, which as in the case of electrical workers, was at times quite radical. As we describe, labor unions in Mexico have often been closely allied to the ruling party, even to the point that their officers have been granted official governmental posts. This cooptation and a lack of internal union democracy has seriously limited the labor movement's success in furthering the interests of workers.

In addition, the organized labor movement has been limited by the fact that the majority of Mexican workers are employed in the informal sector in which the possibility of unionization is basically nil. Yet aside from various peasant and agrarian actions, unions and labor organizations were the first identifiable entities to address the plight of the Mexican laboring classes. The focus of these organizations and the labor movement in general was primarily on improving wages and working conditions, but there was also early concern with other benefits, including pensions. Later, this focus on the conditions of work expanded as other groups, including women, indigenous populations, LGBTQ activists, the elderly, and others extended the discourse to focus on human rights more generally, and on specific group rights in particular.

The gender division among retiree organizations is striking and reflects the economic activity in which men and women engaged during the first half of the 20th Century (González-Guerra and Gutiérrez Castro 2010). Women did not enter into the industrial labor force until the second half of the 20th Century. Their presence in education, though, was quite common at least at the primary levels. Although today women are found in every part of the Mexican economy, those who today are old were socialized in very different historical periods and were less involved in union struggles. Even for those who worked, traditional gender roles prevailed and for them retirement meant returning home to the roles of mother, grandmother, and wife, roles grounded in "Mexican female values" (Gamboa-Suárez and Dario Olivo-Huerta 2018).

As a result of many historical forces then, various groups of retirees and pensioners have unique identities and sources of cultural, social, and political capital that they can potentially leverage to influence public policy to protect their rights. Given the importance of pensions and health care to retirees, protecting these benefits occupies a major place on the agendas of groups of retired union members. Although issues related to quality of life are important, basic social and political rights remain vital in guaranteeing an optimal quality of life. Given the centrality of labor and working-class interests in determining the vitality of civil society and in defining welfare policy generally, we begin with groups with strong ties to the labor movement and those whose memberships possess high levels of social and cultural capital. First, though, we present a story of a unique entrepreneur who without being forced, concerned himself with the welfare of his workers.

The Early 20th Century: An Exceptional and Progressive Entrepreneur

Although our focus in this chapter is on the Mexican labor movement and the experiences of labor activists in defining the rights of retired workers, we begin with the story of a highly respected and progressive Mexican entrepreneur, Eugenio Garza Sada, who provided extensive benefits to his workers, including retirement plans, well before they were extended to other workers in Mexico or almost anywhere else. In many ways this enlightened entrepreneur created an early labor utopia, which like most utopias, was difficult to replicate. The benefits Garza Sada provided to his workers predated the benefits and job protections that are still incompletely guaranteed by the state. We relate this story since it shows what might be possible under enlightened management. It is an idealized picture to be sure, but it illustrates that what laborers struggle for on a daily basis can in fact be achieved given the right circumstances. Since those circumstances rarely exist, class struggle is the only option.

The story begins at the end of the 19th Century, during the Porfirian period, a time not favorable to labor interests. The location was the Cuauhtémoc Brewery that was founded in Monterrey, Nuevo León by businessman Isaac Garza, Eugenio's father. In addition to the brewery, Isaac Garza had interests in many other production enterprises (Haber 1989). During the Mexican Revolution, which began in 1910 and lasted a decade, the brewery closed and the Garza family migrated to the United States (Cavazos 2016). In the 1920s two of the sons, including Eugenio Garza Sada, (Sada was his mother's family name) returned to Monterrey to take over management of the brewery. Despite the difficult economic situation caused by the Great War, Eugenio Garza Sada succeeded in restarting production and building a thriving business (Recio 2007). The company would become an example of successful industrialization and it fostered other companies that produced inputs to the beer making and distribution processes. Garza Sada's objective was to make the Mexican beer industry self-sustaining using products manufactured in the country, rather than being imported from the United States.

Garza Sada sponsored various progressive practices to increase wages and improve working conditions, as well as to foster social and educational development projects at a time when there was little union presence. His legacy in the history of Mexican entrepreneurship is based on his example as a leader who focused on generating jobs and assuring the social security of his workers and their families (Recio 2015). This included medical care at the company's clinic and hospital, a pension plan that would ensure workers' economic security in old age, and education for their children. This was carried out in collaboration with the Polytechnic Institute of Nuevo León that sought to educate the peasants to make them workers in the industry. Eugenio Garza Sada founded the Instituto Tecnológico y de Estudios Superiores (ITESM) (Institute of Technology and Advanced Studies) in Monterrey in 1943. Later, a benevolent society he sponsored funded the construction of housing for brewery workers, and provided them medical care and economic security in retirement.

Garza Sada's private social security and social welfare initiatives can be seen as a model for Mexico's current social security institutions (IMSS and ISSSTE). In the 21st Century, the retirement system plan that Garza Sada developed continues to protect active and retired workers, despite the fact that the Cervecería Cuauhtémoc has been sold to a transnational company. Eugenio Garza Sada took steps to protect workers and retirees in case the company was sold. This episode in Mexico's economic history reveals the best of an entrepreneurial class committed to workers and the well-being of their families. To this day Garza Sada is venerated and respected in Monterrey, which has become a dynamic economic center. In the context of our discussion it is particularly salient since Garza Sada was committed to the security of retired workers. He fostered what today we would term "active aging." Unfortunately, Garza Sada's creation was an ideal rather than a model. His story is an exception to the practice of placing productivity and profit above workers' interests and rights, which informed state labor policy and the behavior of the captains of industry. Garza Sada's model sadly did not become a template for the entire country. In the end he was a victim of the ongoing class struggle. In the official version, he was killed in 1973 in an attempted kidnapping by members of a Communist faction who called themselves the September 23 league, although not everyone agrees with this account. Whoever was responsible for Garza Sada's death, though, as we explain below the weakness of the Mexican labor movement has meant that workers and their families must continue to fight for their rights against rather daunting odds.

Unions and the Struggle for Basic Rights

In Mexico, the figure of the retiree or pensioner is historically quite recent. During most of the country's history, the economy remained predominantly agricultural, and as in most pre-industrial societies, retirement had no meaning. One worked and contributed to the family's subsistence economy until one died or could no longer function. Industrialization lay in the future, as did the possibility of retirement. The sequence of industrialization, unionization, and retirement requires that we briefly summarize the role of unionization in bringing about and defining retirement for workers in the formal sector. For those in the informal sector the story of course is very different. For individuals who spend many years in informal employment retirement, and certainly a comfortable retirement, remains a pipe dream. Nonetheless, the struggle for labor rights was important in and of itself, but in the context of our discussion it is particularly important since it also provided workers valuable experience in the struggle for their rights, experiences that would later fuel social movements focused on human and social rights more generally.

The story begins then with the industrialization that took place in the late 19th and early 20th Centuries (Gutiérrez Castro 2011). Although important organized job actions occurred in mining and textiles during the 19th Century, it was not until the 20th Century that the expansion of transportation, electrical generation and distribution, the petroleum industry, and more gave rise to the Mexican labor movement. During the 19th and early 20th Centuries workers' rights to organize and to demand better working conditions and higher wages were not guaranteed. Neither the Mexican constitution of 1824 nor that of 1857 recognized the rights of workers to form associations or unions (Villegas Rojas 2016). Nonetheless, as Mexicans increasingly became industrial proletariat, they were forced by deplorable working conditions and low wages to struggle for their collective interests (Gutiérrez Castro 2011). During the early 20th Century a growing exasperation with those deplorable working conditions, low wages, and exploitation resulted in more frequent strikes by miners and other workers.

The constitution of 1917 formally recognized the right of workers to organize and make demands of their employers. It also affirmed their right to an eight-hour work day, a living wage, and more (Villegas Rojas 2016). These protections were largely a political ploy to appease labor and they had little practical impact. In 1931the Ley Federal de Trabajo (Federal Labor Law) was passed (Delarbre and Yáñez 1976). This law affirmed and codified the rights of workers to unionize, to form federations of unions, and more (Villegas Rojas 2016). Unfortunately, in practice the law became an instrument for the control of labor since it made the government the ultimate arbiter of all labor demands and disputes (Delarbre and Yáñez 1976). Several subsequent refinements and additions to labor laws provided a formal legal grounding for workers' rights, especially their rights to unionize and strike. Again though, these supposed legal guarantees did not place power in workers' hands and they continued to be at the mercy of the State and factory owners. Unions and the labor movement in fact became instruments for the State control of labor. As a consequence, and as we discuss below, unions remained weak and unable to greatly improve workers' wages and working conditions.

Although the first labor associations emerged after the Mexican Revolution, the real watershed of union activity can be traced to the 1930s and 1940s, when unions arose in new strategic sectors, including petroleum, electricity, and telecommunications (Delarbre and Yáñez 1976; Gutiérrez Castro 2011). As the country industrialized, education became more important and teachers, who still have strong unions, became an important force for the modernization of the country. A prominent educator, José Vasconcelos, who served as Rector of the National Autonomous University of Mexico, and as Head of the Secretariat of Public Education under President Álvaro Obregón in the 1920s, was a great promoter of education at the national level (Krauze 2011, ch 3). In addition to furthering their own interests, educators continue to promote a broad political and human rights agenda.

A Struggle Independent of Political Parties

As a consequence of these early labor rights movements, many workers had gained extensive experience in political activism independently of political parties. Not only were political parties largely oblivious to labor issues and the plight of workers, they are generally viewed as complicit in undermining the limited protections that workers had gained. Against massive odds, though, unions continued the struggle. Among the most proactive unions in this defense of labor rights was the Luz y Fuerza del Centro, LyFC (Light and Power of Central Mexico), a member of the large Sindicato Mexicano de Electricistas, mentioned above.

The union mentality among retired electrical workers emerges throughout our interviews and focus groups. Two quotes from focus group interviews with retirees of the electrical union illustrate the fact that for these retirees their past activities inform their current activist stance:

> I am retired from [a] power and light company that is no longer operating. I belong to the Mexican electrician's union ... we are still participating in the union; we are representatives and we are trying to keep up with the policies that are governing the country and those that concern retirees. Here we engage in different activities including sports and recreational and family events.
>
> (J. A., 66, JPSME)

> What the union has given me and also Power and Light, is a stable life fortunately without serious economic [hardship]. We cooperate with the union; they call us to advise the boys. That helps us to be

active, to participate and to interact with our fellow workers. We are like a family because we all know each other and talk as if we were a family, even though we were from different departments. We met at meetings, and we learned to interact with the young people too.

(R. S., 68, JPSME)

Retired members of the LyFC strongly identified with the union's century-long struggle for worker's rights. José, a retired union member, worked for a power company that was started in 1903 with foreign capital. The LyFC was founded in 1914. At that time, more radical union members saw themselves as part of the global struggle of the proletariat against the domination of capital. Don J. L. explains:

It was not a matter ... of reaching a level of harmony with capital, but rather the opposite, to combat it from the angle of demands, claims, and the needs of [a person] who recognizes that he is an exploited subject, that he is an oppressed subject; [and that] the union is going to give [the workers] the collective strength necessary to be able to confront capital.

(J. L., 58, JPSME)

This adversarial stance prevailed for many years. Given the strategic importance of the power sector of the economy, though, it was eventually nationalized. Don M. D., a retired electrical worker, stated, "we are going to celebrate 101 years as an established union for the defense of workers ... this union first started under a foreign company ... and we ended up working for a state-owned company" (M. D., 57, JPSME). Don M. D. mentioned that there is an identity, a root of "unionism in our blood ... it is an organization that gave us everything and we are very loyal to it."

The adversarial relationship between the government and the electrical workers' unions was exacerbated during the neoliberal period by State attempts to privatize the energy sector and eliminate unions (Comas 2018). In the words of a member of the SME, this union was the "main bastion of resistance" against the reform. The suppression of LyFC and the firing of its 44,000 members did not make the union disappear; rather it fueled an ongoing battle focused on stopping the privatization of the public electrical system. A key strategy of the SME in recent years has been to form alliances with other movements and organizations (Comas 2018). In addition to militant union activities directed toward the government, retirees and pensioners of the union sponsor an ongoing informational program that educates active and retired members concerning important policy issues that affect them.

Although the electrician's union does not frame its objectives in terms of active aging, the members are in fact engaging in it extensively with cultural, social, and health workshops and courses sponsored by the union. Antonio, another retired electrical worker, explained that the union sponsors recreational activities, and holds assemblies in which the workers inform themselves of national politics, and conferences to which informed speakers are invited to educate the members on timely issues (J. A., 66, JPSME, CDMX). Don R. S., another LyFC retiree, explained that the organization engages in ongoing political monitoring to keep abreast of the legislative changes that could affect union life and members' rights. As he noted, "among retirees and pensioners, we have political groups which are dedicated to studying the issues related to the laws ... in order to give an opinion; there are about 15 or 20 groups" (R. S., 68, JPSME).

Until recently the union movement was largely male since women were not employed as industrial workers (Juárez and Quilodrán 1990; Quilodrán de Aguirre and Juárez Carcaño 2009). The conventional wisdom was that women naturally assumed domestic roles and should not work outside the home. This bias was increased by a bias towards workers of productive age. This devaluation of maturity is reflected in the absence of themes related to aging or old age in union discourse. Traditionally, old age was devalued in terms of productive labor by a public portrayal of the body as an engine of youthful masculine productivity (González Cordero 2020). The elderly might have been venerated as elders, but they were not viewed as productive. This bias, in combination with the gender bias, led to the neglect of women's needs as they entered the labor force and as they aged. Older women's unique needs have often been at odds with the objectives of a labor union movement focused predominantly on youthful masculinity (González Nicolás 2012).

As a consequence of this absence of women in the industrial labor force, most currently retired industrial workers are men, whose meeting points and venues for community participation are the groups of retirees and pensioners. Many of these men retained their gender role identity as breadwinners for their families, and as fighters for collective economic benefits. These identities motivate the support networks and self-help groups in which they meet. One sector in which women have been active in dealing with issues of retirement security and the rights of older workers is in basic and higher education. Organizations of retired teachers are powerful political forces in Mexico, but as we explain below, they too have had a complicated relationship with the government.

Sources of Union Weakness

The Mexican labor movement has never been as powerful or influential as the labor movements of European countries, largely because it has always faced crippling opposition from employers and the State (Delarbre and Yáñez 1976; Lenti 2017; Teichman 2009). In addition to lacking independence from the State and powerful employers, Mexican unions historically lacked internal democracy. They became a central political force in the support of the official party, the PRI, and they remained relatively ineffective in improving the wages and working conditions of their members, primarily because of official State policies aimed at increasing productivity and profits by keeping wages low (Bensusán 2004; Caulfield 2004; Greer, Stevens, and Stephens 2007). Mexican society has historically been highly corporatist with a single dominant party and a powerful presidency. Even after the defeat of the PRI in 2000, unions have had difficulty in furthering their objectives (Davis and Coleman 1989; Delarbre and Yáñez 1976; Hermanson and De la Garza Toledo 2005; La Botz 1988; Mayer 2006; Gutiérrez Rufrancos 2016). Nonetheless, the experience that workers gained in even unsuccessful struggles for rights have had longer term effects. They served as venues in which workers in the formal sector engaged in a militant discourse focused on collective rights.

Most unions in Mexico have historically been "official" or company unions, which means that they are sponsored and controlled by employers, with the backing of official state policy (Delarbre and Yáñez 1976; Greer, Stevens, and Stephens 2007). This continues to be the case in *maquiladora* plants, factories owned and operated by foreign corporations that are attracted by the low wage environment in Mexico (Caulfield 2004). In order to attract foreign investment, the Mexican government has been highly motivated to keep wages low. To accomplish this, labor militancy and wage demands have had to be suppressed. That has been accomplished by labor legislation that favors closed shops in which the official union is the only one allowed. Historically, the officers of these official unions have received government posts and other benefits in exchange for supporting official labor policies. Not surprisingly, rank and file union members are not involved. In many cases, workers are unaware that they are even members of the union to which they pay dues. They do not participate in the choice of union leaders, nor do they have any say in union policies.

The Confederation of Mexican Workers

Despite the relative weakness of the Mexican labor movement, major conflicts between management and workers have occurred in many sectors, including petroleum, steel, metalwork, electrical power, automobile manufacturing, mining, insurance, banking, and more (Caulfield 2004; Greer, Stevens, and Stephens 2007; Hermanson and De la Garza Toledo 2005). Many social, economic, and political forces have undermined the ability of Mexican laborers to effectively demand their rights. One major barrier to extensive unionization of the labor force in general is that fact that the majority of Mexicans labor in the informal sector in which they have no contracts or any protection from exploitation. Informal workers have no access to private health insurance, pensions, worker's compensation, or any of the other benefits. Informal workers have no ability to unionize, largely because their employers, who are often themselves, have no resources with which to provide higher pay or benefits.

The *Confederación de Trabajadores de México*, CTM (Confederation of Mexican Workers) is the largest coalition of labor unions in Mexico (Greer, Stevens, and Stephens 2007). The CMT, and other labor confederations that came before it, were largely extensions of the Institutional Revolutionary Party (PRI) (Caulfield 2004; Greer, Stevens, and Stephens 2007). As the result of changes within the PRI, and Mexican society at large, CTM's influence has declined and more independent unions have made some gains, although those remain fairly marginal (Bensusán 2004). Despite recent changes in labor law that increase collective bargaining rights, these have not resulted in significant advances in labor's relative power (Anner 2008). Indeed, rates of unionization have been declining, largely as the result of neoliberal pro-employer labor market policies and globalized economic competition (Alzaga 2018; Greer, Stevens, and Stephens 2007; Hermanson and De la Garza Toledo 2005).

In recent years non-governmental organizations and social movements, including international organizations and unions, have affiliated with and encouraged independent Mexican labor unions to demand better wages and benefits and to become more democratic, changes that represent a major break with the past. Bensusán (2004) offers a useful three-category classification of Mexican unions based on their relationship to the State, their focus on the interests of their memberships, and their levels of internal democracy. The first, "state-corporatist" unions, includes the official unions we described above that are dependent on and cooperate closely with the State to maintain labor peace, to keep wages low, and to increase productivity. As we mentioned, Mexican labor law gives these unions exclusive rights to represent the worker in a plant, excluding independent unions. These unions typically lack internal democracy and have an authoritarian hierarchical structure. Examples of these unions include the CMT, federations representing public sector employees, and national industrial unions, including the Mexican Mining and Metalworker's Union, the Mexican Petroleum Workers Union, and the General Union of Mexican Electrical Workers.

The second category consists of "social trade unions," many of which were previously state-corporatist, but which since the 1980s have begun to distance themselves from the official labor movement. They depend on a broader range of support and resources and have strengthened their bargaining power with employers. They have higher levels of internal democracy, and typically have elected leaders. Unions such as the Mexican Telephone Workers' Union, the Mexican Electricians' Union, and others are of this sort. The third category consists of "movement" trade unions. These unions are characterized by strong opposition to neoliberal economic policies and their open confrontations with the State. They are more democratic than more state-oriented unions and resort to the full range of labor actions, such as strikes, work stoppages, and mobilizations to attempt to improve the wages and working conditions of their members. New organizations in the service sector, unions of university employees, and dissident elements of the National Education Worker Union are of this type. Of particular relevance to our discussion is the fact that movement trade unions also have links to broader social movements and non-governmental organizations, as well as international labor organizations and U.S. and Canadian unions (Bensusán 2004; Caulfield 2004).

The history of the Mexican labor movement and the influence that various political forces have had on it are fascinating and informative, but that history is not a core theme in our presentation. We mention it briefly because the union movement, along with a long history of social movements in Mexico, provided opportunities for activism and political engagement for many of the members of the organizations that today focus on issues related to the rights of marginalized populations, including older persons. Although the union movement in Mexico has not been successful in countering the negative effects of neoliberalism or in greatly enhancing the situation of ordinary workers, it has served as an important training ground for those who are currently demanding their human and social rights.

Unfortunately, developments have undermined the potential for increased union influence in the economy. During the 1980s Mexico's default on its foreign debt and the ensuing severe economic crises along with other social changes resulted in a deterioration of the social image and already limited power of unions (Bortz and Mendiola 1991). Union membership dropped and both government and employers have continued their attempts to undermine labor rights (Fairris and Levine 2004; Zepeda Martínez 2009). Today even the limited gains of the labor movement are threatened by an economic model that focuses on the generation of wealth at the cost of the deterioration of the economic situation of workers in general. The globalized neoliberal economic model that has prevailed since the 1970s, combined with the declining political strength of unions, has greatly undermined the economic rights of workers. Increasingly, the inadequate wages of employed male family members require that females make up for the loss of purchasing power by entering the labor market. In a nation in which the family has traditionally been the sole source of support for elderly parents, this new economic reality has profound implications and brings us back to our basic motivating question. If the family cannot provide the material or instrumental care that older parents need, and the State lacks adequate revenues or policies to deal with the defamilisation of care, what alternatives are there? Again, we ask about the potential of civil society organizations to address at least certain aspects of the problem.

Other Formal Sector Retiree Organizations

While the frames and discourse of retired industrial union members are structured by their struggle for labor and union rights, other retiree organizations frame their objectives in more varied ways. Those whose members have been social activists, employees of federal or State governments, and those whose members have high levels of education or who worked in professions with a history of activism, such as school teachers and university professors, frame their objectives in ways that differ somewhat from those of industrial workers or from those of organizations that we describe in the next chapter whose memberships have little labor market experience. The organizations we deal with in this section are clearly concerned with economic and social rights, but their memberships and approaches, as well as their histories, lead them to focus on other issues as well.

Numerous social movements have actively attempted to improve the lot of marginalized groups in Mexico (Foweraker and Craig 1990; Johnston and Almeida 2006; Stahler-Sholk 2014; Stahler-Sholk, Vanden, and Becker 2014; Stahler-Sholk, Vanden, and Kuecker 2008). These have been central to the emergence of the new human and social rights agenda, which along with the rights of ethnic and racial minorities, abused and neglected children, women at risk of violence, the poor, and others have altered the discourse on older citizens to focus on their human, political, economic, and social rights (Montes de Oca 2000; Montes de Oca et al. 2018; Montes de Oca Zavala 2013; Montes de Oca Zavala 2014; Montes de Oca Zavala and Gutiérrez Cuellar 2018).

Activist Aging

These groups draw upon their members' high levels of education, their experience in government, and their ongoing social activism to further their agendas. We focus on three groups, (1) Jubilados y Pensiondos del Instituto de Seguridad y Servicios Sociales de los Trabajadores del Estado (PISSSTE) (Retirees and Pensioners of the Institute of Security and Social Services of State Workers); (2) Jubilados y pensionados de la Coordinadora Nacional de los Trabajadores de la Educación (JPCNTE) (Retirees and Pensioners of the National Coordinating Committee of Education Workers), and (3) Pioneros Creativos en Libertad (PICRELI) (Creative Pioneers in Freedom) which consists of retirees and pensioners of the Autonomous University of Mexico (UNAM). These retiree organizations are characterized by strong political organization based on their members' high levels of education and their experience in the governmental and public sectors. Although groups of retired industrial workers are predominantly male, these organizations increasingly include women, reflecting the gradual increase in female labor force participation since the 1980s. They also include individuals who retired early and who are highly active.

A retiree of the State Workers Union (PISSSTE) explained his role and the objectives of the retiree's organization of state workers as follows:

> It has been four years since we began this organization of retired persons in order to make two demands of the government t... I worked in the Ministry of Finance for thirty-seven years ... we feel that as workers of this city and in light of the needs related to the third age ... we made two requests of the government that have not yet been granted ... I am the coordinator, I am the leader of everything ... We form commissions ... a group of 200 or 300 members participate and they name a commission so that together with me they identify the problem; the subway workers have a commission ... all the branches of the federal government [are represented].
>
> (A. P., 71, PISSSTE)

A member of the retired teachers' association (JPCNTE) told us the following:

> We are teachers [in] DF. This organization consists of primary, pre-school and special education teachers ... As a democratic organization we have had several ... even within the same union there are different points of view. We are the democratic part, the counterpart is the Revolutionary Vanguard [led by] Jonguitude, then by Elba Esther and now by Diaz de la Torre ... The union [has been functioning] since the forties ... We [have made requests of] several government institutions of ... DF or the ISSSTE, and engage in cultural events, outings, promotions, everything that [can be done to help those co-workers] who are close to retirement.
>
> (E.P., 64, JPCNTE)

Unlike the organizations made up of retired industrial workers that do not frame their missions in terms of quality of life or active aging, these organizations frame their objectives more in terms of those objectives. Given the fact that many of the State agencies these individuals worked for allowed early retirement, many retired when they were quite young. For many the state assured their security in old age, and in retirement they engage in an ongoing struggle to preserve those benefits. State workers were socialized into a traditional patronage model characterized by loyalty and State-provided benefits that characterized the period prior to the neoliberal era. Today, these retired workers organize to make demands with respect to their individual and collective rights that they see as threatened by various reforms to the retirement system. These threats involve important changes to the pension system that affect both current workers and potentially current retirees. Longer periods of required contribution in order to receive a full pension mean that many workers who spent years in informal employment retire with very low incomes. In 1997 the IMSS and in 2010 the ISSSTE replaced their traditional defined-benefit pension plans with defined-contribution plans. The older defined-benefit plans were funded collectively and guaranteed a set retirement income; the new defined-contribution arrangements require that the worker save for his or her own retirement, severing the bond of solidarity between generations. The privatization of the electric power sector and actual and planned reforms in the education sector have also mobilized those workers.

We might observe that although the members of these groups do not frame their objectives in terms of active aging per se, they are actually aging quite actively since they are highly engaged and socially involved. Rather than framing their objectives in terms of aging issues, though, they frame them in terms of the struggle against what they see as unjust social and political conditions, much as they did during their working years. The vast majority of members have higher levels of education, and most are married and have a retirement income. Their health tends to be good, although when they become ill their organizational activity tends to decrease or cease altogether.

Retired State Workers

Retirees of the Instituto de Seguridad y Servicios Socialesde los Trabajadores del Estado, ISSSTE (the Institute for Social Security and Services for State Workers), which was founded in the middle of the 20th Century, were not particularly politically active until the last years of that century. For many years retired state workers received defined-benefit pensions that were paid for by active workers and were guaranteed by the State. During the last decades of the 20th Century this pension scheme, like many others, was converted to a fully-funded defined-contribution scheme in which workers are required to save for their own retirements (H. Cámara de Diputados 2007). These reforms were preceded by similar privatization at Instituto Mexicano del Seguro Social, IMSS (Mexican Institute for Social Security) (Ramírez López and Valencia Armas 2008). This shift places the risk of economic downturns and poor pension fund performance squarely on the worker who may arrive at retirement with inadequate savings. As with other transitions of this sort it introduced problems and confusion associated with transferring workers from the old regime to the new one (Mesa-Lago 2004; Mesa-Lago 2008; OECD 2015; Orenstein 2008). Given the implications of these changes for active workers and for retirees, various subgroups with specific concerns formed. Among these were groups of retirees and pensioners. These groups were greatly concerned about the implications of the complex changes in the retirement systems for their pensions (Ramírez López and Valencia Armas 2008).

Retirees of ISSSTE do not become members of union-sponsored retiree or pensioner groups. Rather, when they retire many organize small groups themselves that remain affiliated with the union. Approximately five thousand ISSSTE retirees participate in these groups. In this way, retirees remain affiliated with the union and politically active in order to protect their economic rights. These groups of retired workers offer mutual support, often including co-residence, and they offer one another advice on the problems one can encounter in obtaining social security. Don M. P., an ISSSTE retiree emphasized:

> that is part of the political–social work that we do. For example, we work with people in treasury and when someone has problems with property, we say to them "Let's see how we can help" … and all that with legal advice … We meet and guide them, if it is necessary to take legal action, we guide them.
>
> (M. P., 79, PISSSTE)

Don A. B., another ISSSTE retiree explained that:

> [a]bove all, we talk about what harms our companions, such as the medical service, for which we continue to struggle, medical service and the judgements that the ISSSTE is not paying for … a lot of work is being done to [assure compliance] with article 147, which requires that the system or ISSSTE must pay the difference that a retiree receives in relation to what an active worker gets. Before, they paid it, now they will not because of the changes that have been made by the federal work commissions. Benefits are insufficient.
>
> (A. B., 71, PISSSTE)

These groups of the old union members have been very active in resisting neoliberal reforms that affect both active workers and retirees. In their public discourses, retirees make the point that the neoliberal argument in favor of these reforms portrays them as a burden on the economy. As this same respondent told us, "we are a burden for the great economic interests of pensions, that is why they privatize the pension, [for which] they changed the ISSSTE law" (A. B., 71, ISSSTE). He went on to explain the objectives of the group:

> There are several objectives. First, that … both the federal and the local [governments] comply with what the federal laws establish, we

all abide by section "b" and by the ISSSTE law that in 2007 was reformed, as a result of the Supreme Court leaving in force the previous law, through a tenth transitory article, which is the one that the majority of active workers chose.

(A. B., 71, ISSSTE)

For many months after the pension reforms were announced there were demonstrations at ISSSTE offices, in the congress, and in other government offices. In addition to protesting, these groups informed themselves of the technicalities of the law and the repercussions of the changes that the government was making. Don J. F. (58, ISSSTE) told us that at the time the national confederation of retirees from all over the Federal District (today CDMX) sponsored assemblies with speakers to inform the public of how the government was trying to change the laws and the consequences that would have for workers.

Although their discourse is highly political and often confrontational, the actions of retirees also reflect personal dimensions. Some retirees had been active in many social causes, in addition to the union struggle, since early in life. Don A. B., one such life-long activist, described the role that struggle had played in his life:

I have participated in the most important social movements here in Mexico. The 68 [student protests], struggles of peasants, settlers ... of everything ... I am a man of convictions ... I like to do social work, fight for people, that is my philosophy of life ... I believe that achieving the goals of the fight because that strengthens you psychologically and emotionally. Those of us who were active workers and struggled to achieve something, that is, remember the time, say, when I was young, we fought ... and we did it! Now we fight ... because it is our responsibility and if we succeed, it will strengthen me psychologically and in many aspects. I believe that we retirees are the great transformers of the country! We made the great transformations of the country ... The rulers do not pay attention, and the young people less because they pay more attention to what the media says.

(A. B., 71, ISSSTE)

Women and Retired Teachers' Unions

Retired teachers, many of whom were State workers, were also active in the political struggle to protect what they had gained as union members. Educators in Mexico are affiliated with one of the largest unions in Latin America and the Caribbean. The Sindicato Nacional de Trabajadores de la Educación, SNTE (National Union of Education Workers), has been active since 1943. The union is made up of state, municipal, and private sector educators and retirees (https://snte.org.mx/). Given the fact that women have been involved in education for decades, a large fraction of union members is women. Since the 1980s, the SNTE and its various factions have faced political attacks from the state, which has sought control over the educational system and the support of the union for government policies. The union's relationship with the federal, State, and municipal governments has varied from cooperation to resistance (Loyo-Brambila 2008).

Under neoliberal governments the union has opposed educational reforms aimed at the privatization of education. These and other changes led many teachers to retire early in fear of losing part of their pensions. A participant in a group interview in Mexico City explained that "[w]hat we do are very small and very significant [acts], a meeting of retirees can be social or it can be political because they are teachers who do not separate themselves from politics" (Group interview section 9, JPCNTE, CDMX). It is important to emphasize that the union is not monolithic and members do not adhere to a prescribed ideology. Members hold many political points of view, some reflecting centrist positions on various issues, and others positions that are farther to the left.

Of particular relevance to our discussion is the fact that the union includes groups that focus specifically on protecting the rights of retired teachers, some of whom retire early. Educators, like workers in the electrical power sector or ISSSTE, qualify for retirement after thirty years of service. A worker who begins working at an early age can retire quite young. For these early retirees, retirement can be long, which makes a predictable and stable pension and high-quality medical care imperative. One individual in a group interview in Mexico City explained that:

> When [we] see that the authority, the agency or in this case the ISSSTE is not treating [someone] adequately, then, we intervene ... requesting that their medical attention be expedited; already being in the hospital, in bed, we intervene to speed up their operation or their studies; and on the other hand, we promote social events, recreational festivals and outings.
>
> (Group interview section 9, JPCNTE)

Their objective is the defense of the economic, social, and cultural rights of older people, who are sometimes forgotten in the larger human rights movement. One respondent in a group interview explained that:

> [t]here are many retirement organizations that meet to ask for greater respect for their participants, sometimes they [the old people] are not seen or do not appear in the media, they are not very present unless they take over the ISSSTE offices or unless they take over an avenue,

so they exist but they do not exist. Unless a serious situation happens in a nursing home or foster care, they don't exist.

(Group interview section 9, JPCNTE, CDMX)

The dominant discourse of this group of organizations, then, emphasizes political action as the basis of self-help. This approach reinforces the struggle for economic and human rights, related not only to the union in question, but to the nation as a whole. This struggle is framed in terms of economic security and demands for the rights of ex-workers, including adequate medical care. These organizations have a clear trade union origin perspective, and while most focus on their own memberships, there are limited attempts to forge bonds with other unions or groups of older people. More than other groups, though, their discourse focuses on the protection of economic rights rather than issues related to the elderly, although the economic struggle has clear implications for older workers and the older population in general. As one respondent noted, "[w]ell, it is what they owe [us] ... the benefits we have [and that we are fighting to retain and improve.] A pension increase ... a bonus, and that they respect us because although we are retired, we are still workers" (S. M., 72, PISSSTE).

Like the electrical workers, retired teachers possess a high level of human and cultural capital. The union of retired teachers (JPCNTE) displays another unique characteristic. It is highly democratic in its approach to furthering the demands of teachers. The organization is the most generative of the associations of older persons in Mexico City. JPCNTE engages in a social justice discourse, emphasizing active engagement and advocacy for educators. In terms of aging, their discourse also reflects a concern for functioning, but above all, for social integration and an active life. These foci reflect the values of the traditional trade union struggle, and a concern for solidarity with younger generations. Yet one must be realistic about the possibilities. As three informants told us:

Above all, think of goals and still be able to realize them. Fortunately, they can be realized, but we also have to be realistic [about] what we can do ... what influence do we have?

(M. P., 79, PISSSTE)

We cooperate with the union, they call us to advise the boys ... that helps us to be active, to participate and to live with our companions; we learn to live with young people too.

(R. S., 68, JPSME)

It means having a project already ... what I'm going to do, what I'm going to dedicate myself to ... [how] I'm going to use my time, how

I'm going to live with my family, how I'm going to integrate with them.

(Focus Group Participant, JPCNTE)

University Professors

One very unusual group of retirees stands out because of the fact that its members have very high levels of education and, consequently, high levels of social and cultural capital. Retirees of the Autonomous University of Mexico (UNAM), named PICRELI (Pioneros Creativos en Libertad: Creative Pioneers in Freedom), clearly have extensive experience in the public sphere. Their educations empower them to deal with the complexities of formal bureaucracies and social policies. As one might expect of a group of retired academics, the group is characterized by a low degree of social organization but a high degree of citizenship. That is, although unlike labor unions, the fact that most of its members have professional and advanced degrees, gives them extensive knowledge of multiple ways of exercising their rights. The members are primarily women with doctorate degrees and a substantial work history. The group's objectives are to engage in group activities and to communicate, but above all to remain informed. As four informants explained, the members feel a high degree of empowerment and generativity:

> We are trying to help the new retirees so that it does not cost them as much work as it cost us ... it cost us from the formalities in the ISSSTE that leave you sitting [for] hours, they bring you back again and again ... At least for me it was a disaster, they want to continue ... at UNAM and suddenly we realize that we arrived at the UNAM and then because our office already disappeared, our job ... [has been given] to another person, we no longer have, we can no longer park because our credentials disappeared, they took them away, then we no longer have a place to ... come and visit, to see, and we feel that [our time has been] wasted because we have more than thirty years of experience ... Ah ... everyone is worth it, right? And when we could consult, we could give tips, we could advise ... give some seminar, give some talk, give some workshop ... most of us have a lucid mind, out there if there are some others that already have begun to have mental problems, but most of us because we have a clear mind ... are struggling to be given a place.
>
> (O. V., 78, PICRELI)

To propose to the University that [it benefits from] our experience to do some things, we have proposed many things that we could do but also that the University, as I understand it, has a place for us and some considerations since many of us, since we [have worked] at UNAM for a long time.

(V. M., 73, PICRELI)

Active aging has a lot to do with transmitting all the experience one has acquired throughout one's life.

(C. H., 74, PICRELI)

I think it's also an attitude of not simply to wait for death or to [wait for visits from] children or grandchildren ... I have a good relationship with my son and my granddaughters. [But that can't be everything. One needs] economic independence, intellectual independence, the ability to make decisions, to own one's own life.

(O. V., 74, PICRELI)

Beneficent Patriarchy: An Elusive Ideal

We return to the story of entrepreneur Enrique Garza Sada that we recounted at the beginning of this chapter. Garza Sada was a wealthy man from an established family, who nonetheless was concerned for the well-being of his employees. He is an example of a progressive and enlightened employer who was concerned with the welfare of retired as well as current workers, at a time when State policy and business practices promoted low wages and labor marginality. The actions of this entrepreneur should stand as an example for what other firms and what government should do. The Cuauhtémoc brewery was a very productive enterprise that was an engine of industrialization in the north of the country. The company provided training and mobility opportunities for its workers, who were mainly men, but it also looked after the well-being of their families by providing housing, education for their children, as well as medical services and retirement plans for workers. The Cuauhtémoc brewery introduced these innovations decades before worker security or even the general welfare of the population became a focus of government policy. A century after Garza Sada's enlightened leadership, the company still ensures the welfare of retirees and their families. Retirees of Cervecería Cuauhtémoc (RCC) continue to be protected by the company's private pension system.

Despite its commitment to its workers the profitability of the company did not suffer, proving that profitability and the responsible and humane treatment of employees are not incompatible. Unfortunately, it is also proof that workers cannot count on the beneficence and enlightenment of bosses, either industrial or union bosses, to guarantee their rights. Those rights must be fought for and for that fight to be successful the entire State apparatus as it affects social welfare and rights must be changed. One unique reason for the Garza Sada's successful pension plan was that not only was it based on sound financial principles, it benefitted from the advice of experts on aging. The concept of an institute focused on the needs of older individuals was first introduced in the state of Nuevo Leon (Carmona Valdés 2016). Obaldo, a retired worker who supervises the company's relations with retirees and pensioners, explained that since the 1970s workers are prepared for retirement through "life and development plan" courses, which they must take at 60, the mandatory retirement age. As part of this program workers are prepared for a new stage of life, which can be rather long given greatly increased life expectancy in the state of Nuevo León. He went on to elaborate:

> the program consists of five phases consisting of various sessions covering a whole year [...] The first phase at is an introduction, then the legal issues, the whole question of the types of pressures that one might experience; they provide an orientation ... then they go on. There is the question of the nature of the changes [that one experiences], of the significance that they have, the question of all those changes [that one experiences at] that stage of life. In the next phase, it is [renewing ties] with the family ... with the wife, with the children, yes, and in the last phase it is [the issue of] the use and enjoyment of free time. All the important aspects of time are [dealt with] and a program and activities are developed concerning the use of time ... The last phase consists of introspection [and an examination] of life and values. It is the final part of consciousness and all [of those phases are] integrated [with the help of] a psychologist who deals with the subject of emotional well-being ... Other aspects of health, including nutrition [are covered by] doctors and specialists who discuss hypertension, diabetes, [and cancer].
>
> (O. J., 57, RCC)

The programs that this company has institutionalized to provide income, training, housing, and retirement security to its workers are truly astonishing since the initiative was carried out without a mandate from the government. The social rights that this company provided voluntarily and in generous amounts were exactly those rights that later workers in other industries would have to fight so hard to acquire, if they ever did. What is so striking is that this private welfare system was established prior to the creation of social welfare institutions. Enrique Garza Sada remains a legend in Monterrey and his legacy is universally admired. A world with more enlightened leaders with Garza Sada's wisdom and benevolence is an ideal, but one that is largely ephemeral in most places. For workers seeking their rights, and for other groups characterized by marginality, poverty, and powerlessness, but even for middle-class workers and individuals, their basic social, as well as their human rights, depend on their own efforts.

Unions and labor mobilization more generally are vital components of an active and vital civil society, one in which individuals, including older individuals, can create venues in which to define their needs and from which to articulate their demands. Unions are among the most important incubators of potential change, just as they can be instruments of repression and weakness for workers. The electrical workers union (SME) is a particularly relevant example. These already politicized workers were forced to deal with the privatization of the industry during the Felipe Calderón administration. In response, the union framed its mission as not only protecting the benefits of its members, but as combatting the adoption of undemocratic labor policies and practices that harm the country's workers generally. The retirees' organization (JPSME) reflects this experience and embodies an identity and mentality focused on the exercise of democratic rights and participation in decision-making related to important social issues. Because of their political experience as union members and the highly politicized discourse in which they engaged, this group and groups like it represent important actors in the political culture of the country. Today the future of the Mexican labor movement and its potential impact on social policy is at a crossroads. The new labor law passed under the new Obrador Administration holds out the promise of a break with the official unions of the past and a greater voice for workers (de la Vega 2019; Gurley 2019). More open and democratic unions could foster a more active civil society generally. Given Mexico's history of serious union repression, though, labor's influence could be seriously diminished in the future if union culture is seriously weakened. Labor reforms and neoliberal economics more generally could weaken powerful traditional unions while blocking the rise of more independent unions. In the next two chapters we will examine groups that are made up of and include older individuals whose discourse and framing of the problems they face have given rise to a new human rights agenda.

References

Alzaga, Oscar. 2018. "Helgas, sindictos y luchas sociales en la historia de México." *alegatos* 99:411–434.

Anner, Mark. 2008. "Meeting the Challenges of Industrial Restructuring: Labor Reform and Enforcement in Latin America." *Latin American Politics and Society* 50 (2):33–65.

Bacon, David. 2019. "The Rebirth of Mexico's Electrical Workers." New York, NY: The North American Congress on Latin America. Retrieved 7/15/2020 from https://nacla.org/news/2019/02/07/rebirth-mexico%E2%80%99s-electrical-workers.

Bensusán, Graciela. 2004. "A New Scenario for Mexican Trade Unions: Changes in the Structure of Political and Economic Opportunities." Pp. 237–285 in *Dilemmas of Political Change in Mexico*, edited by Kevin J. Middlebrook. London, UK: Institute of Latin American Studies.

Bortz, Jeffrey L., and Salvador Mendiola. 1991. "El impacto social de la crisis económica de México." *Revista Mexicana de Sociología* 53 (1):43–69.

Briggs, Asa. 1961. "The Welfare State in Historical Perspective." *European Journal of Sociology* 2 (2):221–258.

Carmona Valdés, Sandra. 2016. *Historia de una pasión. La dignificación de la vejez en México.* Monterrey, México: Editorial Font.

Casas-Patiño, Donovan, Sergio Reséndiz-Rivera, and Isaac Casas. 2009. "Reseña cronológica del movimiento médico 1964–1965." *Boletín Mexicano de Historia y Filosofía de la Medicina* 12 (1):9–13.

Caulfield, Norman. 2004. "Labor Relations in Mexico: Historical Legacies and Some Recent Trends." *Labor History* 45:445–467.

Cavazos, Gabriela Recio. 2016. *Don Eugenio Garza Sada: Ideas, acción, legado.* Monterrey, Mexico: Editorial Font.

Comas, Júlia Martí. 2018. "Las luchas contra la privatización de la energía en México." Madrid, Spain: Pueblos – Revista de Información y Debate. Retrieved 7/27/2020 from http://www.revistapueblos.org/contacto/.

Davis, Charles L., and Kenneth M. Coleman. 1989. "Structural Determinants of Working-Class Politicization: The Role of Independent Unions in Mexico." *Mexican Studies/Estudios Mexicanos* 5 (1):89.

de la Vega, Oscar. 2019. "MEXICO – An Overview of the Recent Labor Law Reform in Mexico." American Bar Association. Retrieved 7/21/2020 from https://www.americanbar.org/groups/labor_law/publications/ilelc_newsletters/issue-may-2019/an-overview-of-the-recent-labor-law-reform-in-mexico/.

Delarbre, Raúl Trejo, and Aníbal Yáñez. 1976. "The Mexican Labor Movement: 1917–1975." *Latin American Perspectives* 3 (1):133–153.

Fairris, David, and Edward Levine. 2004. "Declining Union Density in Mexico, 1984–2000." *Monthly Labor Review* September:10–17. Retrieved 5/24/2020 from https://www.bls.gov/opub/mlr/2004/article/declining-union-density-in-mexico-1984-2000.htm.

Foweraker, Joe, and Ann L. Craig (Eds.). 1990. *Popular Movements and Political Change in Mexico.* Boulder, CO: Lynne Rienner Publishers.

Gamboa-Suárez, Julieta, and Omar Dario Olivo-Huerta. 2018. "La perspectiva sobre el trabajo femenino y el lugar social de las mujeres en el semanario Ceteme, órgano informativo de la Confederación de Trabajadores de México, 1959–1968, núm. 12, Universidad de Antioquia." *Trashumante. Revista Americana de Historia Social* 12:89–119.

González-Guerra, José Merced, and Antonio Gutiérrez Castro (Eds.). 2010. *El sindicalismo en México. Historia, crisis y perspectivas.* Mexico City: Plaza y Valdés.

González Cordero, Francisco Javier. 2020. "Masculinidades y vejez. Cuerpos, trabajo y curso de vida en Axotlan, Edo. Mex." Doctoral thesis. Mexico City: UNAM.

González Nicolás, Inés. 2012. "Participación sindical de las trabajadoras en México." *Nueva Sociedad* 184:14–149.

Greer, Charles R., Charles D. Stevens, and Gregory K. Stephens. 2007. "The State of Unions in Mexico." *Journal of Labor Research* 28 (1):69–92.

Gurley, Lauren Kaori. 2019. "Is Mexico on the Brink of a Labor Revolution?" *The New Republic.* Retrieved 7/21/2020 from https://newrepublic.com/article/153467/mexico-brink-labor-revolution.

Gutiérrez Castro, Antonio. 2011. "Breve recorrido histórico del sindicalismo mexicano." Pp. 17–42 in *El sindicalismo en México. Historia, crisis y perspectivas*, edited by José González Guerra Merced and Antonio Gutiérrez Castro. Mexico City: Plaza y Valdés.

Gutiérrez Rufrancos, Héctor Elías. 2016. "What Do Mexican Unions Do?" PhD Thesis, University of Sussex. Brighton, UK. Retrieved 4/9/2020 from http://sro.sussex.ac.uk/id/eprint/68412/1/Guti%C3%A9rrez%20Rufrancos,%20H%C3%A9ctor%20El%C3%ADDas.pdf.

Haber, Stephen H. 1989. *Industry and Underdevelopment. The Industrialization of Mexico, 1890–1940*. Stanford, CA: Stanford University Press.

H. Cámara de Diputados. 2007. "Aspectos Relevangtes de la Reforma al ISSSTE." Mexico City: Centro de Estudios de las Finanzas Públicas. Retrieved 7/28/2020 from https://www.cefp.gob.mx/notas/2007/notacefp0102007.pdf.

Hermanson, Jeff, and Enrique de la Garza Toledo. 2005. "El Corporativismo y las Nuevas Luchas en las Maquilas de México: El Papel de las Redes Internacionales de Apoyo." Pp. 181–213 in *Sindicatos y Nuevos Movimientos Sociales en América Latina*, edited by Enrique de la Garza Toledo. Buenos Aires, Argentina: CLACSO.

Johnston, Hank, and Paul Almeida (Eds.). 2006. *Latin American Social Movements: Globalization, Democratization, and Transnational Networks*. New York, NY: Rowman & Littlefield.

Juárez, Fátima, and Julieta Quilodrán. 1990. "Mujeres pioneras del cambio reproductivo en México." *Revista Mexicana de Sociología* 52 (1):33–49.

Krauze, Enrique. 2011. *Redentores: Ideas y Poder en América Latina*. New York, NY: Vintage Español.

La Botz, Dan. 1988. *The Crisis of Mexican Labor*. New York, NY: Praeger.

Lenti, Joseph U. 2017. *Redeeming the Revolution: The State and Organized Labor in Post-Tlatelolco Mexico*. Lincoln, NE: University of Nebraska Press.

Loyo-Brambila, Aurora. 2008. "Sindicalismo magisterial." *Revista Mexicana de Investigación Educativa* 13 (37):345–349.

Mayer, Jean-François. 2006. "Changes in Relations between the State and Independent Unions? Mexico Under the Fox Presidency." *Canadian Journal of Latin American and Caribbean Studies / Revue canadienne des études latino-américaines et caraïbes* 31 (61):9–35.

Mesa-Lago, Carmelo. 2004. "An Appraisal of a Quarter-Century of Structural Pension Reforms in Latin America." *CEPAL Review* 84:57–81.

Mesa-Lago, Carmelo. 2008. *Reassembling Social Security: A Survey of Pensions and Health Care Reforms in Latin America*. New York, NY: Oxford University Press.

Montes de Oca, Verónica. 2000. "Experiencia institucional y situacíon social de los ancianos en la ciudad de México." Pp. 419–456 in *Las políticas sociales en México al fin del milenio. Descentralizaíon, disenño y gestión*, edited by Rolando Cordera and Alicia Ziccardi. Mexico City: Coordinación de Humanidades/Facultad de Economia/Miguel Angel Porrúa.

Montes de Oca, Verónica, Mariana Paredes, Vicente Rodríguez, and Sagrario Garay. 2018. "Older Persons and Human Rights in Latin America and the Caribbean." *International Journal on Ageing in Developing Countries* 2 (2):149–164.

Montes de Oca Zavala, Verónica. 2013. "La discriminación hacia la vejez en la ciudad de México: contrastes sociolpoliticos y jurídicos a nivel nacional y local." *Revista Perspectivas Sociales/Social Perspectives* 15 (1):47–80.

Montes de Oca Zavala, Verónica. 2014. "Cuidados y servicios sociales frente a la dependencia en el marco del envejecimiento demográfico en México." Pp. 169–181 in *Autonomía y dignidad en la vejez: Teoría y práctica en políticas de derechos de las personas mayores*, edited by Sandra Huenchuan and Rosa Icela Rodríguez, under the coordination of Alicia Bárcena and Miguel Ángel Mancera. Mexico City: CEPAL.

Montes de Oca Zavala, Veronica, and Paola Carmina Gutiérrez Cuellar. 2018. "La discriminación entre la población mexicana: una revisión para pensar avances y desafíos." Pp. 285–302 in *Por la igualdad somos mucho más que dos. 15 Años de lucha contra la discriminación en México*, edited by Mario Alfredo Hernández Sánchez, Yoloxóchitl Casas Chousal, and Marcela Azuela Gómez. Mexico City: CONAPRED and SEGOB.

OECD. 2015. "OECD Reviews of Pension Systems MEXICO." Retrieved 8/10/2020 from http://www.oecd.org/pensions/private-pensions/OECD-Mexico-Pension-System-Review-2015.pdf.

Orenstein, Mitchell A. 2008. *Privatizing Pensions: The Transnational Campaign for Social Security Reform*. Princeton, NJ: Princeton University Press.

Quilodrán de Aguirre, Julieta, and Fátima Juárez Carcaño. 2009. "Las pioneras del cambio reproductivo: un análisis desde sus propios relatos." *Notas de Población* 87:63–94.

Ramírez López, Berenice Patricia, and Alberto Valencia Armas. 2008. *La Ley del ISSSTE ¿y las pensiones? Distrito Federal, México*. Mexico City: Universidad Nacional Autónoma de México.

Recio, Gabriela. 2007. "El nacimiento de la industria cervecera en México, 1880–1910." Pp. 155–185 in *Cruda realidad: producción, consumo y fiscalidad de las bebidas alcohólicas en México y América Latina, siglos XVII–XX*, edited by Ernest Sánchez Santiró. Mexico City: Instituto Mora.

Recio, Gabriela 2015. "Empresas y empresarios: la importancia de las biografías." *Boletín Virtual Red de Estudios de Empresa* 20:2–6.

Stahler-Sholk, Richard. 2014. "Mexico: Autonomy, Collective Identity, and the Zapatista Social Movement." Pp. 187–207 in *Rethinking Latin American Social Movements: Radical Action from Below*, edited by Richard Stahler-Sholk, Harry E. Vanden, and Marc Becker. New York, NY: Rowman & Littlefield.

Stahler-Sholk, Richard, Harry E. Vanden, and Marc Becker (Eds.). 2014. *Rethinking Latin American Social Movements: Radical Action from Below*. New York, NY: Rowman & Littlefield.

Stahler-Sholk, Richard, Harry E. Vanden, and Glen David Kuecker (Eds.). 2008. *Latin American Social Movements in the Twenty-first Century: Resistance, Power, and Democracy*. New York, NY: Rowman & Littlefield.

Teichman, Judith A. 2009. "Competing Visions of Democracy and Development in the Era of Neoliberalism in Mexico and Chile." *International Political Science Review* 30 (1):67–87.

Villegas Rojas, Pedro S. 2016. "Fundamentación legal del sindicalismo mexicano." Pp. 43–62 in *El sindicalismo en México. Historia, crisis y perspectivas*, edited by José Merced, González Guerra, and Antonio Gutiérrez Castro. Mexico City: Plaza y Valdés.

Zepeda Martínez, Roberto. 2009. "Disminución de la tasa de trabajadores sindicalizados en México durante el periodo neoliberal." *Revista mexicana de ciencias políticas y sociales* 51:57–81.

Chapter 7

Improving the Quality of Life

In the last chapter we began our examination of specific retiree organizations by reviewing the role of the Mexican labor movement as the original source of wide-spread organized struggles for basic rights. Although the Mexican labor movement has never been a major force in Mexican politics, and many unions are little more than fronts for the owners of enterprises or the government, collective job action has been common. This labor militancy has led workers to recognize that they can organize to further their own interests. As we saw, that mentality and militancy is often carried into retirement. Many union retirees remain active in protecting the rights they earned through collective action. Other groups we studied are quite different in terms of their members' backgrounds and characteristics, as well as their objectives. Many are made up primarily of women who have been lifelong homemakers who have not worked, or done so only informally or sporadically. They have lower levels of education and little experience in unions or social movements. For the members of these organizations the group is less a venue for demanding rights, and more an extension of the family where they enjoy social interaction and emotional support. Emilia Buendía Saavedra told us of what the organization she belongs to means to those who participate.

EMILIA: I am Emilia Buendía Saavedra. I am 66 years old. I was born in Guadalajara Jalisco but I've been here (Mexico City) for fifty-two years ... I come to the active aging class where they give us talks, that is, they give us tips on how to age, on how to take responsibility ourselves for our medical appointments, for the medications that we have to take. In my case, I take medications for high blood pressure. I have celiac disease and I have been on a special diet for about eight years ... For the past three years here, I suffered from hyper-thyroidism, which is also controlled ... I have osteoporosis, which they are treating me for ... I am aware of myself, of my person, of my individuality and also of my family ... I am very happy with this program and all it offers to help us take responsibility for ourselves and to help each other as we do in our family.

DOI: 10.4324/9781003205609-7

INTERVIEWER: Could you tell me about some of the activities that you engage in here?

EMILIA: Our group is called [name] active aging. We have a project with the National University of Mexico, which is called "active aging" in which we attend lectures and practice tai chi ... which from what I understand and what I have read does not cure any disease but it helps with the quality of life ... I have been coming here two and a half years, almost three, and I'm doing very well ... The talks are once a week for two hours, and on the remaining four days we have an hour of tai chi. What is tai chi? Tai chi, as far as I understand it and seen it, is a martial art with round, slow, long movements, that has made us very well. At least it has been great for me because it has helped me to be a little more flexible than before. At the same time, they also give us a bit of Chi Kung, which is a light self-massage on the whole body so that wakes up our cells and our tissues so they become more flexible, and although it may seem unbelievable, little by little they become more supple and less rigid. It doesn't happen overnight so you have to keep at it ... It is a very, very beautiful group because there is a lot of camaraderie between the teachers and us ... We are very well integrated, the teacher Araceli is doing a monumental job and I thank her a lot.

INTERVIEWER: What would the concept of active aging mean to you?

EMILIA: For me, active aging is aging in the best possible way, being aware of it and doing what we have to do, without straining. At the same time this group "renewal" personally produces great benefits. Active aging is aging in the best way with zest because that also helps us ... understand ourselves and others. We help ourselves and help others. For me active aging also means being aware of yourself and taking care of yourself, because there are people who are a bit isolated and they get angry at everything because they are confined and have no other vision, they don't leave their house ... or maybe they can't because they already have some disability ... But this aging is a process that occurs little by little ... It's slow and we accept it and how better than with a certain courage?

INTERVIEWER: And from your point of view, why do people come? What is the motive that would make them come here?

EMILIA: I believe that everyone wants to do it. When I was working, I asked God frequently that after I retired, I would find a place like this, because I did not want to stay at home confined by four walls. It's worse that I am not a grandmother. My daughter said to me "now that you are retired, I don't want you to stay in the house. Let's see now that you to have something, that you have a plan of life." I asked her, what do you mean by a "plan of life"? Because I had been very immersed in my work ... she said, "yes, what are you going to do now?"

INTERVIEWER: What are the benefits of coming to the group?

EMILIA: Well we are more empowered, I feel more empowered, freer, I am more stable when I walk and I do not fall so much, because here they even teach us how to walk. The group allows us to age with dignity, so that nobody need feel sorry for us. We want respect and not pity.

Stronger and Healthier

These excerpts from an interview with a very active and engaged older woman illustrate some of the activities typical of what is probably the most common type of voluntary CSO in Mexico. This organization's core objective is to provide emotional and instrumental support to older individuals who would otherwise be at high risk of isolation and loneliness, as well as malnutrition, illness, and serious injury. Emilia speaks of feeling empowered by her participation and her involvement with others; she identifies socializing as a major benefit of the group's activities. From her perspective, her physical and emotional health have improved as the result of these social interactions. This is an example of an organization that is focused primarily on improving the quality of life of participants. Such groups are clearly important and complement, even if they cannot replace, the emotional and instrumental supports that have traditionally been the responsibility of families.

Emilia's interview directly addresses one of the questions that we address in this book, related to whether and in what ways non-governmental and faith-based organizations can fulfil at least some of the functions of the traditional family, or compensate for an incomplete welfare state. This function may seem less important than the objectives pursued by the more militant groups engaged in the struggle for a more just social and economic order, but improving the quality of life of older individuals is far from trivial. Engagement with others, and the educational activities that such organizations often sponsor, potentially contribute to a greater civic consciousness among their participants. In addition, organizations focused on the quality of life play an extremely important practical role. As we have argued, the dramatic and rapid social and demographic changes that accompany modernization, urbanization, and globalization are making it increasingly difficult, if not impossible, for the family to provide all of the support and care that older parents need. Although defamilisation has shifted many of those responsibilities to the State, it too is limited in what it can do, especially in the case of low and middle-income countries. Historically, faith-based communities have served many of those family functions. The strong ties that one forms with co-religionists and members of communities of faith make it clear that under the right circumstances, strangers can indeed become family.

The organizations we dealt with in the last chapter were made up of individuals with union backgrounds, high levels of education, a history of public and government service, or involvement in social movements, experiences that provided them with the social and cultural capital for more effective collective action. Their framing discourses centered on political power and the preservation of rights gained through strikes and social activism. They did not, for the most part, frame their objectives in terms of active aging or improving the quality of life of their members, although that would clearly be the result of successful attempts to guarantee pensions, health care, and the rest of their activist agenda. The organizations we deal with in this chapter have very different memberships and they engage in different discourses. They are found primarily in marginalized districts of urban centers, and their participants are predominantly female. These women tend to have little education and most spent their lives as homemakers. As a consequence, few have retirement incomes of their own. They tend to be old and in poor health. For these women the group is an extension of the family that provides social supports that are not provided by the State. These organizations do not frame their objectives in terms of militant attempts to protect human and social rights. For the most part, their discourse focuses specifically on improving the quality of life of their members, most of whom have experienced physical hardships and suffer from significant health problems.

Autonomy

While one's quality of life clearly depends on access to the material goods and services that sustain health and vitality, it also depends on optimal autonomy, by which we mean the ability and freedom to self-actualize, that is, to make important life decisions for oneself, and to make the most of one's capacities and opportunities in accordance with one's own desires. Autonomy is a concept that can apply to collectivities or organizations, such as the Autonomous University of Mexico, or an autonomous state. Such a concept emphasizes the independence of the entity referred to and the fact that its members or its directors act without undue interference by the government or outsiders The concept of autonomy is also highly individualistic, referring to the ideal situation in which the individual acts as a fully unencumbered agent who makes decisions and life choices in accordance with her or his free will. It is this aspect of the concept of autonomy that we address in this chapter. Clearly one's degree of autonomy is constrained by external political, economic, and social forces, as well as by one's own physical and cognitive capacities. Optimizing autonomy, then, means overcoming those constraints to the extent possible. In addition to affirming one's personal rights, a useful concept of autonomy also involves recognizing one's obligations and duties to others.

We focus on the efforts of CSOs to optimize individuals' autonomy within the constraints that structure their lives.

In this context it would be useful to elaborate briefly on the meaning of autonomy, and relate it to the actions of CSOs who deal with older persons in Mexico and elsewhere. Autonomy represents a core concept in moral theory and in the medical, social, and behavioral sciences, and it relates directly to the moral independence and rights of older persons (Kuhse, Schüklenk, and Singer 2016). The concept lies at the core of the principles codified in the international conventions on the right of older persons that we discussed in Chapter three. The basic principle is codified in the Belmont Report, in which the federal government specifies the basic ethical principles that govern all research involving human subjects in the U.S. (Beauchamp and Childress 2012; U.S. Department of Health and Human Services 1979). Similar principles apply to research involving human subjects in Mexico and other nations.

Although the idea of autonomy may seem clear at first glance, the meaning and sources of autonomy are far more complex than they might initially seem. Since at least the Enlightenment, our individualistic Western liberal tradition has strongly privileged the rights of the person, and it places an ultimate value on one's freedom to pursue his or her personal goals with minimal interference. Such a conception of autonomy, though, is historically recent and foreign to many cultures. It remains highly contested even in Western nations where an excessive focus on individual freedom is strongly criticized for giving insufficient weight to the social, cultural, and historical contexts that place duties and expectations on individuals (Etzioni 1993; Ho 2008; Jennings 2016; Lévinas 2016; MacIntyre 1981; Mackenzie and Stoljar 2000). Autonomy conceived of in terms of a radical self-determination and self-governance raises serious concerns related to human interdependency and the social origins of the self and identity. Although values related to freedom and the right to express oneself as one wishes are widely held, the notion of complete autonomy is frequently and often strongly rejected. Feminists, for example, criticize the standard view of autonomy as being excessively masculine and for ignoring its relational nature (Donchin 2001).

The concept of autonomy, as well as those of entitlements, rights, and duties are clearly life-course dependent. Young children by definition possess limited autonomy. Parents or their legal surrogates must make important decisions for them. Similarly, individuals who are seriously cognitively impaired have limited autonomy. For many older individuals serious physical and cognitive impairments undermine autonomy. Yet, while some degree of decline might be inevitable, the complete loss of autonomy is not. It is, in fact, a core aspect of "active" or "successful" aging. While one's capacity to live independently may decline with age, other cultural, social, and organizational factors interact with physical and cognitive capacity to determine one's degree of autonomy.

Civil Society and Autonomy

Civil society organizations are a crucial part of social life in Mexico. They range from informal collectivities with no formal organization to more formally structured groups focused on improving the quality of life, or advancing the rights, of the populations they serve. Certain of these organizations, like those we examined in the last chapter, are affiliated with unions or political parties, while others are closely tied to the government or religious groups. Others have ties to transnational social movements and organizations. Today one observes a growing diversity of organizations that reflect not only a concern for the physical and emotional well-being of older individuals, but increasingly encourage political mobilization and foment citizen demands for basic rights. These organizations mobilize around demands for public services, access to adequate health care, and basic pensions which have not been democratically or universally accessible. The political struggle for human rights and for greater equity and democracy, which we describe in greater detail in the next chapter, has encouraged political and social participation and the emergence of demands for both redistribution and recognition. With the aging of the population, older people have become much more active participants in this discourse.

In this chapter, though, we focus on organizations devoted largely to improving the quality of life of those who participate. Their missions primarily involve increasing individuals' autonomy and control over their own lives. Occasionally they help older individuals access social resources, and some engage in educational activities, particularly related to improving health and psychological resilience. As we have mentioned, it is important to understand how the objectives and activities of the wide range of civil society groups we deal with in this book reflect the economic and social profiles of the populations they represent, as well as the economic and occupational sectors in which they operate, the problems they address, and the historical activism of the particular occupational and social sectors from which they emerge.

As we discussed in Chapter one, the relatively recent evolution of civil society and the increase in the number of civil society organizations is not unique to Mexico. These organizations have emerged in many nations where they focus on improving the quality of life of older persons, as well as promoting the exercise of their rights through new ways of conceptualizing and constructing citizenship (Wanderley 2009). International organizations, such as *HelpAge International* (https://www.helpage.org/who-we-are/about-the-global-network/), which has branches in many nations, works to address the human and social rights of older individuals globally. In Latin America they work to help older individuals in Bolivia, Colombia, and Peru claim their rights and access the benefits they are entitled to. This new approach includes a completely different perspective on aging, more focused on active aging and social and political participation, but also one that affirms autonomy and the ability of older citizens to act as effective agents in the defense of their individual as well as their collective political and social rights. Increasingly, older individuals play a determining role in building institutional connections between social actors and government.

In Mexico, older people are increasingly empowered with the support of CSOs and the academy and are increasingly forcing governments to recognize their needs and their rights (Das and Poole 2004). Older citizens are coming to recognize their capacity to control important aspects of their lives and those of their communities. Such insights can begin with interactions among individuals who support one another in improving the quality of their lives. Increasingly, but to varying degrees depending on the various factors we have alluded to, older people are consolidating themselves collectively as competitive and dynamic social actors who demand specific rights (OAS 2017). Ultimately, though, only the State can guarantee such rights, but their actual implementation requires the constant prodding of non-governmental, faith-based, and other civil society organizations.

Critiques of Active Aging

As positive as the concept of active, successful, or healthful aging might at first glance seem, it is important to remember that, much like the concept of civil society itself, active aging has been criticized for being what we might refer to as insufficiently political. Such criticisms arise from the implication or indeed the overt claim that is often made that an individual has nearly complete control over her or his own health and well-being. We might characterize this perspective as focused on a level of autonomy that does not in fact exist. From an extreme perspective, one need not age since decline, disability, and disease reflect lifestyle choices that are under one's own control (Lamb 2017; Lamb 2020). Such a perspective misattributes responsibility for negative outcomes and situations to the individual rather than to structural factors, such as poverty, inadequate welfare state support, low levels of education, unhealthy work environments, political unrest, and more.

Although we focus on organizations that foster autonomy and active aging, our use of the concept of active aging focuses more on political, economic, and social aspects of aging and less on individual-level factors over which individuals supposedly have control. This conception is based on the proposition that the physical, emotional, and social well-being of individuals of all ages depends on their social position and the resources to which they have access. Although organizations whose formal agendas focus largely on the quality of life may not directly frame their objectives in political or activist terms, the objective of improving the quality of life cannot be completely divorced from political and economic processes that limit individuals' autonomy and ability to optimize their health and well-being.

Improving Quality of Life

Our observations led us to conclude that perhaps the most common type of CSO focused on issues related to aging in Mexico consists of those whose core missions focus on improving the quality of life of those they serve. Their specific organizational dynamics and structures differ significantly among states and municipalities, reflecting their individual origins and philosophies, the dominant political parties that rule the state in which they operate, as well as the characteristics of the populations they serve. We differentiate between private and public organizations that deal with some aspect of aging and divide them further into two major categories, based largely on the nature of the degree of dependency and marginality of the older individuals they serve. The first group deals with older individuals who are highly dependent in terms of social isolation, economic insecurity, functional incapacity, and psychological vulnerability. These organizations provide supports that allow vulnerable older individuals to function as well as possible given the reality of their situations and their high level of dependency. The largest sub-category among this group consists of non-State CSOs, both secular and faith-based, who receive little or no State support.

The second group is much smaller and consists of organizations sponsored and supported by federal, State, and local governments. These links emphasize the fact that distinctions between non-governmental and government-sponsored or supported organizations are not always clear. In the United States, many non-governmental organizations receive support and even sponsorship from different levels of government. This second group of organizations deals with older individuals who are less dependent and marginalized. For these individuals support is intended to enhance individuals' independence and allow them to function on their own.

In this discussion we focus on the first large grouping, those CSOs whose core objectives are improving the quality of life of those older individuals at highest risk. Figure 7.1 offers a graphic representation of the hierarchy of the organizations in this first group, which comprises the majority of organizations that deal with older persons. Within it we include both public and private organizations, although the latter is much smaller than the first. The pyramid reflects the relative number of each type of organization, as well as the relative size of the populations that each serves. At the base, addressing the needs of the largest population of

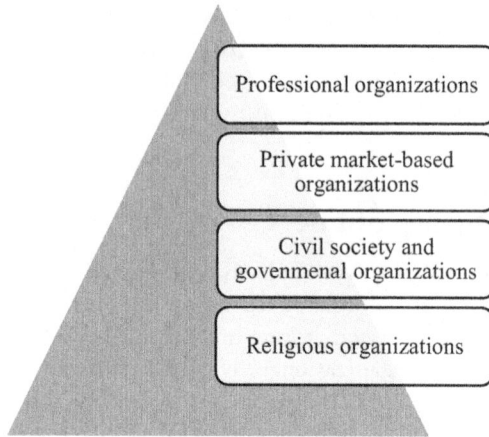

Figure 7.1 Hierarchy of organizations that promote quality of life among the most disabled.
Source: Authors' classification based on field research.

the most vulnerable, are faith-based, civil society, and governmental organizations. Higher up are private market-based organizations that provide services to individuals who can afford to pay at least some amount for the services they receive. Their number is limited by the fact that relatively few individuals can afford to do so. At the top of the pyramid are professional organizations, such as the *Sociedad Jalisciense de Gerontología y Geriatría* (Jalisco Society of Gerontology and Geriatrics), the *Asociación Mexicana de Geriatría y Gerontología* (the Mexican Association of Geriatrics and Gerontology), that provide specialized services to a small number of older persons.

The Most Vulnerable

Although we do not have a census or even a partially complete count of organizations whose missions are to improve the quality of life of older individuals and others, we begin with brief examples of the sorts of organizations we are dealing with. The *Comunidad Participativa Tepito A.C.* (Participatory Community Tepito: https://movimientodeaccionsocial.org.mx/organizaciones-mas/comunidad-participativa-tepito-a-c) emerged after the September 1985 Mexico City earthquake in order to deal with the extensive needs of vulnerable older individuals, many of whose family members were lost or killed in the earthquake. This CSO receives funding from international donors and local contributors. These resources are used to strengthen neighborhood social networks in order to permit vulnerable older individuals to remain in their homes. This support includes assistance in dealing with health problems and other daily needs. An interesting feature of this organization's approach is that it owns residences in which certain individuals are allowed to live during their lifetime, after which someone else moves in. Social workers provide assistance and case management in order to enhance the autonomy and quality of life of the older residents.

A new and unique civil society organization that focuses on a particular segment of the aging population is the *Xochiquetzal House* in Mexico City (http://casaxochiquetzal.wordpress.com/). This organization has taken on a very important mission. It provides care to sex workers who have reached old age without family or financial resources. Many of these individuals have been sexually exploited and many have been trafficked, and although they have survived their ordeal, they have no place to turn. These individuals are survivors, and their life experiences have often made them combative and difficult to deal with in other care contexts. Xochiquetzal house receives both government support and private donations.

Many other unique organizations exist in all Mexican cities. Recently established organizations in Jalisco include a group of volunteers, *Voluntariado Estamos Contigo* (Volunteers, We Are with You: http://www.vec.org.mx/), that began operations in 1993, and the *Entre humanos* (Among Humans) that began operations in 2010. These organizations promote an intergenerational support model at the family level and promote that philosophy through the media. We encountered other groups focused on improving the lives of older people in the states of Nuevo León, Oaxaca, and Yucatán. What is clear is that the creation and dynamics of these organizations are determined by the social and political history of the state and municipality in which they operate, as well as local and State government policies, the organization's own political position and philosophy, and the level of activism and involvement of the local movement for human rights of older persons.

Contexts of Caregiving

The sample of organizations which were the objects of the study are from large urban areas. These are listed in the methodological appendix. We focused on urban areas since in Mexico 61% of the population 60 and older is concentrated in urban areas of greater than 15,000 inhabitants. Our sample therefore reflects an urban perspective on aging and the ways in which active aging is defined. The neighborhoods in which these organizations operate are often the poorest and most marginal. Although the majority of older individuals in modern Mexico live in cities, a large number of older individuals remain in the small villages and rural areas and their experiences are no doubt quite different than those of urban dwellers. Those individuals are aging in more traditional contexts, which today are often extremely poor areas which young people have abandoned in search of greater opportunities. Unfortunately, we can shed no light on their unique experiences of aging.

The urban areas we selected represent very different social and cultural contexts with different sociodemographic profiles that may affect the perception and treatment of older people. These differences also affect older individuals' motivations and opportunities to act to defend their rights and the types of activities in which they engage. Several economic, political, demographic, and social characteristics of Mexico City and the states in which we worked are presented in Table 7.1. Most of the measures are self-explanatory. The level of marginalization is based on a measure developed by the *Consejo Nacional de Población*, CONAPO (National Population Council) based on several indices related to average levels of education, housing quality, income, and more (Bustos 2011). We will not go into the details of this complex measure but only affirm that it clearly differentiates between poor southern states and more affluent northern states. We categorize the locations as varying from a very low degree of marginalization to a high level.

Table 7.1 Characteristics of Mexico City and states in which interviews were conducted

Indicator	Mexico City	Jalisco	Nuevo León	Oaxaca	Yucatán
Level of marginalization	Very low	Low	Very low	Very high	High
Year of laws protecting aged	2000	2010	2004	2014	1999
Population 2015 (Thousands)	8,919	7,845	5,120	3,968	2,097
Population 60 and older	1,004	671	407	406	196
Percentage of population 60 and older	11%	9%	8%	10%	9%
Life expectancy at birth 2015	76.2	75.7	76.7	73.2	75.6
Aging index 2015	71.7	37.1	38.0	40.4	43.0
Percentage of the population 60 and older who are indigenous	4%	2%	2%	48%	61%
Percentage of the population 60 and older with a pension	45%	37%	58%	16%	37%

Source: Computations based on data from INEGI 2015, CONAPO 2016, and SEDESOL and INAPAM 2015.

The aging index is a ratio of the population over 60 to that 15 and younger multiplied by 100. It shows that the population of Mexico City is clearly older than that of the state of Oaxaca in the south. Other measures include the year in which laws protecting older peoples' rights were adopted, the percentage of the population 60 and older, the percentage of the population that is indigenous, and pension coverage.

As the table reveals, states in the south of the country, and especially Oaxaca, are characterized by high levels of marginalization. Jalisco and Nuevo León, on the other hand, have lower levels of marginalization. The states differ in other respects. Only 8% of the population of Nuevo León, a richer and economically dynamic area, is 60 or older. States vary considerably in the proportion of older individuals who receive a pension. Nearly 60% of residents 60 and older in Nuevo León receive a pension, whereas only 15% in Oaxaca receive a pension. States also differ in the year in which they adopted laws to protect older individuals. Jalisco and Oaxaca were quite late. Unfortunately, the existence of state laws protecting the rights of older persons is no guarantee that those rights are in fact protected. The situation is in many ways worse for indigenous populations than for others. Again, states differ significantly in the size of their indigenous populations. Nearly half of the older population of Oaxaca and over 60% of the population of Yucatán are indigenous.

The phrase "quality of life" refers to those dimensions of physical, mental, and social functioning that facilitate social connectedness and interaction with others. Enhancing one's quality of life, then, requires reducing the risk of loneliness and encouraging physical and social functioning (Fernández-Mayoralas and Rojo Pérez 2005; Rojo Pérez, Fernández-Mayoralas, and Pozo Rivera 2000). The focus on quality of life defined in these terms has a clear motivation. The new urban experience in aging can be traumatic, especially for those older individuals with few material or social resources. Dependency, poverty, helplessness, and personal insecurity among older people are common. A minority lose their family or are abandoned. CSOs are among the few options offering assistance to this population of older individuals who in old age are left totally dependent on the State or charity. Civil society institutions were pioneers in developing an assistance approach which had to be implemented with limited resources, few trained personnel, and no scientific knowledge. The first innovations were in fact developed by religious organizations affiliated with the Catholic Church. These were motivated by the Christian principle of charity and a calling to care for those forgotten by society (Quintanar Olguín 2000).

Religious Groups

As part of their basic philosophy of ministering to the needy and helpless, religious groups and institutions have historically provided charity to the most vulnerable segments of the population. The Catholic Church has been dominant in Mexico since colonial times and, despite some excesses practiced in converting native populations, it has ministered to the poor and rejected. Faith-based groups are for the most part not revolutionary, but rather assume a charitable stance in providing care directly, rather than demanding that the State provide services. One of these organizations is the *Pastoral del Hermano Mayor* (Pastoral for the Older Brother) in Nuevo León, where it attends to individuals with serious material needs. One volunteer explained that:

> [w]e in the Pastoral have a section that provides support … we have identified people who do not have anything to eat nor anything to wear. So, a group of people takes them food … it is a very interesting ministry, there are many people who are in bad shape.
>
> (H. A., male, 52, Pastoral del Hermano Mayor)

For the most part, these organizations carry out their activities with little formal training in mental health services, but seek to support the physical and mental functioning of older individuals by providing spiritual comfort in order to enhance emotional health. The informant we just quoted went on to explain that "in many cases, people are disappointed in life, so they arrive looking for me to listen to them, to attend to them, to talk to them. There we give them that attention and they feel very welcomed and happy."

Marginalization and exclusion are the consequences of inequalities among individuals and groups in important life domains. Göran Therborn (2016), a sociologist, elaborates three manifestations and sources of different forms of inequality among individuals. The first is vital inequality, which refers to socially-conditioned differences in such well-being indicators as mortality, life expectancy, morbidity, and infant and child health. The second is existential inequality, which refers to deficits in domains of life that provide meaning and hope, such as autonomy, dignity, freedom, respect, and the capacity for self-development. The third is resource inequality, which is how the term is commonly used. It refers to differential access to material resources. The objective of such a classification is to emphasize important dimensions of inequality, as well as their complex, pervasive, and interactive nature, and their dire consequences for all aspects of well-being. Each of these sources of inequality, and certainly their intersection, constitute not only threats to physical and emotional health, but together they place one at elevated risk of existential despair, a classical concept in existential philosophy and therapy that relates to the loss of a sense of life's meaning (Schneider and Krug 2017). The concept relates directly to the realms of meaning and spirituality, domains that are quintessentially religious.

The issue of existential despair goes directly to basic issues of human existence and the tragic nature of life. A sense of meaning and purpose can be as salient as basic physical needs, perhaps even more so. For humans, hope and a sense of justice are basic to health. For many older individuals, especially those steeped in traditional cultures, spirituality and faith are central to a meaningful existence. As the volunteer at the Pastoral we quoted above explained:

> The most important thing for the elderly, after the basic needs, perhaps before the basic needs, is the issue of hope, spirituality, and faith. An older adult who has these issues well strengthened is calmer and more comfortable with himself. That is my own experience and it is the experience of when we began to read from different areas and from different universities and many of the reflections go in that sense, of course, many things determine their warmth or well-being.
>
> (H. A., male, 52, Pastoral del Hermano Mayor)

Although charity lies at the core of Catholic and religious philosophies more generally, some groups and organizations go further, as in the case of liberation theology that directly confronts the structural basis of inequalities of all types (Andrade 2017). More generally, though, faith-based organizations seek to diminish resource inequality by providing food and creating social support networks. Improvements in nutrition and medical care can greatly reduce vital inequality, and ultimately reductions in resource and vital inequality can help reduce existential inequality and greatly improve the lives of individuals and communities.

The historical mission of religious institutions to tend to the spiritual welfare of their parishioners increasingly extends to their physical and emotional welfare. One serious possibility for at least partially addressing the needs of destitute older individuals is to involve faith-based organizations more formally. State sponsored programs designed to train volunteers in topics related to the instrumental and social support needs of older individuals could be introduced at a modest cost. Some might object to any cooperation between the Church and the State, but the reality is that Mexico is a Catholic country with a large population living in poverty. Addressing their needs must take precedence over other considerations. In recent decades Pentecostal Protestantism has made extensive inroads into Latin America generally, largely through active support of individuals in need (Lindhardt 2016). To address objections to State sponsorship of religion, government support could be contingent on an organization's agreement not to proselytize in exchange for providing government-sponsored support. Religious institutions are highly trusted in Mexico. Their influence is simply too important to ignore when it comes to dealing with major social problems.

Secular Groups

Although historically faith-based groups may have been among the first to cater to the needs of the poor and infirm, today many secular organizations carry out very important work in providing assistance to individuals with very specific problems, such as dementia or homelessness. Although they are formally secular, in a highly religions nation like Mexico many receive some assistance from the Catholic Church and other denominations. In Guadalajara the organization *Plenitud y Demencias A.C.* (A Full Life with Dementia) provides support to people with some degree of cognitive impairment. They work with individuals and their families, and are financed by the Institute for Social Development (INDESOL), which falls within the Secretariat for Social Development (SEDESOL) of the federal government. This organization competes with others to obtain financing. One of those in charge is Mtra. Irais Bonilla, a psychologist and gerontologist, who told us about the profile of the people she cares for in their homes:

> A year and a half ago we carried out a census and we managed to identify around 100 older adults, who had no food ... they live in houses made of tarps, held up by sticks, mere shells, totally precarious. So, we said we are going to help ... Well, what are we going to do? We already talked to them; they already trusted us to give them information. We administered a mini-mental status exam and a mini-nutritional exam to get some idea of their condition ... So what we did was monthly visits and we provide support, people suddenly want to help, a lot of goods arrives, we bring them food, we spend a little time with them ... we identify needs, for example, there are people who live alone.
>
> (I. B., female 33, Plenitud y Demencias A.C.)

The goal of this organization, then, is to make life as joyous and involved as possible for individuals with serious cognitive impairments. This philosophy and the organization's approach represent a very novel perspective. Iris Bonilla went on to explain that:

> something very important is to provide information and training to the family, to raise awareness that this elderly adult can have a good quality of life even if he or she has some type of cognitive impairment ... with good information and training this can be accomplished ... Now our next project [is to] support them with cognitive therapy workshops for which we do not have funds yet, but we are looking for them. It is a project that is already in place and I think we are going to make it work as soon as we need to in order to

achieve the goal of making their behavioral symptoms decrease, making them calmer.

(I. B., female 33, Plenitud y Demencias A.C.)

One of Plenitud's core objectives is to educate families concerning important aspects of the quality of life of their family member with dementia. This aspect of the care of older individuals is central, but is often not taken into account in long-term care institutions run by the State. Active family support networks for people with cognitive impairment can greatly improve the quality of life of an older person. Again, given the fiscal limitations of the State and the fact that families are unaware of the course and nature of cognitive decline, organizations like Plenitud provide an invaluable service. Iris Bonilla went on to explain that:

> it is something, it is impressive to see how the same family that is not aware of what can be done, of the need for support, of issues related to the older person's quality of life, of what it means to be well can deal with it if they have a little information and a little training.

As a charitable organization, Plenitud makes no profit and continuously seeks financial resources to carry out its mission.

Caring for Those with Leprosy and Tuberculosis

Another unique organization with a very important mission is the *Asociación Jaliciense de Protección al Leproso A.C.* (Jalisco Association for the Protection of Lepers) in Guadalajara, Jalisco. This organization was founded to deal with the leprosy epidemic of the mid-20th Century (Torres-Guerrero et al. 2011). Later the organization turned to the isolation and care of tuberculosis patients. Currently their mission has extended to providing shelter to older people without a home or family who are living on the street. It is ironic that the objective of isolation for transmissible diseases such as leprosy and tuberculosis, once largely eradicated, would serve as a paradigm for the care of older people. One of the administrators explained the organization's objectives. She said that "We care for the indigent elderly, provide for all their needs for food, medicine, shelter. We provide a clean bed, warm meals, and we try to maintain their quality of life within the limitations of the place and their health" (R. G., female, 53, Jalisco Association for the Protection of Lepers A.C.).

This organization depends on a board of trustees that supports it financially. The staff is minimal, but they manage to attend to their homeless population and to improve the quality of their lives at least marginally by adopting a healthcare paradigm, and providing shelter, hygiene, and food. Social assistance of this sort has been the objective of many supportive organizations since the 1970s. This social support approach has been adopted by government agencies as a model for their own efforts. These sorts of social assistance organizations serve as the lifeline of last resort for the most marginalized populations who are victims of the three inequalities summarized by Göran Therborn (2016) who we mentioned earlier. They suffer the accumulated disadvantages of intersecting resource, vital, and existential inequalities. As the administrator we mentioned before went on to explain:

> We welcome them, no matter what condition they are in. Rather here it is need that matters they no longer have a place to go then we welcome them. They come to us in wheelchairs, 90% of them have a mental situation, Alzheimer's, senile dementia. We have several in wheelchairs as the result of age-related deterioration ... we have people who have amputations, diabetes, people who have been struggling, living on the street. I can't tell you that everyone is in that condition, no, it varies.
>
> (R. G., female, 53, Jalisco Association for the Protection of Lepers A.C.)

Even though it is unaffiliated, many of the organization's activities are supported by the Church. It also depends on volunteers, and it receives support from other organizations, such as the Red Cross and the Civil Hospital of Guadalajara, an organization that itself serves those without rights or resources.

Luis Elizondo Asylum

Another example can be found in Monterrey in the *Luis Elizondo Asylum* (https://www.asiloluiselizondo.org/es/) founded in 1956, but in which religious sisters had provided services since the beginning of the 20th Century. This institution provides residential services and is supported by businessmen and other private funders. The residents pay nothing. The organization is overseen by a Council that includes businessmen from Monterrey. The focus of this nursing home is on rehabilitation. It employs twenty-four nurses and caregivers, a geriatrician, a psychologist, a social worker, a nutritionist, as well as administrative staff. The people who are served are 60 and older and are functioning well, but wish to live in that institution. One administrator explained:

> we serve 100 residents ... we have 114 beds and we do not occupy all of them, we have a special geriatric care area together with the little hospital for residents who have a disease and require special care and need hospital care.
>
> (B. M., female, 45, Luis Elizondo Asylum)

Other Organizations

These organizations provide basic services to the poorest and most vulnerable segments of the population, those without family, support networks, resources, or shelter. As we have noted, many similar organizations have religious origins and their missions retain a religious focus on charitable support. Without these services it is unclear what would happen to the individuals they serve. It is clear, though, that the need is far greater than what the State could provide. The extent of the needs of this population for whom physical and mental illness accompany extreme poverty and social marginalization poses major challenges to all levels of government and the community.

One organization that we encountered has an extremely interesting program that addresses a very specific need. *Estamos Contigo* (We Are With You) is a volunteer organization that emerged in the 1990s. It focuses on the needs of the most disadvantaged sectors of the population. Georgina Monge, its Director, explains that since it began in 1995 the organization has provided support to other organizations that assist marginalized segments of the older population. The services they support include social assistance, institutional care, nursing homes, and more, including both financial and in-kind support. This group is motivated by a philosophy that does not focus solely on the older person, but rather on families with few resources that often live in marginal neighborhoods. The organization was formed during a decade in which Mexico was addressing the consequences of a period of crisis and difficult economic adjustments. This complex but highly efficient organization works directly in the community in a comprehensive manner to reduce the negative consequences of poverty. A social worker explained aspects of the organization's mission. She noted that:

> in addition to the program for older adults ... we have a Human Training project that serves women under 60 years of age ... by age group and we give them a two-hour class every week ... they are integrated into the different groups and at the end of the month if the person attends their four classes, at the end they are given a food basket ... with basic items for which, in addition to paying with the hours of attendance they pay a symbolic fee of 40 pesos.
>
> (G. M., female, 56, We Are With You)

In attempting to address the negative consequences of poverty, this organization and others with similar missions confront the reality of the need to employ mental and physical therapy to preserve, and hopefully improve older individuals' quality of life. Estimates from the Mexican Health and Aging Study indicate that as many as 45% of Mexicans 65 and older need assistance with basic activities of daily living or with instrumental activities of basic living (Arroyo, Montes de Oca, and Garay 2017). Again, given the rapid aging of the population the need will only increase. It is clear that there is great demand for these sorts of services that delay dependency as long as possible. How effective they are at significantly reducing serious incapacity is unknown, but it is clear that they provide an extremely important service. A social worker told us of the nature of training she and others were receiving:

> Well right now they are giving us training, a teacher from ITESO, a psychologist from ITESO with topics from aging, the acceptance of aging, health care and many ... mental exercises, from playful games, physical activities, practically two hours in which the elderly are working on their mind, their body, also what is part of their personal growth.
>
> (M. G., female, 42, We Are With You)

This type of social assistance has a very important positive impact on the quality of life of older people in Jalisco, not only because it preserves physical and mental health of the older person him or herself, but also because the training covers family dynamics, as part of an attempt to alter dysfunctional family behaviors in ways that enhance older parents' autonomy.

Fundación Oportunidades A.C.

Another interesting group is *Fundación Oportunidades A.C.* (Opportunities) that introduced a program named "Entre Hermanos" (Among Brothers) in Jalisco, which since 2008 has paired young students with older adults who have some academic or relevant background that qualifies them to teach. For example, they may have a degree, or have worked in education, business, commerce, or have some experience that qualifies them to serve as mentors for young people. These mentors tend to have middle-class backgrounds, but despite this, they require training to bring them up to speed on pedagogy. One 72-year-old female mentor explained:

> There are basic competences, including listening, openness to change, resilience and more. There are also thematic topics including sexuality, being young, grief. There is also the subject of thanatology ... Another part that is important are the workshops that have been offered to them – reading, art therapy, dance classes, yoga, English, contemporary art ... some they can choose and others are mandatory. Many resist art therapy, but it is mandatory.
>
> (C. C., female, 72, Entre Hermanos)

Among Brothers seeks to build links between generations based on education for youth, but it has a far broader impact for the older mentors themselves. The educational training that they receive allows many to improve their academic skills and to gain a greater capacity to support themselves, and also to maintain their social involvement and improve their physical and mental health. The older volunteers who take part in this program as facilitators or mentors receive a monthly fee for forming a bond with the young person. Between Brothers does not depend on the government for support. Rather, it receives funding from Fundación Oportunidades A.C., which distributes private funds, largely from one sponsoring family, whose purpose is to foster intergenerational interactions and support.

Amanecer Veracruzana

In Mexico City, many organizations focused on older persons emerged at the beginning of the new century during the administration of the current President Andrés Manuel López Obrador. The new president is particularly concerned with the situation of older Mexicans. One such organization is *Amanecer Veracruzana* (Dawn in Veracruz, AMV), located in the Iztapalapa district on Mexico City's east side. This organization focuses on quality of life and self-help. The Iztapalapa district is marginal, which is reflected in the low level of physical, cultural, and social capital of the organization's participants. AMV is composed mainly of women 75 and older. They are mostly widows; many are migrants; and almost none are in good health. The vast majority suffer from diabetes and hypertension. Most spent their lives as homemakers, have extremely low levels of education, and have no pension income. Despite these physical and social limitations, though, the aging experience of the AMV women can be described as active. Their activities are centered in the neighborhood, and focused on recreational activities that are intended to maintain optimal physical functioning in the face of the rising incidence of chronic disease and disability among its members. An older female participant told us of the activities offered:

> Well, before we made handicrafts, we decorated dishes, did ceramic painting, but then many did not want to anymore. Then a teacher came and after she left another woman came, the one who is now coordinator, to teach us sewing and activities of that sort ... before we had many more teachers because there were more of us, they taught us those paper things for the Day of the Dead or to make flowers.
>
> (J. G., female, 83, AMV)

For these types of organizations that cater to a large public with few resources and often marginal health, enhancing physical functioning is very important in maintaining the domestic economy, reducing drug expenses, and allowing older individuals to continue participating in family life. Physical and mental stimulation is vital in maintaining an older person's individual and social quality of life. As a consequence, the organization's conception of active aging emphasizes physical activities and the stimulation of the body and mind as one ages. From interviews and focus groups it became clear that physical and artistic activities are not only forms of entertainment and social participation, they protect against the negative effects of isolation. Perhaps most importantly, though, the organization's emphasis on participation and active aging is intended to transform the public image of old age, as well as the self-image of participants, from that of a time in life characterized by disease and serious functional decline to the recognition that older individuals can be active agents in control of important aspects their lives. Although the organization's activities clearly reflect frame realignment, they do not involve direct political action. As one 83-year-old woman explained:

> Active aging? It means that we are active and we are proud to be active ... we are not letting ourselves go; I always tell my girls, we have to move, as long as God keeps us standing we are going to do the rest, give thanks to God who gives us life and to be able to do something here.
>
> (M. H., female, 83, AMV)

One aspect of the program that draws attention is that it includes no educational component nor training in human rights. All of the organization's efforts focus on the need to maintain physical and mental functioning, to deal with the stress experienced at home with children and caregiving responsibilities, but also it emphasizes the need to get out of the house and away from the problems of family life. The same older woman spoke of why people participate:

> They are motivated to come for the same reason, because they leave their problems at home and come here to de-stress, to talk, to do their work, for example, crafts, exercise, dancing, whatever ... they leave their problems at home for a while and that is what helps them a lot too, because being at home they shut themselves up and problems grow for them.
>
> (M. H. female, 83, AMV)

The organization clearly enhances the quality of life of its members, but their low levels of education and income, and consequently of human and cultural capital, result in limited capacity to influence the State. Amanecer has applied for government support but its applications have not been successful. The organization depends on multiple sources for funding. With the new Obrador Administration, the government is more of a possibility. Given the organization's focus on the old and infirm, younger generations are not involved, perhaps contributing to the organization's difficulty in obtaining governmental support. Similar groups with little ability to influence governmental policy or actions are common in Mexico City. Their powerlessness derives from the particular condition of the older population itself, but also from the high degree of marginality of many districts and neighborhoods in the city, and a general lack of programs targeted to older people.

Un Granito de Arena

Amanecer serves a population with clear needs for support. Yet the participants do enjoy some level of autonomy. At some point, though, some older individuals lose all autonomy and become totally reliant on others. One organization that we have mentioned before, *Un Granito De Arena A.C.* (A Grain of Sand, http://www.hogarungranitodearena.org.mx/), caters to this highly needy population. This non-profit voluntary organization provides services to individuals with serious functional impairments in Mexico City. It has been in operation for fifteen years and is affiliated with the Network of Associations of Senior Citizens in Mexico City. Currently the organization provides residential and other services at four locations. Given the serious impairment and lack of autonomy of most of their clients, the administrators and staff function basically *in loco parentis*, that is, as parents. They are adamant defenders of the human rights of the older individuals they care for. The organization works to put the reality of the need for long-term care and the needs of seriously dependent older people on public and political agendas. Their social activism in the political sphere is complemented by their association with the Network of Associations of Older People in Mexico City. Through this collaboration they address the challenges faced by civil society organizations and their need for financing. They are active in emphasizing the importance of a societal level response to the growing needs of impoverished and functionally impaired older people.

Private For-Profit Organizations

Although our focus in this book is primarily on organizations that provide care to and advocate for older persons with few or no resources, we must mention that for-profit organizations that provide support services to certain older individuals operate in Mexico. Given the fact that few older individuals can afford to pay for the highest quality care, their market is limited. Nonetheless, although private for-profit nursing and day care are unlikely to become the norm, these organizations basically define the state of the art in eldercare. Certain of these organizations require a monthly payment for the purchase of specific services for disabled and cognitively impaired older persons. Among these we again find several institutions with religious origins and affiliations. We can offer only a few examples.

Pro Dignidad Humana A.C. Asilo Juan Pablo II

Pro Dignidad Humana A.C. Asilo Juan Pablo II (Pro Human Dignity A.C. John Paul II Asylum: https://www.calle.es/pro-dignidad-humana-ac-asilo-juan-pablo-ii-P48465.htm), which is located in Guadalajara, Jalisco, has been operating for thirty-four years. It is registered as a civil association whose objective is to provide older individuals with comprehensive care, ranging from basic needs to spiritual support. However, in order to operate it requires donations from other foundations and resources from its almost sixty residents, who are mostly women. In addition, in the past it was affiliated with the *Instituto Jalisciense de Asistencia Social, IJAS* (Institute of Social Assistance of Jalisco), which ceased operations in 2019, together with the *Instituto Jaliciense de las Mujeres* (Institute for Women of Jalisco), which provided training to the staff in fundraising, human rights, institutional development, and geriatric care.

The residents of Juan Pablo II are over 65, are functioning adequately, and have some family ties. In general, in order to be accepted an applicant must want to reside there, she cannot suffer from mental illnesses or contagious diseases, and she must be able to walk or at least support herself, so that she is not totally dependent. The residents are clearly unique. Their ability to pay for long-term care makes them stand out. The residents include women whose children have migrated and people who do not want to live alone and prefer to pay for a place where they can live with other people and carry out supervised daily activities. Many are religious and enjoy participating in services with others. In addition to dining services, the organization offers such amenities as hairdressing, podiatrist services, and a cinema. Two residents told us of their experiences:

> I was working for the federal government, from there I retired. With my retirement I am paying for my stay here, so my daughter ... comes and visits me here.
>
> (A. C., male, 82, resident of the Juan Pablo II Asylum)

> Five years ago I became a widow, for that reason I was very lonely and then one of my five daughters went to live in Germany. ... I want to be completely independent, where I can go alone and be comfortable, and they looked for me in various places and I came here to give glory to God.
>
> (M. M., female, 77, resident in the Juan Pablo II Asylum)

Improving the Quality of Life 181

Casa Loyola A.C.

Another faith-based institution, the Casa Loyola A.C., better known as the Ignatian Center of Spirituality, provides services and training to another sector of the population that adheres to a Jesuit version of Catholicism, which is basically progressive. One female instructor explained that certain individuals do not feel comfortable with the approach. She noted that:

> If they are very conservative or religious people, they leave, because we don't promote ... let's say a conservative religiosity, rather the other way around. On a personal level I can tell you that a large part of our job is to try to help people take off some religious prejudices, and they even have the opportunity to review their images of God.
>
> (C. A., female,71, Casa Loyola)

This institution is not a residential facility. The membership are people linked to Jesuit universities who seek to engage in spiritual reflection, and conforming to Jesuit tradition education is central to this agenda. The organization is private and is financed by class fees, room rentals, and other income-generating activities. The female instructor continued and explained that:

> the socioeconomic level does influence, why? Because we charge. People who ask us, we give them help. The center lives by renting the rooms, the spaces and some courses that are given, but nothing else, we have to be self-supporting. Look, we are aware ... it has been elitist, no way, I don't like it ... We have accepted people without resources, we deny no one.
>
> (C. A., female, 71, Casa Loyola)

Fundación Mano Amiga Mano Anciana

These are only a few of the wide range of organizations that provide care to older people with varying degrees of dependency. Another notable example is the *Fundación Mano Amiga Mano Anciana* (Helping Hand, Old Hand) I.A.P, which serves seriously dependent people in the south of Mexico City. This institution began operation in 1982 with the objective of serving people with primarily mental rather than physical limitations. The population served is 65 and older and includes fifty people with chronic diseases, dementia, or Alzheimer's. The environment of this institution is very pleasant with gardens and ample spaces for wheelchairs. Residents are able to enjoy themselves with the assistance of specialized caregivers. As the director explained:

most of them are in wheelchairs, they can no longer walk, they can no longer fend for themselves and those who care for them have to walk behind them because since they have their mental problem they are not aware of the danger, so you have to be very watchful.

(M. B., female, 56, Mano Amiga Mano Anciana, IAP)

The caregivers are primarily volunteers. A doctor is available from Monday to Friday from 11:00 a.m. to 7:00 p.m. Another doctor is available on weekends and holidays. The organization maintains a portfolio of psychiatrists and psychologists. Nurses work in four shifts and assistance is always available.

Day Care

Many older individuals with limited autonomy could benefit from something short of institutional or residential care. Adult day care provides an alternative that allows an older person to interact with others of similar age and experiences, while allowing other adult family members to work. Indeed, many of the organizations we have mentioned in fact provide similar services. Among private institutions that provide adult day care we encountered *Grandes Personas A.C.* (Grand Adults) that provides day home service to older persons in Monterrey, Nuevo León (https://www.facebook.com/grandespersonasmty/). This organization serves older individuals with a medium to high socioeconomic profile. Its director is a specialist in the sorts of trauma, including falls, that older people experience. This enterprise was established in 2016 with support from entrepreneurs in Nuevo León who had business ties in Spain. The program consisted of a day care facility with a clientele limited to twenty-two people. The organization is a private company that has its own non-pharmacological rehabilitation treatment model that seeks to stimulate the functional capacity of older persons. The entrepreneurial and academic dynamism of Monterrey and Nuevo León contribute to the program. Universities in Nuevo León offer specialties in gerontology and in aging psychology. Experts from these programs, some of whom have studied in Spain, offer an exceptional level of professional care.

Gericare A.C.

Another example of private home-based care is *Gericare A.C.* (https://www.gericare.com.mx/), which has developed a unique program of home care for dependent older people that is divided into three levels of care based on the older person's level of functioning. The managers and care providers of this organization maintain a broad range of contacts with professionals in many countries outside of Mexico, expanding their professional capacities beyond what is available locally. The company has introduced activities that are pioneering innovations in the treatment of dependent older persons. These are designed for a sector of the population with economic, educational, and cultural resources. The organization employs an intergenerational model, and old and young people participate mutually gratifying musical activities. As one teacher in the organization explained:

> a six-year-old project that I love, it's called "vintage people" which is a rock forum for older adults. Right now, I teach them ... and they have more than 100 presentations, they have gone to Mexico and Guadalajara, but the interesting thing ... is the intergenerational idea. It is a school for kids, so the director is a friend of mine and you have to do something in music ... for the older people it is stimulation and getting into an exercise.
> (B. D., female, 40, Gericare, https://blog.gericare.com.mx/conoce-a -vintage-people/)

As this example reveals, the services provided in this institution are very innovative, they provide home care, but they also operate a day center which provides services to a maximum of sixty people. Their services are focused on people with some form of dependency and the rehabilitation program is focused on improving physical health. The organization has a gym with equipment and an instructor. Classes in yoga, meditation, and fitness are available. Classes in French, psychology, and other topics are offered. Monterrey has a very affluent and engaged business class, and it is a state with a high life expectancy, which increases the demand for this type of service. In the future the poorer and more ethnic states will have to find some compromise between state support and the private market. CSOs will no doubt play an important role.

Professional Gerontology and Geriatric Associations

At the top of Figure 7.1 we placed professional associations, which provide limited, but clearly professional-level services to certain older individuals. These consist of gerontological and geriatric professionals, with specialized gerontological and geriatric knowledge that complements medical and clinical treatments. These associations promote greater professionalization in the care of older persons, but in addition to increasing the scientific basis of care, they have had to integrate a clear understanding of the role of older persons in Mexican society and the ways in which social processes affect the aging process. As of yet specialization in geriatrics and the application of gerontological knowledge does not inform public policy in all states. Many of these professionals are in private practice or provide services through the for-profit arrangement we mentioned earlier. Although these professional associations do not deal with the vast majority of older individuals, they introduce an important professional scientific perspective into the care of older persons. To the extent that their knowledge and insights can be incorporated into the system for the care of older persons more generally, the overall quality of care of older persons could be improved. Once again, certain CSOs are in ideal positions to assist in the dissemination of such professional knowledge to a far larger population.

Three such organizations at the national level are the *Sociedad Mexicana de Geronto-Geriatría A.C.* (Mexican Society of Geronto-Geriatrics) (https://www.facebook.com/someggi/), the *Asociación Mexicana de Gerontología y Geriatría*, AMGG (Mexican Association of Gerontology and Geriatrics) (https://www.amgg.com.mx/), and more recently the *Colegio Nacional de Medicina Geriátrica* (National College Geriatric Medicine) (https://conam eger.org/). These and similar associations and organizations carry out training and ongoing education for doctors and other health professionals specializing in the care of older persons. Currently many have extended that mission to provide training for lay caregivers of older persons.

These professional organizations are more common in certain areas. In Guadalajara, Jalisco, the *Jalisco Geronto-Geriatrics Society* (SGGJ) is affiliated with the Jalisco Medical Association and the local medical college. This society was founded in 1990 by Dr. Ángel Felipe, a visionary doctor. It is the only interdisciplinary organization in the country focused on the care of older persons. Although it has formal funding, many of the services and help that it provides older people is by volunteers. The current President of the Society, María G. Salvatierra, is a female gerontologist. She told us of some of the charitable activities that the Society carries out annually:

> In these health days we go specifically with people with limited resources, those who do not have the opportunity to pay for a specialist, there they will be treated within the health day. We invite the community to join this cause. The beauty of this health day is that we do it without a peso, everything is in donation in time or in kind.
>
> (M. S., female, President, SOGEJAL)

We Must Care for One Another

Perhaps the most obvious role of volunteers, community groups, faith-based organizations, and other civil society organizations is to care for the less fortunate. Such a mission emerges directly from traditional religious teachings of charity and ministering to the poor and infirm. Such organizations appear to make up the majority of organizations dealing with older individuals in Mexico, or we might say that care designed to preserve or enhance the quality of life makes up a large fraction of the activities of the organizations we observed. Indeed, even those organizations we mentioned in the last chapter whose objectives were more political and activist were concerned with improving the quality of life of their members, if not so directly or explicitly as those we dealt with in this chapter. The memberships of those organizations were younger on average, and their participants had experience in union-sponsored job actions and other social movements aimed at the protection of labor and citizenship rights.

The organizations we described in this chapter for the most part cater to individuals with far less social or human capital. They are older and lack the sorts of backgrounds that would lead them to engage in more adversarial or confrontational actions. For the most part, they attempt to complement the family, or even compensate for its absence, in providing care and support to older individuals. A major theme that pervaded our interactions with these organizations was their desire to further active aging and avoid isolation through social interaction. For the most part, these organizations follow a social assistance paradigm, designed to address the material, social, and emotional needs of the most marginal segments of the older population. With few exceptions, they do not rely on professionally trained staff nor do they draw on an established body of scientific knowledge. Many of those involved bring extensive experience in community activism and years of experience in dealing with older individuals in need, some with substantial physical and cognitive impairments.

Although unpaid volunteers play a central role in providing care to older individuals, these organizations draw upon a wide range of funding, from grants from the State and international funders, to domestic philanthropic organizations and businesses. The involvement of the business sector was particularly evident in Monterrey, Nuevo León, an economically dynamic northern city with an engaged business community. What is clear is that the need is already greater than municipal, state, or federal governments can address. The rapid aging of the Mexican population, in combination with mounting state fiscal limitations means that this burden will grow as individuals live longer with more serious physical and cognitive limitations. Although improved living conditions and better medical care have extended life expectancy, they have not brought about a significant compression of morbidity. Families and the State must draw upon whatever cultural, social, and economic resources are available to address this problem. For all of their clear weaknesses, civil society organizations and their hybrid forms that may evolve in the future, including perhaps the emergence of social enterprise focused on the care of older persons, will be an essential part of the care mix.

In the next chapter we examine a set of organizations that builds upon the experiences and missions of the organizations we have dealt with in the previous and this chapter. These organizations' frames and missions go beyond a concern for the quality of life and are informed by a revivified human and social rights agenda, the outlines of which are embodied in the several international conventions on the rights of older persons that we discussed in Chapter three. These organizations not only focus on the rights of older individuals, but that of citizens more generally. Their focus on rights represents an awakening of a more dynamic civic consciousness as previously marginalized and silent groups stand up to demand their basic human and social rights.

References

Andrade, Luis Martinez. 2017. "Liberation Theology: A Critique of Modernity." *Interventions* 19 (5):620–630.

Arroyo, Concepción, Verónica Montes de Oca, and Sagrario Garay. 2017. *Los cuidados en el envejecimiento. Ponencia presentada en el 4° Congreso de Latinoamericano y Caribeño de Ciencias Sociales.* Salamanca, España: CEPAL.

Beauchamp, Tom L., and James F. Childress. 2012. *Principles of Biomedical Ethics.* Oxford, UK: Oxford University Press.

Bustos, Alfredo. 2011. "Niveles de marginación: una estrategia multivariada de clasificación. Realidad, datos y espacio." *Realidad, Datos y Espacio Revista Internacional de Estadística y Geografía* 2 (1):169–186.

CONAPO. 2016. "Índice de marginación por entidad federativa y municipio 2015." Retrieved 5/22/21 from https://www.gob.mx/conapo/documentos/indice-de-marginacion-por-entidad-federativa-y-municipio-2015.

Das, Veena, and Deborah Poole. 2004. *Anthropology in the Margins of the State.* Santa Fe, NM: School of American Research Press.

Donchin, Anne. 2001. "Understanding Autonomy Relationally: Toward a Reconfiguration of Bioethical Principles." *Journal of Medicine and Philosophy* 26 (4):365–386.

Etzioni, Amitai. 1993. *The Spirit of Community: Rights, Responsibilities, and the Communitarian Agenda.* New York, NY: Crown Publishers.

Fernández-Mayoralas, G., and F. Rojo Pérez. 2005. "Calidad de Vida y Salud: Planteamientos Conceptuales y Métodos de Investigación." *Territoris. Revista del Departament de Ciències de la Terra (Número: monográfico sobre Geografía de la Salud)* 5:117–135.

Ho, Anita. 2008. "The Individualist Model of Autonomy and the Challenge of Disability." *Bioethical Inquiry* 5:193–207.

INEGI. 2015. "Encuesta Intercensal 2015." Retrieved 5/22/21 from https://www.inegi.org.mx/programas/intercensal/2015/#Tabulados.

Jennings, Bruce. 2016. "Reconceptualizing Autonomy: A Relational Turn in Bioethics." Hastings Center Report.

Kuhse, Helga, Udo Schüklenk, and Peter Singer (Eds.). 2016. *Bioethics: An Anthology.* Malden, MA: Wiley Blackwell.

Lamb, Sarah (Ed.). 2017. *Successful Aging as a Contemporary Obsession: Global Perspectives.* New Brunswick, NJ: Rutgers University Press.

Lamb, Sarah. 2020. "'You Don't Have to Act or Feel Old': Successful Aging as a U.S. Cultural Project." Pp. 49–64 in *The Cultural Context of Aging: Worldwide Perspectives*, edited by Jay Sokolovsky. Santa Barbara, CA: Praeger.

Lévinas, Emmanuel. 2016 [1961]. "Totalité et Infini: Essai sur l'extériorité." *Encyclopaedia Universalis*. Boulogne-Billancourt, France: Encyclopaedia Universalis.

Lindhardt, Martin (Ed.). 2016. *New Ways of Being Pentecostal in Latin America*. Kindle Edition. New York, NY: Lexington Books.

MacIntyre, Alasdair. 1981. *After Virtue: A Study in Moral Theory*. Notre Dame, IN: University of Notre Dame Press.

Mackenzie, Catrina, and Natalie Stoljar (Eds.). 2000. *Relational Autonomy: Feminist Perspectives on Autonomy, Agency, and the Social Self*. New York, NY: Oxford University Press.

OAS. 2017. "Inter-American Convention on Protecting the Human Rights of Older Persons (A-70)." Retrieved 12/6/2017 from http://www.oas.org/en/about/who_we_are.asp.

Quintanar Olguín, Fernando. 2000. *Atención a los Ancianos en Asilos y Casas Hogar de la Ciudad de México. Ante el Escenario de la Tercera Ola*. Mexico City: Plaza y Valdéz.

Rojo Pérez, F., G. Fernández-Mayoralas, and E. Pozo Rivera. 2000. "Envejecer en casa: los predictores de la satisfacción con la casa, el barrio y el vecindario como componentes de la calidad de vida de las personas mayores en Madrid." *Revista Multidisciplinar de Gerontología* 10 (4):222–233.

Schneider, Kirk J., and Orah T. Krug. 2017. *Existential–Humanistic Therapy*. Washington, DC: American Psychological Association.

SEDESOL and INAPAM. 2015. "Perfil Demográfico, Epidemiológico y Social de la Población Adulta Mayor en el País, una Propuesta de Política Pública." Retrieved 5/22/2021 from http://www.inapam.gob.mx/work/models/INAPAM/Resource/918/1/images/ADULTOS%20MAYORES%20POR%20ESTADO%20CD1.pdf.

Therborn, Göran. 2016. *Los campos de exterminio de la desigualdad*. Mexico City: Fondo de Cultura Económica.

Torres-Guerrero, Edoardo, Felipe Martínez, Carlos Enrique, Atoche Diéguez, Jisel Arrazola, Blanca Carlos, and Roberto Arenas. 2011. "Lepra en México. Una breve reseña histórica." *Dermatología Revista Mexicana* 55 (5):290–295.

Trouillot, Michel-Rolph. 2001. "The Anthropology of the State in the Age of Globalization: Close Encounters of the Deceptive Kind." *Current Anthropology* 42 (1):125–138.

U.S. Department of Health and Human Services. 1979. "The Belmont Report: Ethical Principles and Guidelines for the Protection of Human Subjects of Research." Office for Human Research Protections. Retrieved 8/20/2020 from https://www.hhs.gov/ohrp/regulations-and-policy/belmont-report/read-the belmont-report/index.html.

Wanderley, F. 2009. "Prácticas estatales y el ejercicio de la ciudadanía: encuentros de la población con la burocracia en Bolivia." *Íconos* 34:67–79.

Chapter 8

The Expanding Human Rights Agenda

Although most civil society organizations that deal with issues of aging actively foster an improved quality of life, if only by providing older individuals a place to interact with others and to learn about healthful lifestyles, some take a more activist approach that includes clearly politically motivated objectives. Among these are the protection of human and social rights. The members of these organizations are not necessarily veterans of the labor movement, nor are they the retired government workers or unionized teachers and university professors we dealt with in Chapter six. Many, though, have participated in the wide range of social movements, protests, and citizen actions that have been common in Mexico. In many ways, they are the vanguard of a new transnational social phenomenon that represents a rejection of the more repressive aspects of tradition, and looks to a future in which the rights of individuals are seen as preeminent and universal. Many of these organizations have been influenced by the international women's movement, the environmental movement, the movement against human trafficking, the human rights movement, and others. Margarita Aragón Fabiola is one such individual and she explained to us how she became an activist fighting for the rights of older people.

MARGARITA: Good afternoon, I am Margarita Aragón Fabiola. I am 75 years old and I have lived in these pedregales (popular zones) in the periphery of the Coyoacán delegation (borough in Mexico City) for 50 years. ... I studied accounting ... many years ago, and later I trained in human rights. I was in the interdisciplinary human rights academy ... I have earned different diplomas, including one in successful aging from the National School of Social Work ... I represent the human rights committee of Ajusco, which is a grassroots committee that was founded by the Jesuits ... We first began to fight for economic, social, cultural, and environmental rights – the right to have a place to live, then the right to education, schools for boys and girls, and then health services. We ... requested and finally have a deed, to these plots that began as squatter encampments.

DOI: 10.4324/9781003205609-8

The committee turned 30 ... on November 7 ... The founding
documents were signed by eighty-four organizations that were part of
the national network of human rights organizations ... This network
works with children, with abused women, and those who are victims
of violence ... I was a co-founder ... before I was on the committee I
was influenced politically and spiritually by the Jesuits and my
training is Christian and inspired politically by liberation theology ...
I was a supporter of seventy associations in these seven colonias ...
The basic objective was first to raise the residents' awareness of their
rights ...

MARGARITA EXPLAINS HOW SHE BECAME ACTIVE IN ELDER RIGHTS: ... I
began to dedicate myself to the rights of the elderly ten years ago
because ... there are people my age who have been evicted by their
own families ... Two years ago in Aztecas Svenue in the camellón, a
man was found on a grass mat at two in the morning. There are cases
right now in which the committee, together with the Miguel Agustín
Pro committee, are bringing criminal charges against individuals who
have dispossessed elderly people. It is very serious ...

Right now, we have ten cases of older people who have been ejected from their homes ... The ejected parents are afraid to denounce
their sons and daughters ... I am an old person, but fortunately I do
not have that problem, which is particularly serious for women in
these poorer zones.

MARGARITA EXPLAINS THE ORGANIZATION'S CONSCIOUSNESS-RAISING
OBJECTIVE AND THE WAY THE MESSAGE IS SPREAD: The central objective is
to sensitize and raise awareness among the people of this popular
area ... so that they know their human rights and know how to
defend them. The number involved multiplies ... ten people tell
another ten and that is how we ... link with each other ... We work
with people from youth groups, boys' and girls' groups, and also with
gay groups, both gay boys and girls from the area ... We have already
spread the message and sensitized people because many of those
youngsters are rejected by their own parents ... We meet in public
places, sometimes the church lends us a multipurpose room, sometimes we meet in a high school, sometimes in some space like the
house of culture ... but many times in private homes.

INTERVIEWER: Where does the desire to work in committee come from?

MARGARITA: My goodness ... well, we arrived here over fifty years ago,
right ... but when we arrived, we had no water, we had no light, this
was a place of invasion (squatter settlement). Well we (Margarita's
family) didn't invade, someone else sold us half of the lot that they
had invaded, but the needs were the same for all of us ... and as I
told you at the beginning we had to find places for schools and more
and this led us to organize ourselves and then to articulate our

demands, but it was a process of about ten to twelve years to achieve. Now it is well established and it works just like a little machine, a little clock. It is very pleasant, I love it.

INTERVIEWER: How do you finance your activities?

MARGARITA: The Jesuit Noyola foundation provided help with projects focused primarily on older people for two years from 2014 to 2016 ... we had to form a Civil Association to be able to ... have legitimacy and for more than money ... we had to have legitimacy with the authorities ... Currently we have no government money but we are carrying out a project promoting ... non-discrimination against older people for which we are seeking funds.

INTERVIEWER: Can you tell us what you consider to be the most important of rights of the elderly?

MARGARITA: Well, for me the most important ones relate to the convention. It is an inter-American international legal instrument that has a gender and rights approach in relation to economic, social, cultural, and environmental rights ... For us, the elderly, the right to work is very important, the right to health, the right to food, the right to education because despite being older people, I believe that we all have the right to continue and progress in our studies. Or if we are illiterate, we have the right to become literate ... the right to life and dignity in old age, the right not to be subjected to torture or cruel, inhuman, and degrading treatment, the right not to be discriminated against – in this area where I live old people are seriously discriminated against. The right to political participation is important ... and I also think it is important to have access to specialized care in risky situations and emergencies.

... Another very important right is access to justice and that the desires of the older person are not undervalued ... Unfortunately, not all of us have a pension ... I think that another very important right is to long-term care ... and for that we must form community groups and organize families.

The Ongoing Struggle for Basic Rights

Margarita Aragón Fabiola is a truly inspiring woman. She was not a union activist, nor has she been a government or party official, although she has worked for non-governmental human rights organizations on highly politicized issues. As she explained, her approach to rights and to social activism was influenced by Jesuit theology, particularly liberation theology, which takes the welfare and rights of the marginalized and powerless victims of social injustice as the core of its mission. Our interaction with Margarita also revealed her commitment to involving her neighbors and others in the struggle to improve their collective well-being. Together over the years these individuals were able to acquire ownership of the land they occupied illegally, and they were able to create communities that developed the collective ability to demand water and other social services from municipal authorities. Margarita is unique in other ways. Both her son and daughter are human rights activists who have been involved in many of Margarita's struggles.

Although Margarita is clearly an exceptional individual in terms of her commitment to social activism, she embodies a spirit that has influenced many Mexican social movements, some of which we have described in previous chapters (de la Garza Toledo 2005; Escobar and Alvarez 1992; Johnston and Almeida 2006; Monsiváis 1987; Stahler-Sholk, Vanden, and Becker 2014; Stahler-Sholk, Vanden, and Kuecker 2008). One particularly important phenomenon to which Margarita's narrative draws our attention is the large number of urban popular movements that emerged after the major student protest movement of 1968. Many of these movements involved land invasions of the sort that Margarita mentioned as the origin of her own community (Delgadillo 2016; Ward 1976; Ward 1998). The rapid urbanization of the country as individuals moved from rural areas to Mexico City, Monterrey, Guadalajara, and other major metropolitan areas was accompanied by a massive housing shortage (Bennett 1992). The problem was compounded by traditional land tenure laws that concentrated land in the hands of a few large landowners (Albertus et al. 2016; Assies 2007; Lombard 2015).

Out of necessity many of the new arrivals took over vacant land owned by large landowners, often at the periphery of urban areas or on old *ejido* plots (communal farmland) that had been incorporated into growing urban areas. Without titles to the land these families were illegal squatters, and although evictions occurred, in order to deal with the potentially explosive situation the government often recognized the squatters' rights and granted them title to the occupied terrain (Lombard 2015). In her book *Fuerte es el Silencio* (Silence is Strong), Elena Poniatowska, a prolific writer and sensitive chronicler of the lives of marginalized Mexicans, recounts one such invasion that took place in Cuernavaca, the capital of the state of Morelos, south of Mexico City:

> The invasion took place at seven in the evening. By the early morning of March 31, 1973, they had taken the land. In Güero Medrano's notebook, seven hundred families were listed – he himself wrote them down – but at the appointed time only six appeared. At nine, two hours later, some people arrived with their belongings in tow. They approached timidly, dragging their feet. Irritated, Güero Medrano yelled "What happened to the others?"
>
> Aquileo Mederos Vásquez, alias Full, his second in command, speculated, "It seems that they were scared by the numerous police patrols around here!"

...

Realizing that the men did not respond as he had expected, Güero Medrano took a motorcycle and that same night he set out to visit all the slums of the city of Cuernavaca. In every quarter he would shout out, "Remember the commitment you made to me, now we are going to carry it out!" The families looked at one another with fear (after all, land invasion is an illicit, criminal act), but they were the same people who had cheered him six days earlier at the ANOCE (National Student Peasant Workers Association) assembly, in which they decided to invade on Saturday, March 31. It was the last meeting and everyone formally committed to being at the Villa de las Flores at seven at night with their belongings. During that week Güero Medrano held meetings of three, four men and women urging them to action: "If we delay, we will lose the land." It had been days that Güero had distributed flyers in the slums of Cuernavaca announcing the invasion of Villa de las Flores and that those who arrived first would be given the best lots.

On Sunday until dawn more colonists arrived: they stood on the ground, numb with fear, they did not even put down their odds and ends so as not to become attached, not to say that this piece is mine. They remained standing embracing a hen, grasping a grocery bag: "We are assessing it all, it's not going to be that bad," until Güero returned with the deafening noise of his motorcycle:

"There isn't a moment to lose. What are you waiting for?"

"It's just that we came to take a look ..."

"What look, if you come as onlookers, go away. If you want land, grab it."

"But Güero."

"Don't be assholes."

Güero Medrano shouted over the din of his machine "Perk up and get to work, I'll be back soon."

And so, pushing them, he distributed four hundred meter lots to each of the first thirty families, with the condition that they build at top speed ... With everything and his shouts, his "hurry up," and his power of conviction, the invaders could not shake their fear. There is no lesson harder than that of freedom. They had brought the most essential things, their casseroles, trinkets, the odd little pot, their dogs and cats ...

Thus, at dawn on March 31, they took the land. Thirty families terrified by their own actions settled in a neighborhood called Villa de las Flores, almost directly in front of the Temixco beach resort, on the road that leaves Cuernavaca towards Taxco.

(Poniatowska 1980, pp. 181–183, author translation)

Over the subsequent years individual families built their homes on the invaded land using their own resources and labor. This scene was repeated in many other places. The huge number of invasions clearly reflected the absence of policies to address the needs of the rapidly growing homeless population. The phenomenon also resulted in strong criticism of the ruling party and fed into a growing social movement with multiple facets. Although the situations in Morelos, Guerrero, and Oaxaca, states characterized by great social inequality, are well known, invasions also occurred in the country's capital, but faced less serious repression. Margarita Fabiola, with whose story we began this chapter, lived through those times and with her family built her home and community on invaded land in the outskirts of Mexico City.

In Chapter six we dealt with organizations whose members had union experience, had worked for governmental agencies, or had experience in politics or education. These experiences provided them human and social capital that they could bring to bear in making collective demands in the hope of improving their lot. Given Mexico's historic clientelism and corporatism, it has been an uphill battle, and until recently largely unsuccessful. Yet those previous experiences represent a clear advantage. They molded expectations and made it clear that even against heavy odds, individuals can act as effective collective agents. The organizations we deal with in this chapter frame their missions more in terms of the new human and social rights agenda. In many ways they are outgrowths of the struggles for workers' rights and the earlier social movements and protests by indigenous peoples, students, landless peasants, and others. They are manifestations of a transition in civil society in Mexico, and perhaps elsewhere, in which the activist lessons of the past are incorporated into a revivified sense of the ability of local groups to influence larger processes and institutions. These organizations draw upon the experience and commitment of a wide range of activists and members of different ethnic groups, with different religious affiliations, and different levels of education and experiences as social activists. They are part of a more dynamic civil society in Mexico that will hopefully increase citizen input into a traditionally corporatist political culture.

Union struggles, student protests, and increasing middle class rejection of the old ways has fueled demands for basic rights and for recognition, in addition to redistribution. Squatter settlements and land invasions are a particularly powerful example. In these cases, ordinary people with little political or union experience or with little education engaged in collective action, in many cases inspired by dynamic personalities like Margarita Fabiola or Güero Medrano who led the invasion of Villa de las Flores, to demand the basic necessities of a dignified life. In Margarita's case, the experience in demanding the rights of squatters fueled a mission to advocate for older individuals and their unique needs. In what follows we examine the frames these organizations employ to further the cause of the rights of older Mexicans.

Social Uprisings and the "Dirty War"

Given the high stakes, the struggle for social rights and the social movements that furthered that agenda have not always been peaceful. Although Mexico may not have experienced the same level of State violence against political opposition that occurred in other Latin American nations, the decades of the 1960s and 1970s were characterized by often violent protests and equally violent State repression. As in other Latin American countries this unrest was fueled by massive social inequalities, widespread poverty, and completely inadequate State policies and institutions. In addition to widespread protest, the period saw the emergence of numerous guerrilla movements that fought for the rights of workers and other groups (Mendoza García 2011). These included teachers, railroad workers, doctors, copper miners, landless peasants, university students, and others. Most of these movements were aggressively repressed (Minetti 2017). The official state response focused on the elimination of opposition to the ruling party, the PRI, through violently repressive actions that became known as the "dirty war" in which thousands of individuals were killed (Aviña 2016; McCormick 2017; Mendoza García 2011). The 1968 student protests in the Plaza de las Tres Cultural in Tlatelolco that we mentioned at the beginning of Chapter one ended in the massacre of hundreds of students.

The resort to guerilla tactics reflected the fact that opposition parties were weak and any criticism of the ruling party was forced underground and stigmatized as communist. Although the Communist Party did exist and groups such as the 23 September League, a communist cell, engaged in violent actions, such as the attempted kidnapping and murder of Enrique Garza Sada who we introduced in Chapter six (Illades 2017), most movement members were driven by desperation rather than political motives. The administrations of Gustavo Díaz Ordaz (December 1, 1964–November 30, 1970) and Luis Echeverría (December 1, 1970–November 30, 1976) stand out for their high levels of repression and for their serious unwillingness and inability to alleviate widespread poverty or address the problems caused by massive migration from the countryside to large cities. Teachers Rubén Jaramillo (1900–1962), Genaro Vázquez (1931–1972), and Lucio Cabañas (1938–1974), heirs of the Emiliano Zapata struggle, were leaders of one of the many guerrilla uprisings against injustice and the concentration of wealth in just a few hands (Glockner 2007). During the Echeverríia administration their movement faced violent repression punctuated by the murder of activists.

An Evolving Human and Social Rights Discourse

Our categorizations of CSO frames and discourses is clearly somewhat arbitrary and the different categories overlap to varying degrees. As we have noted, nearly all CSOs at some level share aspects of the quality of life frame since assuring the highest quality of life possible for older individuals is a common, if not specifically stated goal. While neither retired union members nor their organizations frame their objectives in terms of active aging or improving the quality of life of their members, their focus on guaranteeing retired workers the material and social rights they earned through union membership clearly furthers that objective. Although maintaining or even improving an older person's physical and mental health is clearly central to fostering active aging and assuring a high quality of life, reaching that objective cannot be accomplished without altering the social reality within which older individuals' health and well-being are determined (Estes 2001; Estes 2011). Individuals age in unique cultural, economic, and political contexts in which their access to the necessities of active aging are determined. Along with age, one's gender, race, ethnicity, religion, sexual identity, and more interact to place certain individuals and groups at particularly high risk of disadvantage and marginalization throughout the life course (Collins and Bilge 2016; Estes 2001).

A core characteristic of the organizations we deal with in this chapter is that they are focused on the structural sources of active aging. In addition, they specifically include human rights in their explanatory frames. We see them as representing a new phase in the development of civil society in Mexico in which large numbers of previously disengaged individuals and groups become more aware of the political, social, and economic factors that constrain their freedoms and keep them marginalized. They are part of a growing awareness of individuals' ability to act collectively to change the status quo.

An International Social Movement

As we noted in Chapter three, the conception of human rights as basic, inviolate, and universal gained widespread support only in the 1970s (Moyn 2010). After World War II, the United Nations General Assembly adopted the *Universal Declaration of Human Rights*, the first international statement affirming the existence and universality of such rights (United Nations 1948). However, the Declaration did not immediately protect the rights of many groups of people, including racial, religious, and ethnic minorities and others, among which were older people who faced serious risk of discrimination, poverty, and social marginalization. Progress in defining and protecting their rights and interests was slow and involved decades of effort by organizations that brought the plight of vulnerable older individuals to the public's attention. In Chapter three we summarized the major international forums and conventions that established the basic principles concerning the rights of older individuals. These international conventions, which were particularly important in Latin America, reflect what is in fact a new transnational social movement motivated by many previous movements dealing with the rights of older persons and others. The objective of this movement is to reframe the ways in which older persons and society at large view the aging process. The ultimate objective, as we have emphasized throughout, is to change the image of old-age from that of a period of decline and disengagement, to one of active citizenship and participation. In this chapter we emphasize the role of CSOs in fostering these international conventions and their growing role in furthering the recognition of the human rights of all groups

Parallel Forums of CSOs

It is important to note that the official government-sponsored meetings on the rights of older persons that have taken place during the last twenty years did not occur in a political vacuum. In all cases, parallel forums of civil society organizations met at more or less the same time and made their opinions known to the official government representatives. These independent organizations clearly influenced the principles that were affirmed and the recommendations that were made (Díaz Oramas et al. 2019; Montes de Oca et al. 2018). These parallel forums were similar to those that feminist organizations have held in conjunction with the major international conferences on women's rights (United Nations 2020).

Although we provided a general overview of this series of conferences in Chapter three, we reiterate their major objectives here in terms of the actions of specific civil society organizations, given their relevance to new initiatives at a local level. The first of the major conferences was the NGO World Forum on Aging that took place in April 2002 in Madrid, Spain (World NGO Forum on Aging 2002b). That conference signaled the beginning of a new era in the public discourse on older people; it introduced their marginalized status as a major focus of the international human and social rights movement. An important aspect of the Madrid meeting was that it drew particular attention to the serious problems faced by older persons in developing countries (Montes de Oca 2003). The conference produced a document entitled "Development and the Rights of Older People" that framed the many specific issues addressed in terms of basic rights and the appropriate response of governments and other social institutions. The clear message was that the plight of the world's impoverished and marginalized older population could no longer be ignored. The Forum's proposals fueled academic interest and stimulated scientific research into the serious needs of older persons that local, state, and federal governments were not addressing. Of particular importance for low and middle-income countries was the Forum's emphasis on the importance of adapting development initiatives and goals to include older individuals. The final report notes that:

> One of the most important challenges is integrating aging into development processes and international commitments to enable older people to escape chronic poverty. The international community must take steps to ensure lifelong health care and sufficient means to age with dignity, with the aim of creating fully integrated societies in a more just and united global world.
>
> (World NGO Forum on Aging 2002b)

The final report also emphasizes the potential role of non-governmental organizations when it states that:

> Most particularly, we must conclude that NGOs are legitimate channels for civil society to be able to demand the achievement of a special dimension in the construction of a new society through their actions, which attempt to remedy the culture of indifference, exasperated individualism, competitiveness and utilitarianism which currently threaten all realms of human fellowship, and, in order to avoid all rupture between generations, NGOs are destined to promote a new mindset, new customs, news ways of being, a new culture based on solidarity. For all these reasons, the NGOs assembled in Madrid at the II World Forum on Ageing proclaim the need to build not only a society for all ages, but a society that pursues social justice and welfare without forgetting to place individuals and their dignity at the centre of its goals.
>
> (Official translation: World NGO Forum on Aging 2002a)

Many issues were discussed in the multiple meetings of the CSOs that converged in Madrid. Those that stand out include economic development and humanitarian aid, human rights, the right to health, the right to housing, the fostering of public policies favorable to older persons, the right to social participation, and more. Human rights, together with gender, pervaded the recommendations and represented major intersecting foci. The Forum also called for ombudsmen for the elderly, and it focused on age discrimination, poverty, the situation of ethnic minorities, migration, legal protections, and more. One hundred seventeen recommendations were grouped into three priority areas: (1) older people and development, (2) the promotion of well-being and health, and (3) the creation of favorable environments for older people.

Following the Madrid meeting, a series of regional forums organized by the Economic Commission for Latin America and the Caribbean (ECLAC) were held to begin the implementation of the Madrid recommendations and to assess the situation of older people locally. These meetings brought together academics, regional CSOs, and government officials. The first meeting was held two years after Madrid in Santiago de Chile in 2003, from which a document entitled the *Declaration of Civil Society* emerged (https://consultora cec.files.wordpress.com/2015/08/sociedad-civil-declaracion-de-santiago-2003. pdf). This meeting brought together seventy-four national civil society organizations and thirteen international networks and agencies. Again, this meeting focused on the human and social rights of older persons, and the need to alleviate poverty and to defend their dignity. By this point the international human rights agenda had taken on an aging aspect. The following paragraph conveys the tone of the final document. It states that the:

> poverty, discrimination, and exclusion in which older adults live are incompatible with human dignity, with the mandate of our Constitutions that consecrate the person as the end of society and the State, with the principles and international commitments that the States have signed regarding the universality, integrality and interdependence of Human Rights.
>
> (Declaration of Santiago de Chile, 2003)

In 2007 the next regional forum took place in Brasilia. For the most part, it was a repeat of Santiago and expressed many of the same demands, but it went a step further. The forum suggested the adoption of an international convention as a mechanism for guiding the actions of State governments (https://www.un.org/esa/socdev/ageing/documents/regional_review/ Declaracion_Brasilia.pdf). Among the twenty-nine proposals included in the final report were the following:

> 24.Recommend that account be taken of older persons in the efforts under way to achieve the internationally agreed development goals, including those adopted in the Millennium Declaration; 25.Agree to request the member countries of the United Nations Human Rights Council to consider the possibility of appointing a special rapporteur responsible for the promotion and protection of the human rights of older persons; 26.Pledge to make the necessary consultations with our Governments to promote the drafting of a convention on the rights of older persons within the framework of the United Nations.
>
> (Declaration of Brasilia, 2007)

Along with these international discussions and a growing consensus on human rights that had evolved to include economic, social, cultural, and environmental rights, something extremely important for the political and social extension of human rights occurred in Mexico. In 2011, a major reform to the Constitution was introduced designed to guarantee the human rights of all citizens and to bring the Mexican Constitution into conformity with the highest international standards (Ek 2012; García-Castillo 2015). This change was particularly important since it accompanied the creation of several autonomous publicly funded agencies that are charged with defending human rights and monitoring the actions of the Mexican government's public policy institutions. The constitutional reform was a somewhat belated response to the serious violations of human rights that had been common in the past. This reform largely reaffirms the Constitution of 1917, which represented a legal watershed in the defense of the human rights of women, children, the elderly, migrants, and people with disabilities. Despite the 1917 guarantees, serious violations of basic rights continued. The 2011 reforms were an attempt to address these shortcomings and reflect a changing public awareness of human rights.

In 2012, ten years after Madrid, another Regional Meeting of Civil Society on Aging was held in Costa Rica, resulting in the Declaration of Tres Ríos, which was largely focused on Central America. The most striking aspect of this forum was an extensive focus on migrant, indigenous, and Afro-descendant populations. These groups had suffered serious violations of human rights in the region. For the first time in the series this forum pointed out the problem of multiple discrimination, that is discrimination based on two or more characteristics, as well as the unique mistreatment and abuse inflicted upon the old. Among the main proposals appears a clear call for policies that recognize and promote respect for the diversity of old age that exists in rural areas, especially in less developed countries. It states that:

> The focus of public policies and programs directed at the elderly has not been accompanied by the development of a vision of old age that accounts for the diversity of ways of aging. They lack intergenerational and gender perspectives and make rural, indigenous, and Afro-descendant people invisible.
>
> (Red Latinoamericana de Gerontología 2012)

The Declaration of Tres Ríos is also unique in that it includes a more elaborate analysis of the problems faced by old people in Latin America and the Caribbean based on scientific evidence. This includes information on important aspects of the labor market, including informality and precariousness that result in inadequate social security coverage in old age. The Declaration reflects a very important evolution in the discourse on human rights, that continues in the Charter of San José, which emerged from the third regional intergovernmental conference on aging in Latin

America and the Caribbean held in San José, Costa Rica in 2012 (CEPAL 2012; Huenchuan 2013), as well as the Montevideo Consensus on Population and Development (CEPAL 2013). Montevideo covered all population groups from a human rights and gender perspective, but integrated new dimensions focused on culture and the life course. These documents were important antecedents of the Inter-American Convention for the Protection of the Human Rights of Older Persons, which in 2015 was adopted by the Organization of American States and embodied in the Yapacaraí declaration of 2017.

The Montevideo Consensus

In order to provide some sense of the significance of these accords let us briefly describe the Montevideo Consensus on Population and Development, which consists of ten chapters that address different issues related to population policy. A notable aspect of this document was the degree of consensus that resulted in more than thirty-three countries in the Latin American and Caribbean region signing on to a document which introduces a rights-based and gender-based approach to population policy. The first chapter addresses the integration of populations and their dynamics in sustainable development with equality and respect for human rights. It promotes respect for the human rights of children, adolescents, young adults, and the old. It specifically underscores the importance of the rights of women, people with disabilities, as well as migrants, LBGTQ individuals, indigenous peoples, and Afro-descendants. It also addresses the specific situation of rural residents, that is those who live in the countryside or the jungle, and well as the unique needs of those who live in urban territories and spaces. Although this consensus will hopefully eventually be superseded by even more inclusive agreements, to date it is the most inclusive document dealing with culture, gender, and human rights. In addition, it also recognizes the importance of civil society organizations and social movements in furthering the human rights agenda.

Section C. is entitled "Aging, social protection and socioeconomic challenges," and identifies older people as subjects with specific rights as well as needs related to their unique cultural, gender, and population groups. This section recognizes the importance of the participation of older people in development and recognizes their potential contribution. It also condemns the stigmatization of older people and promotes a philosophy of active aging and the maintenance of an intergenerational exchange that contributes to overall social welfare and development. Another central issue addressed in this section that was echoed in subsequent conventions is a clear condemnation of age discrimination in all its multiple forms including physical, sexual, economic, and psychological. This document is linked to other conventions that deal with human rights, such as the Women's Platform for Action of the Fourth World Conference on Women, the convention on the rights of persons with disabilities, the permanent forums for indigenous issues, the International Decade for People of African Descent, the Durban Declaration and Program of Action adopted at the World Conference against Racism, Racial Discrimination, Xenophobia and Related Intolerance, and the High-level Dialogue on International Migration and Development, among others. For all these reasons and more, the Montevideo Convention represents one of the most important legal instruments in the world in terms of the progress it represents in the definition, conceptualization, and proposed responses to age-based discrimination.

A recent addition to this series of CSO forums and declarations was the Ypacaraí Declaration, named after the Paraguayan city where a meeting of more than 350 older people, primarily leaders of civil society organizations from eighteen countries in Latin America and the Caribbean region, was held in 2017. Each participant traveled hours by bus and used their own resources to participate in the event. Never before had so many issues been addressed at so many meetings organized by older persons themselves. Several accomplishments stand out. Among the most important was strong support for the signing of the Inter-American Convention for the Protection of the Human Rights of Older Persons. This strong sentiment also informed discussions in several of the panels represented and reflected an unprecedented evolution in the defense of human rights, especially with reference to older individuals.

The impact of Ypacaraí and of the previous regional meetings organized by ECLAC is clearly revealed in the increased references to human rights in publications produced by the region's CSOs and the official documents of the intergovernmental forums that clearly responded to CSO pressure. An ATLAS.ti word count of the various official multilateral pronouncements revealed an increase in the occurrence of the word "rights" from nineteen in the Santiago declaration of 2003 to 741 in the Declaración de Asunción in 2017.

The Paraguayan forum also dealt with international migration and the unique experiences of aging characteristic of the islands of the Caribbean and the Antilles. It also addressed new concerns such as sexuality among the elderly and their post-reproductive health. The rights that were identified as in most urgent need of recognition were the rights to economic security, health care, work opportunities, personal care and support for caregivers, institutional care, participation in social life, and more. The seriously negative effects of violence, abuse, poverty, multiple discrimination, and ageism were strongly condemned. The activism of civil society organizations demanding prompt action by governments almost immediately resulted in the Declaration of Asunción in 2017.

A New Perspective

The spirit and objectives of these new international conventions on human rights generally, and the rights of older persons in particular, reflect a recent and profound transformation in the public conception of human and civil rights of specific groups. They also testify to the important role of civil society organizations in bringing about major change in public policies. Today, inequality and discrimination, and the entrenched social mechanisms that perpetuate them, remain serious problems in Latin America, as they do elsewhere. It would be easy to become cynical about the possibilities for change. The 1970s and 1980s in Latin America were a period of dictatorship and widespread and shocking human rights abuses. As we have documented, that period led to protests and social activism against the grotesque inequalities and injustice that have historically characterized Latin America. However slow or incomplete the evolution of this new discourse may be, it reflects a new reality in which human rights abuses can no longer be completely hidden from public view. This progress represents an evolution of the spirit of the Mexican constitutional amendments of 2011 related to human rights, and the statements of principle of the conventions we have described. It is also clear that any hope for an invigorated civil society is heavily dependent on the collective action of organizations committed to that end.

In terms of civil society organizations we identified four large groupings that employ different frames with reference to human rights and older persons. This four-group classification is again primarily for the sake of discussion. Clear distinctions between groups are impossible since their boundaries remain fuzzy. Based on our observations these four groups consist of: (1) those that provide care to older people without a specific focus on human rights; (2) those that advocate for human rights generally, without a specific focus on the rights of older persons; (3) CSOs in transition that did not previously concern themselves with human rights, but are increasingly doing so; and (4) those that take protecting and extending human rights as a core mission. In this chapter we focus on the second, third, and fourth categories.

Human Rights without a Focus on Aging

Let us begin with those organizations that struggle for human rights generally, but do not specifically focus on aging or the needs of older people as part of their core explanatory frame or agenda. Later we will examine organizations that advocate for the rights of older persons, often in the context of a more general struggle for social, economic, cultural, and environmental rights. The dynamic of an organization's adoption of the rights agenda can be convoluted. Many organizations that today further a general human and social rights agenda began their efforts in defense of a particular right, such as the right to education, to housing, to economic security, and more. Often, as part of this process they became aware of the particular plight of older persons.

We encountered organizations that have been somewhat out of the public eye, but that have become increasingly vocal in furthering a human rights agenda, although again while not specifically addressing the unique rights of older persons. These organizations operate in an environment in which federal, State, and municipal governments have established bureaus and agencies that address the human rights of women, indigenous populations, and Afro-descendant peoples. We located several civil society organizations of this sort in Oaxaca. This more general view of the rights of vulnerable individuals can be seen in groups of lawyers who are dedicated to defending the rights of indigenous women and other traditionally marginalized groups. As of yet, though, they do not view age as an independent dimension of disadvantage. Although the discourse on rights is evolving, the role of age as an intersecting dimension of disadvantage that undermines the welfare of indigenous, afro-descendent, and other groups has not been fully articulated. The absence of a human rights perspective with reference to the elderly was evident in the statement by a public servant who told us that she did not have the resources to identify or address the special needs of older persons. She noted that:

> Oaxaca has a care system made up of municipal agencies ... I cannot change it, nor is there going to be an extra provision for adults, the elderly, or for changing mental conceptions so that people can think of themselves not as helpless, but as people with rights and a lot of wisdom that they contribute.
>
> (B. G., female, Councilor for Human Rights and Gender Equity)

In Oaxaca a public and governmental affirmation of the human rights of specific groups, including women, has emerged, but the city has no office or specific agency to deal with human rights issues related to older individuals. This lack of an institutional mechanism at the state level for dealing with the unique needs of older citizens is common in Mexico, as it is elsewhere. The existence of formal governmental recognition of a group's human rights of course does not necessarily translate immediately into effective action to protect them. Although a public discourse and agenda focused on gender equality has evolved in recent years, sexism remains a serious problem. The agenda focused on aging is more recent, and is in reality only beginning to take shape. The reasons for this lack of attention to aging issues is clear, as we have noted in earlier chapters. The pace of population aging presents Mexico with serious challenges, but it is a fairly recent phenomenon. As one human rights official told us:

The Mexican state is overwhelmed by this reality of older people they have not been able to deal with and have taken actions, pure assistance actions with very few human rights actions ... The challenge we have is to make a diagnosis because we do not have data. The other is that we do not have mapping of structural needs, which have to do with work, which have to do with physical integrity, which have to do with housing, which have to do with intrafamily violence ... and also have to do with autonomy.

(J. S., Ombudsman for Human Rights of the people of Oaxaca)

Although a focus on the rights of older persons has emerged only recently, as we note a clear agenda is forming and more organizations, including those in our third group, that were not focused on older persons before, are expanding their missions to include advocacy for and service delivery to older persons. CSOs in Mexico, as elsewhere, operate in complex organizational and political environments that include other organizations, governmental agencies, and institutions of higher learning, many of which are involved in research and advocacy related to issues of central interest to CSOs. As the old-age agenda emerges these organizations communicate and share insights, motivating further action. Public universities are important actors in furthering this agenda. Their faculties engage in research sponsored by the government and other organizations, and they collaborate with CSOs in the definition and defense of the human rights of older people. These collaborations are particularly important in identifying the structural factors that undermine the welfare of older people and in conveying that information to other professionals and to the public at large.

Oaxaca again provides a useful example. The General Directorate of Population Studies of Oaxaca conducted a study of the situation of older people in the state. It was the first in-depth study of older persons carried out in this culturally, linguistically, and ethnically diverse area. The findings provided important information concerning the situation of older persons from different subgroups as well as insights into threats to their human rights (Dirección General de población de Oaxaca 2020; Rea Ángeles and Montes de Oca 2020). Unfortunately, although research on human rights has increased at other universities, few studies address the human rights of groups that face particularly serious threats, including older people, individuals with disabilities, or even middle-class women who experience physical, psychological, and economic abuse (Vilar-Compte et al. 2018). Again, though, concern for the rights of older people is growing, often as a result of their own militancy.

The Struggle for the Human Rights of Older Persons

The struggle for the human rights of the elderly accompanies the emergence or recommitment of those organizations that seek to extend the rights of all groups, our fourth category. Among these are research institutions and institutions of higher learning in which the new agenda is emerging. Various organizations address issues related to the human rights of older persons from different perspectives. An interesting and informative case is that of the *Unión de Posesionarios Tierra y Libertad A.C.* (Union of Landholders and Liberty) located in Monterrey, Nuevo León. This organization's mission is based on a community perspective that reflects the student struggles of the 1970s. Its mission focuses on addressing basic needs of those in distress. A concept of human rights as basic and inviolate represents a core frame that informs and structures the organization's actions and its struggle to provide food and shelter to those in need. It provides food in communal dining areas to individuals of all ages, but it pays particular attention to the needs of older persons. In addition to food and clothing the Union provides housing, as well as other services. It does not receive government aid, but relies on donations from a range of donors to finance its operation. In terms of rights, it actively defends general social, economic, cultural, and environmental rights, but again it pays particular attention to the specific rights of older persons. One participant explained that for older individuals:

> [t]he first thing is the right to a pension ... that helps you to be a human being who can enjoy your old age, and ... not only food, home, shelter, clothing, but traveling ... we have it in a real way, Human Rights ... the right to ... medical care, the right to a dignified old age, the right to housing, indeed the right to a quality education.
>
> (E. D., male, Unión de Posesionarios Tierra y Libertad,
> Monterrey, NL)

The organization's location in Monterrey, Nuevo León is clearly one reason for its success. Nuevo León is Mexico's most economically dynamic state with many enterprises and entrepreneurs. This is the state in which the fight for labor and civil rights began and which was the home of human rights activist Rosario Ibarra de Piedra who formed the *Comité Nacional Pro-defensa de Presos, Perseguidos, Desaparecidos y Exiliados Políticos* (National Committee for the Defense of Political Prisoners, the Persecuted, the Disappeared and Political Exiles) in 1977 after her activist son disappeared at the hands of the police (Negrín 2020; Poniatowska 1980, pp. 138–180). Her mission was similar to that of the Madres de la Plaza de Mayo in Argentina that we presented in the first chapter, and it reflected and contributed to a nascent human rights activism that continues today. Ibarra de Piedra was Mexico's first female presidential candidate and served in Congress during the 1980s. This history provided fertile ground for the Unión de Posesionarios Tierra y Libertad and for other human rights advocates. As we mentioned, the Union provides community dining rooms, groceries, health care, vaccinations, legal advice, support for early pregnancy, education, and more to individuals of all ages. The organization also instills a clear sense of rights in those it serves. Another participant explained her understanding of rights:

> Everyone has the right to an adequate standard of living, which ensures, to herself and to her family, health and well-being, especially food, clothing, housing, medical assistance and the necessary social services; you have the same right to insurance in cases of unemployment, illness, widowhood, old age, other cases of loss of means.
>
> (E. D., male, Unión de Posesionarios Tierra y Libertad, Monterrey, NL)

Academic Activists

In the modern world universities, public and private research institutes, and the governmental agencies and private foundations that fund their research are increasingly central to economic development and to an equitable and efficient welfare state. Research into the structural causes of the marginalization of specific groups is vital if one is to attempt to create a more just world. Certainly, politics plays an important role in perpetuating or alleviating human misery, but knowledge is power and it lends a moral force to attempts to change the status quo. Today in Mexico as elsewhere research by academics and independent research institutes is expanding rapidly, as is a growing collaboration between these institutions and civil society organizations in joint efforts to understand and address the plight of older persons with few resources and serious health care and other needs. In many cases activist retiree organizations are established by academics themselves.

Among the most important participants in the human rights debate and struggle are organizations of retired academics who come together to maintain their academic ties, but also to provide some continuity between the intellectual work they pursued during their working years and their activities in retirement. These groups of retirees are highly educated and for the most part physically and mentally sound. In many ways they represent the very definition of active aging. From their perspective, education forms the core of successful aging. An appreciation of the importance of life-long education represents a profound development in gerontology. Education early in life appears to significantly increase one's cognitive reserve, and intellectual and social engagement later in life may allow one to maintain a higher level of certain cognitive abilities longer than might otherwise be possible (Thow et al. 2018; Zarebski 2011; Zhou, Wang and Fang 2018).

This philosophy of lifelong learning is put into practice in different ways. On the one hand, groups of retired professors, teachers, and researchers at public and private institutions maintain an active presence in these institutions. In many cases they continue with union activities and do not form independent organizations of retirees. Other initiatives are aimed at older individuals without academic or research backgrounds who may have less education, but who wish to engage intellectually and to further their understanding of important issues, including human rights. Retired professors provide important educational opportunities to these individuals at a point in life in which education was traditionally irrelevant. This is a substantial change in the traditional philosophy of education that focuses on the quality of life itself and not just on preparation for the job market.

Mexico lags behind other Latin American nations in the introduction of these sorts of programs, but they are growing at a rapid pace. This new philosophy of lifelong education comes with new labels, "geragogy" or "gerontagogy," terms which emphasize the fact that the education of older individuals must pursue appropriate objectives and employ pedagogical methods suited to their needs (Fernández-Portero 1999). Several groups are pursuing variations of these objectives. An interesting experiment was begun in 1988 at the Autonomous University of Nuevo León, which in 2003 gave rise to the Regional Center for the Study of the Elderly. The program introduced a service at the university hospital, the goal of which was to reduce the consumption of medications, especially inappropriate drugs. The program's philosophy treats the patients' human rights as paramount, even when they are undergoing medical treatment. The approach is a reaffirmation of the basic principle of autonomy that we discussed previously which places the respect for an individual's basic right to choose for him or herself above all other considerations. The program draws on the expertise of a multidisciplinary team that includes geriatricians, nurses, social workers, gerontologists, rehabilitation therapists, and psychologists. As one administrator explained:

> In the area of human rights there is more and more awareness because with the participation of INAPAM and the DIF it has become more and more salient, and since the protection of human rights is part of the attorney general's mandate, we see the beginning of respect for the human rights of the elderly.
>
> (R. S., male, Administrator, Regional Center for the Study of the Elderly of the UANL, Monterrey, Nuevo León)

The program's location in Monterrey gives it access to charitable funding by local businessmen among other sources. Its financing strategy assures sustainability and offers a very valuable resource for universities and their staffs. This same administrator told us that patients are charged nothing:

[t]he patient is not charged a penny, all his visits, all his consultations are free. The center receives a remuneration that allows it to continue working and giving service to those who do not have resources. We take from the rich to give to the poor.

(R. S., male, Administrator, Regional Center for the Study of the Elderly of the UANL, Monterrey, Nuevo León)

The mission of the regional center complements that of the University of the Elderly of the Autonomous University of Nuevo León. This program, created in 2011, serves the segment of the city's population we mentioned above that consists of older individuals who wish to continue their educations. The popularity and success of this program clearly demonstrates a concern for older individuals in Monterrey, which is aging rapidly given long average life spans of its residents. The core foci of the program are optimal social functioning, cultural awareness, and health. This broadened perspective of the program is striking in light of the fact that given high rates of old-age poverty, income adequacy has always been an overriding priority for CSOs and others, often resulting in a narrow focus that excludes middle-class individuals with needs such as education and intellectual engagement (Garay Villegas and Montes de Oca Zavala 2011).

Because of their high average levels of education and previous experiences, many of these associations of teachers began with a concern for human rights in their explanatory frames. This perspective is revealed in their official communications, which emphasize citizenship and social participation as important aspects of the exercise of rights in old age. As one 58-year-old women stated, "We take a course ... and it focuses on that, it is literally called 'Human Rights and the culture of peace,' there you see the human rights of the elderly" (Lourdes Sánchez Márquez, Universidad del Adulto Mayor, UANL, Monterrey, Nuevo León).

The focus on education is highly progressive in that it rejects an instrumentalist or pragmatic conception of education that treats it as appropriate only for the young and only for the purpose of preparation for the labor market. As one instructor explained:

In fact, our program is based on the theory of successful aging, from there this arises and I am fully convinced, although there are those who debate and have said no, they have told me and I am fully convinced that if we keep older adults and not just older adults, the entire population, we keep it active in mind and body, they will better develop their abilities and skills and obviously they will last longer, but with quality of life, that is, this is what we ensure that they have a better quality of life in old age.

(L. S., female, Universidad del Adulto Mayor, UANL, Monterrey, Nuevo León)

Another clear benefit of these sorts of initiatives is the support networks they foster and the organizations themselves that provide the sort of emotional support that makes them similar to family. These organizations and their educational focus and their emphasis on intellectual engagement clearly contribute to a higher quality of life, even if that is not the stated objective. When they identify their common interests older people find ways of interacting with each other. These interactions take many forms, including taking group trips, attending events together, learning about new topics and more. The most important outcome, though, is that they begin to take control of their own lives. As Lourdes Sánchez explained:

> With us a student arrives and another totally different one comes out, apart from the academic growth it is a lot, yes, but apart from that, the personal growth that this gives them is enough in that they meet, they continue and thus they form groups of everything, they organize, yeah? They go to parties they celebrate.
> (L. S., female, Universidad del Adulto Mayor, UANL, Monterrey, Nuevo León)

Another notable example is Adultos Mayores en Acción, or Older Adults in Action (*AMA y Trasciende A.C.*: https://silo.tips/download/envejecimien to-exitoso-una-tarea-de-responsabilidad-individual). This organization formed at the Instituto Tecnológico y de Estudios Superiores de Monterrey, ITESM (Technological Institute of Monterrey), a private institution, in 2009. It was made up of retired professors who continue to contribute to the educational and service missions of the university. It has expanded to include businessmen and other employees of businesses in Monterrey. Perhaps most importantly, though, it embodies a uniquely active perspective on aging. The members of this association work with companies and also respond to government requests to assist with projects in communities. Given the wide range of academic backgrounds of its members, these contributions are primarily interdisciplinary and many deal with education. The association represents a valuable source of training and service to the community. It also serves as a clear lesson of the potential loss to society were these still productive older professors relegated to a life of idleness. One female participant told us of their origin. She explained that:

> the first thing we did is hold a seminar on challenges ... for the elderly in the 21st Century. So, what we did was ask ourselves what are you going to be about? We focused on four areas: physical, psychological-mental, spiritual, and patrimonial. So, we invited experts in each one ... we asked them to participate from the heart and we wanted to ask for a modest fee to make an *ambigu* (snack), and

diplomas and others, Since then, as we are teachers here at Tec, they provide us with facilities ... and in January 2009 we constituted ourselves as a Civil Association.

(M. F., female, AMA and Trasciende, Monterrey, Nuevo León)

Given the high level of education of its members, the association has a well-articulated conception of human rights and further a human rights agenda as part of its core mission. In order to promote the cause of human rights more broadly the association has formed links with state agencies that are responsible for the enforcement of the human rights of the elderly. These collaborations promote gradual progress in the consolidation of human rights in Monterrey and the nation as a whole. The same female participant explained that:

we are working there, hand in hand, even now that the Human Rights Commission of Mexico has come, let's plan another project for the citizen laboratories, the issue of disability comes up, but it extends to the elderly. I do not know if you have heard about citizen laboratories ... it is very good because it is to involve citizens, it is a project we value, you need people to implement it, we get the people ... that is very cool ...

(M. F., female, AMA and Trasciende, Monterrey, Nuevo León)

Since the association originates from a private university it largely reflects the values and addresses the needs of a middle-class population whose unique needs are often not taken into account by public policies, many of which of necessity focus primarily on the poor. For this more resourced group a lack of basic needs is less of a problem, and other considerations take precedence. Their focus goes beyond basic needs to emphasize the centrality of human rights more generally. This association represents a segment of the older adult population that worked for many years in the formal sector in public or private companies in which they enjoyed a relatively high standard of living, even as they experienced the inevitable transitions of life such as widowhood, retirement, and illness.

Following much the same logic as AMA y Trasciende, an association was formed by retired academics of the Universidad Nacional Autónoma de México, UNAM (the National Autonomous University of Mexico) in Mexico City. The organization adopted the name *Pioneros de Creatividad en Libertad*, PICRELI (Pioneers of Creativity in Freedom). Its members consist of professors and researchers who have dedicated their lives to research and teaching. For them retirement from active duty represents an opportunity to experiment with other ways of contributing to future generations of students, to the University, and to the nation at large. Although this organization has a sophisticated understanding of the human rights of the elderly, there are few innovative initiatives generated by the members themselves, and as hopeful as these initiatives might be, they remain limited since participation by older professors is limited. In each program between thirty and fifty people participate. This limitation restricts the potential reach of these retiree organizations.

In Yucatán, as in Oaxaca, there are other initiatives or programs centered in private universities such as the Universidad Marista de Mérida, A. C. in Mérida, Yucatán, and the Universidad Del Adulto Mayor, UNIDAM (University of the Older Adult) in Oaxaca. Both are programs that seek to promote education among older people, many of whom left school early and in later life wish to resume their studies as part of the growing emphasis on human development and the right to self-realization and education throughout life. These opportunities compensate to some degree for the educational and training deficits that these older generations experienced in their earlier lives. For them technology is very important given recent developments and the fact that older generations did not have the opportunity to learn about and use new communications and other technologies in their youths leads many to wish to gain some basic mastery even in old age. Mastering these new skills, at least to some degree, is not only useful in linking individuals from different generations, it also conveys an element of status that many aspire to.

We do not want to end this chapter without mentioning two important instances in which older people have assumed the role of organized political actors in defense of their human rights. The first is related to the production of various documents that reflect the new activist philosophy that motivates these organizations. It includes the work of *HelpAge*, an international organization with branches everywhere that advocates for the rights of older persons. The HelpAge Latin American branch has promoted an examination of the conditions that civil society organizations face in their attempts to convince nations to approve the Inter-American Convention for the Protection of Human Rights of Older Persons that we mentioned earlier. This examination reveals the diversity of social and political conditions that foster or impede the adoption of major initiatives to benefit older persons. It also reveals how strategic alliances and effective appropriation processes can have positive effects.

The investigation also concluded that the recognition of civil society by the State is vital, as is the support of the government, including legislatures, for adoption of the Convention. The investigation also concluded that the media plays a very important role in shaping the public agenda and raising social awareness about the condition of old age as well as the aging process. The active role and participation of CSOs in advocacy and institutionalization draws attention to the benefits of ratification (Díaz Oramas et al. 2019).

Another important event that included civil society organizations with a focus on older persons took place on the same dates in the city of Puebla de Zaragoza. That meeting addressed a series of highly relevant topics for the situation of older persons in Mexico. The document that was produced "Envejecer con dignidad y derechos humanos en México: Nuestra meta" (Aging with dignity and human rights in Mexico: our goal), was prepared by working groups in an event that brought together twenty-four groups sponsored by the Mexican National Human Rights Commission. This document addresses specific thematic dimensions, such as: (1) health, (2) economic security, (3) gender, stereotypes, and discrimination, (4) social participation, and (5) civil protection. The latter dimension was motivated by the recent earthquake that caused serious damage in Oaxaca, Puebla, and Mexico City. Based on these thematic dimensions, objectives and commitments were proposed to further the objective of the full realization of the human rights of older persons, with a gender and non-discrimination perspective as suggested by international experts who attended the event.

Currently, and for the first time in its history, Mexico has a government that takes the plight of the most disadvantaged citizens, and especially that of older persons, seriously. Yet its approach does not foster or make full use of civil society. Indeed, a populist approach to social welfare can downplay or even exclude civil society organizations in order to make the State the ultimate benefactor to the needy. Of course, convincing or shaming the State to assume such responsibilities is ironically a major objective of such organizations. Today, in Mexico individuals 68 and older with no other source of income receive a non-contributory pension. In this context the role of CSOs is to extend the right to such pensions and to ensure that older individuals who are entitled actually apply and receive benefits. This new policy conflicts with the refamilisation that is advocated in many of the international conventions and many Mexican public policies. As we noted, that affirmation consists of the statement that older persons have the right to support from their families. This apparent conflict underscores the complexity of addressing the social rights of older persons, especially in the context of the renewed human rights agenda.

To an unknown extent refamilisation policies can conceivably limit the exercise of human rights of the older population. Rather than empowering them to make demands of the government, such policies reaffirm their dependency on the family. It is not clear what the changes introduced by the new federal government will mean for older people and the CSOs that fight for their rights and interests. The government's paternalistic stance toward the older population clearly has benefits, but it may fail to enhance their autonomy. The Covid-19 pandemic has undoubtedly affected the work of CSOs, reduced activism in the streets, and reinforced the role of families as protectors of elderly parents, potentially further reducing their autonomy and independence. The pandemic puts the population with multiple morbidities at greater risk and requires that social support networks exercise the greatest caution in the face of the real possibility of contagion.

During the last two decades, many groups have struggled to bring the human rights of the elderly in the Latin American and Caribbean region into the public view and to enhance the ability of older individuals to advocate for their own interests. Unfortunately, as a result of the confinement required by the Covid-19 pandemic, there is a risk of a regression in the struggle for the institutionalization of a perspective on the human and social rights of particular groups, including the elderly, women, migrants, children, adolescents, people with disabilities, members of the LGBTQ community, indigenous peoples, Afro-Mexicans, and others.

Limitations and Future Hopes

Our focus on CSOs in the context of the ongoing struggle for human rights has been motivated by two considerations. The first is that increasingly the family cannot bear all of the practical and financial responsibility for aging parents. Life expectancy in Mexico, as in most of the world is increasing rapidly and what was a relatively short segment of the life course in previous eras is now rather long. Unfortunately, as we discussed in previous chapters, longer lives have not been accompanied by a compression of morbidity (Angel, Angel, and Hill 2015). As a consequence, a large fraction of those additional years of life are often characterized by poor health and dependency. At the same time, changes in the family including fewer children, higher divorce rates, the need for women to work, and more limit the ability of daughters to care for dependent parents.

The response to this new reality generally has been the defamilisation of the responsibility for aging parents. In the United States Social Security, Medicare, and Medicaid for the poorest older individuals are part of that defamilisation. In Mexico universal non-contributory pensions and publicly-funded health care are core aspects of the Mexican old-age welfare state. Yet, as we have argued there are very real fiscal and practical limits to what the State can provide even in affluent nations. This new reality opens up the possibility for civil society organizations, both as advocates who pressure governments to live up to their duty to all citizens, including older persons, and as direct providers of support and assistance.

As we have been careful to emphasize, civil society is not a magical solution or the only means of addressing the needs of marginalized individuals and groups. As we mentioned, only a few retired academics, as is the case among other retirees, engage in organized civil society action. Most enter into a traditional retirement focused on the home and personal activities. Nonetheless, such movements are growing and they form a vanguard that promises to change the public discourse concerning human and social rights for all citizens. Ultimately, in order to bring about significant change, it is necessary to restructure the basic mechanisms of power that perpetuate the domination of the world's richest inhabitants at the expense of the disadvantaged and dispossessed. Since at least the 19th Century political parties, ideological, and activist movements have been seen as the only possibility. Yet, as we have discussed, in Latin America and elsewhere the belief in revolutionary theories and movements has waned as they have been swept aside by dominant neoliberal policies and administrations, and as those places in which revolutionary parties have seized power have failed to deliver on the promise of full democratization and a more equal distribution of wealth. The rejection of power and hierarchy, and the refusal to engage in politics – characteristics of the horizontal philosophies and policies we discussed in the first chapter – may seem hopelessly naive, but they clearly reflect a serious disillusionment with traditional radical agendas that offer forceful critiques of the status quo, but offer few practical or viable alternatives.

Which leaves us with civil society, with all of the ambiguity of the term and doubts about what disorganized and lower-level approaches can offer. Mexico serves as an interesting example that illustrates the complexity of the environment in which civil society organizations attempt to further the human and social rights of older persons and improve the quality of their lives. Since the middle of the last century clear advances have been made. Although human rights abuses continue, they are a far cry from the torture and murders that occurred during the military dictatorships in many countries. What is indisputable is that such atrocities can no longer be carried out in total secrecy, a fact that can be largely attributed to the efforts of civil society organizations that forced governments to establish truth commissions and to take action against the perpetrators of State-sponsored violence (Keck and Sikkink 1998). Civil society organizations are hardly likely to lead to the sort of communicative utopia envisioned by certain normative theories (Habermas 1970), but they hold the promise of providing venues from which individuals can begin to at least define their common interests.

References

Albertus, Michael, Alberto Diaz-Cayeros, Beatriz Magaloni, and Barry R. Weingast. 2016. "Authoritarian Survival and Poverty Traps: Land Reform in Mexico." *World Development* 77:154–170.

Angel, Ronald J., Jacqueline L. Angel, and Terrence D. Hill. 2015. "Longer Lives, Sicker Lives? Increased Longevity and Extended Disability Among Mexican-Origin Elders." *The Journals of Gerontology Series B: Psychological Sciences and Social Sciences* 70 (4):639–649.

Assies, Willem. 2007. "Land Tenure and Tenure Regimes in Mexico: An Overview." *Journal of Agrarian Change* 8:33–63.

Aviña, Alexander. 2016. "Mexico's Long Dirty War." *NACLA Report on the Americas* 48 (2):144–149.

Bennett, Vivienne. 1992. "The Evolution of Urban Popular Movements in Mexico between 1869 and 1988." Pp. 240–259 in *The Making of Social Movements in Latin America: Identity, Strategy, and Democracy*, edited by Arturo Escobar and Sonia E. Alvarez. Boulder, CO: Westview Press.

CEPAL. 2012. "Carta de San José sobre los derechos de las personas mayores de América Latina y el Caribe." Retrieved 9/27/2020 from https://repositorio.cepal.org/handle/11362/21534.

CEPAL. 2013. "Consenso de Montevideo sobre población y desarrollo3Consenso de Montevideosobre población y desarrollo." Retrieved 9/27/2020 from https://repositorio.cepal.org/bitstream/handle/11362/21835/4/S20131037_es.pdf.

Collins, Patricia Hill, and Sirma Bilge. 2016. *Intersectionality*. Malden, MA: Polity Press.

de la Garza Toledo, Enrique (Ed.). 2005. *Sindicatos y Nuevos movimientos Sociales en América Latina*. Buenos Aires: Consejo Latinoamericano de Ciencias Sociales – CLACSO.

Delgadillo, Víctor. 2016. "Ciudades iletradas: orden urbano y asentamientos populares irregulares en la ciudad de México." *Territorios*:81–99.

Díaz Oramas, A., A. Ortiz Hoyos, L. González Ballesteros, M. Bustamante Torres, and S. López Zuluaga. 2019. *El papel de la sociedad civil en el proceso de firma y ratificación de la Convención Interamericana sobre la Protección de los Derechos Humanos de las Personas Mayores (CIPDHPM)*. Bogota, Colombia: Fundación Saldarriaga Concha.

Dirección General de población de Oaxaca. 2020. "Población Adulta Mayor." *Revista Oaxaca Población Siglo XXI* 45:1–99. Retrieved 10/6/2020 from http://www.digepo.oaxaca.gob.mx/recursos/revistas/revista46.pdf.

Ek, Víctor Manuel Collí. 2012. "Improving Human Rights in Mexico: Constitutional Reforms, International Standards, and New Requirements for Judges." *Human Rights Brief* 20 (1):7–14.

Escobar, Arturo, and Sonia E. Alvarez (Eds.). 1992. *The Making of Social Movements in Latin America*. Boulder, CO: Westview Press.

Estes, Carroll. 2001. *Social Policy and Aging: A Critical Perspective*. Thousand Oaks, CA: Sage.

Estes, Carroll L. 2011. "Crises and Old Age Policy." Pp. 297–320 in *Handbook of Sociology of Aging*, edited by Richard A.SetterstenJr. and Jacqueine L. Angel. New York, NY: Springer.

Fernández-Portero, Cristina. 1999. "La gerontagogía: una nueva disciplina." *Escuela Abierta* 3:183–198.

Garay Villegas, Sagrario, and Verónica Montes de Oca Zavala. 2011. "La vejez en México: una mirada general sobre la situación socioeconómica y familiar de los hombres y mujeres adultos mayores." *Perspectivas Sociales/ Social Perspectives, Universidad Autónoma de Nuevo León – Universidad de Tennessee* 13 (1):143–165.

García-Castillo, Tonatiuh. 2015. "La reforma constitucional Mexicana de 2011 en materia de derechos humanos. Una lectura desde el derecho internacional." *Boletín Mexicano de Derecho Comparado* 48 (143):645–696.

Glockner, Fritz. 2007. *Memoria roja. Historia de la guerrilla en México (1943–1968)*. Mexico City: Ediciones B Grupo Zeta.

Habermas, Jürgen. 1970. "Towards a Theory of Communicative Competence." *Inquiry* 13(1–4):360–375.

Huenchuan, Sandra. 2013. "Los derechos humanos de las personas mayores." Santiago de Chile: CEPAL. Retrieved 9/25/2020 from https://www.fundacionhen rydunant.org/images/stories/biblioteca/derechos-personasmayores-ppublicas/Dere chos_PMayores_M2_SHuenchuan.pdf.

Illades, Carlos (Ed.). 2017. *Camaradas: Nueva Historia Del Comunismo en México*. Mexico City: Secretaria de Cultura and Fondo de Cultura Económica.

Johnston, Hank, and Paul Almeida (Eds.). 2006. *Latin American Social Movements: Globalization, Democratization, and Transnational Networks*. New York, NY: Rowman & Littlefield.

Keck, Margaret, and Kathryn Sikkink. 1998. *Activists beyond Borders: Advocacy Networks in International Politics*. Ithaca, NY: Cornell University Press.

Lombard, Melanie. 2015. "Land Conflict in Peri-urban Areas: Exploring the Effects of Land Reform on Informal Settlement in Mexico." *Urban Studies* 53 (13):2700–2720.

McCormick, Gladys. 2017. "The Last Door: Political Prisoners and the Use of Torture in Mexico's Dirty War." *The Americas* 74 (1):57–81.

Mendoza García, Jorge. 2011. "La tortura en el marco de la guerra sucia en México: un ejercicio de memoria colectiva." *POLIS* 7 (2):139–179.

Minetti, Mariana Mas. 2017. "A Victory for the Truth about Mexico's 'Dirty War'." Washington, DC: Open Society Justice Initiative. Retrieved 6/16/2020 from https://www.justiceinitiative.org/voices/victory-truth-about-mexico-s-dirty-war.

Monsiváis, Carlos. 1987. *Entrada libre. Crónicas de la sociedad que se organiza*. Mexico City: Era.

Montes de Oca, Verónica. 2003. "El Envejecimiento en el Debate Mundial: Reflexión Académica y Política." *Papeles de Población. Universidad Autonoma del Estado De México, Toluca, México* 35:79–104.

Montes de Oca, Verónica, Mariana Paredes, Vicente Rodríguez, and Sagrario Garay. 2018. "Older Persons and Human Rights in Latin America and the Caribbean." *International Journal on Ageing in Developing Countries* 2 (2):149–164.

Moyn, Samuel. 2010. *The Last Utopia: Human Rights in History*. Cambridge, MA: Belknap Press.

Negrín, Edith. 2020. "Testimonios sobre los hijos: Rosario Ibarra de Piedra, a través de Elena Poniatowska, y Javier Sicilia." *Otras Modernidades: Revista de estudios literarios e culturales, Università degli Studie di Milano* 23:193–205.

Poniatowska, Elena. 1980. *Fuerte es el silencio*. Mexico City: Era.

Rea Ángeles, Patricia, and Verónica Montes de Oca. 2020. "Las vejeces en Oaxaca." *Revista Oaxaca Población Siglo XXI* 34:20–32. Retrieved 10/6/2020 from http://www.digepo.oaxaca.gob.mx/recursos/revistas/revista46.pdf.

Red Latinoamericana de Gerontología. 2012. "Declaración de Tres Ríos, Costa Rica." Retrieved 5/18/2021 from https://www.gerontologia.org/portal/informa tion/showInformation.php?idinfo=2402.

Stahler-Sholk, Richard, Harry E. Vanden, and Marc Becker (Eds.). 2014. *Rethinking Latin American Social Movements: Radical Action from Below*. New York, NY: Rowman & Littlefield.

Stahler-Sholk, Richard, Harry E. Vanden, and Glen David Kuecker (Eds.). 2008. *Latin American Social Movements in the Twenty-first Century: Resistance, Power, and Democracy*. New York, NY: Rowman & Littlefield.

Thow, Megan E., Mathew J. Summers, Nichole L. Saunders, Jeffery J. Summers, Karen Ritchie, and James C. Vickers. 2018. "Further Education Improves Cognitive Reserve and Triggers Improvement in Selective Cognitive Functions in Older Adults: The Tasmanian Healthy Brain Project." *Alzheimer's & Dementia: Diagnosis, Assessment & Disease Monitoring* 10:22–30.

United Nations. 1948. "Universal Declaration of Human Rights." Retrieved 7/22/2019 from https://www.un.org/en/universal-declaration-human-rights/index.html.

United Nations. 2020. "Conferences | Women and Gender Equality." Retrieved 9/26/2020 from https://www.un.org/en/conferences/women.

Vilar-Compte, Mireya, Liliana Giraldo-Rodríguez, Adriana Ochoa-Laginas, and Pablo Gaitan-Rossi. 2018. "Association between Depression and Elder Abuse and the Mediation of Social Support: A Cross-Sectional Study of Elder Females in Mexico City." *Journal of Aging and Health*, 30 (4):559–583.

Ward, Peter M. 1976. "Intra-city Migration to Squatter Settlements in Mexico City." *Geoforum* 7 (5):369–382.

Ward, Peter M. 1998. *Mexico City*. Hoboken, NJ: Wiley.

World NGO Forum on Aging. 2002a. "Final Declaration and Recommendations of the World NGO Forum on Aging: 'The Development and Rights of the Elderly'." Retrieved 9/26/2020 from http://www.cruzroja.es/pls/portal30/docs/PAGE/SITE_CRE/ARBOL_CARPETAS/BB_QUE_HACEMOS/B10_INTERVENCION_SOCIAL/PERSONASMAYORES/FORO_ENVEJECIMIENTO/TR02%20138_%20DOCUMENTO%20FINAL_ENG.PDF.

World NGO Forum on Aging. 2002b. "Memoria del Foro Mundial ONG sobre el envejecimiento." Retrieved 9/25/2020 from https://fiapam.org/wp-content/uploads/2016/02/Memoria-Foro-Mundial-ong-Madrid.pdf.

Zarebski, Graciela. 2011. *El Futuro se Construye Hoy. La Reserva Humana*. Buenos Aires, Argentina: Editorial Paidós.

Zhou, Zi, Ping Wang, and Ya Fang. 2018. "Social Engagement and Its Change are Associated with Dementia Risk among Chinese Older Adults: A Longitudinal Study." *Scientific Reports* 8 (1):1551–1551.

Chapter 9

Illiberal Democracy and the Future of Civil Society

The Future of CSOs

Civil society is clearly not new. Humans are social beings and have lived collectively since before the species became identifiably *Homo sapiens*. That fact has given rise to the need to organize our collective existence, which has resulted in various forms of governance and ongoing debates over the natural or most just and efficient State structure. Various versions of the concept of civil society have been debated from the Greeks through the Middle Ages until today (Edwards 2014; Ehrenberg 2011). For the most part, civil society has been synonymous with the State, or at least some idealized version of the just and beneficent State. It is only relatively recently that the term has come to be used to refer to the non-governmental and non-market, but also non-family, sector of collective activity.

What is perhaps most intriguing about current conceptions of civil society is that for political theorists of both the left and the right, and others including communitarians, the State, or at least the State as it is currently configured, is suspect. For the left it is seen as favoring the rich and powerful and acting as an impediment to an equitable and just distribution of wealth and power. For the right it is seen as an impediment to the efficient operation of the market and a threat to individual freedom. For communitarians of various persuasions, the paternalistic State usurps functions that should be the responsibility of lower levels of social organization, as embodied in the Catholic principle of subsidiarity. All of these perspectives place great trust in the economic and political potential of local groups. For the left, local mobilization and organizations can lead to the empowerment of previously marginalized groups and foster individual and group autonomy. For the right, the devolution of centralized power and functions to more local actors and to the market results in greater economic efficiency. Both perspectives reflect the recent fascination with Alexis de Tocqueville's view of the basic value of small-scale American civic life (de Tocqueville 2000 (1835,1840)). As we have noted, this

DOI: 10.4324/9781003205609-9

perspective is gaining traction elsewhere as center and center-left political positions lose appeal in favor of nationalist right-wing positions.

Our investigation and that of many other researchers clearly document the rapid and broad emergence of secular and faith-based civil society organizations. Our focus was primarily on secular organizations, but many of the motivations and activities of faith-based organizations and groups are similar. Both secular and faith-based initiatives share certain proselytizing objectives in that they wish to change people's perceptions or understandings of some aspect of current social reality (Grzybowski 2000). They both seek to bring about conversion experiences, a concept not unlike that of frame realignment. What was perhaps most informative about our investigation of CSOs is the extent to which they differ in their attempts and ability to influence governmental agencies at various levels.

In addition to differences in stated missions, CSOs differ in terms of their membership's gender, previous employment experiences, their previous union and political activities, and their ongoing affiliation with other powerful groups. For purposes of discussion, we grouped CSOs into three large overlapping categories based largely on these characteristics. The first consists of those organizations that emerged from the Mexican labor and other social movements. These were the first organized groupings of individuals to demand their rights. The second consists of more recent organizations, many of which emerged with the election of Andres Lopez Obrador as Mayor of Mexico City in 2000. As Mayor, and now as President, his administration focuses on improving the quality of life of poor Mexicans, as do many independent CSOs. The third category consists of more recent organizations that combine aspects of the previous two categories to bring greater attention to demands for the human and social rights of older persons.

The first group is unique and important since its members had union experience gained as part of a long history of labor mobilization and union activity. As we discussed in Chapter six, the labor union movement in Mexico was largely coopted by the dominant party, the PRI, and faced fierce employer and state resistance. Nonetheless, they provided the first organized venue for any form of collective action and their experiences and example helped give rise to many social movements during the 20th Century. As a result of the oppositional stance of many of these unions or subsets of their members they are perhaps the most politically knowledgeable and active groups of retirees in Mexico. Collectively, they had the most knowledge of government bureaucracies and potentially effective ways of pressing their demands.

This first group includes organizations that represent pensioners of the Institute of Security and Social Services of State Workers, retirees of the Mexican Electrical Union, and former employees of the National Coordinating Committee of Education Workers. These retiree organizations have strong internal organization, again reflecting their members' experience in the governmental and public sectors. Many, especially those consisting of retired teachers and professors, have high average levels of education. Except for the educational sector, in which women have dominated for decades, these organizations are predominantly male, but they increasingly include women, reflecting the gradual increase in female labor force participation since the 1980s. Certain organizations, such as the electrical workers union include many individuals who retired early while they were still relatively young.

An important observation was that organizations composed of retired electrical and other industrial workers do not frame their objectives in terms of active aging. Their discourse is informed by labor struggles and focus on the rights of workers. Although they do not frame the issues they address in terms of active aging, their approach clearly subsumes active aging as part of their stated objective of active engagement and even confrontation. Certain of these organizations are extensions of currently active unions and occupational groups, rather than independent groups of retirees. Their discourse is plainly political and focused on social and political rights, with a major focus on economic security. Of all of the organizations we studied these are the closest to political parties, or at least they have the most developed discourses related to social rights. Unlike groups such as the Zapatistas or the Piqueteros in Argentina that we discussed in the first chapter who reject organizational hierarchy or contacts with the government, these organizations are more conscious of the need to foster structures and capacities to confront government agencies when necessary in order to achieve concrete goals, although they face formidable obstacles.

This group of organizations comes perhaps closest to adopting the sorts of power strategies that the CSO sector often lacks. As we discussed earlier, CSOs have been criticized for their general inability to address the structural causes of economic inequality and other forms of injustice. Some of these organizations overtly reject power and refuse to engage in politics or deal directly with the State. Many refuse to, or simply do not work with or coordinate their efforts with other groups. This stance reflects a philosophy and structure labeled "horizontalism" to emphasize their rejection of hierarchy. In the absence of hierarchy all members have an equal right to express themselves and none has more influence than others. Such a position clearly insulates an organization or movement from cooptation or undue influence, and maybe shields it from the iron law of oligarchy, but it also cuts it off from the sort of organized, broad, and sustained exercise of power that is required to confront forces that do not reject power and that can muster effective resistance.

Our second category of CSOs consists of organizations whose core mission focuses primarily on their members' quality of life, conceived of largely in terms of physical and mental health. For these groups, active aging involves the preservation or restoration of optimal physical functioning and the encouragement of social engagement with others in one's local community. These groups tend to consist of women who have not worked or worked episodically and who are mostly homemakers. They have little union or labor force experience. Unlike the first group, their members lack any experience in the workers' rights movement and they have no experience in government or any other sector. They typically have low levels of education, have lived in marginal neighborhoods, and have low incomes. Their focus on quality-of-life issues informs their definition of active aging. The members of these organizations clearly enjoy and benefit from the social and support activities that these organizations sponsor, but these activities do not promote active engagement in politics or the struggle for human or social rights.

Our third group of organizations, like the second group, focuses on quality of life issues, but includes a more active focus on human and social rights. Their agendas and framing of the problems they address is informed by the new social movements focused on identity politics and the human rights agenda that entered public discourse in the latter part of the 20th and early part of the 21st Centuries. These organizations have a clear quality of life focus, but they also foster intellectual and physical development based on a philosophy of active aging that emphasizes engagement and participation. These organizations' framing of active aging emphasizes the individual's own ability and responsibility for controlling the aging process to the extent possible. In addition to optimal physical and social functioning, though, the protection and exercise of rights is central. Many of these organizations were successful in pressuring governmental authorities into providing various resources to further their members' objectives. Through their own fund-raising efforts and with resources they obtain from the authorities they sponsor workshops, talks, recreational activities, conferences, cinema clubs, and more. The membership of these groups have more education than those in the second group, and they have more work experience and generally more human and social capital.

Post-Traditional Society

We began our excursion into the realm of civil society, active aging, and citizenship with the observation that the number and activity of CSOs increased dramatically during the 20th Century in most nations of the world. That growth continues and is even accelerating as we move further into the 21st Century. A basic question is whether that expansion in the non-State sector is a passing phenomenon or a permanent change in how society functions. CSOs are involved in almost all domains of human activity, sometimes in an overtly political manner, and at other times working in the background at the grass roots level to better the lives of the individuals they serve. As the title of our book suggests, and as we described in earlier chapters, they have assumed many of the functions that in more traditional times were the sole responsibility of the family, and more recently of the welfare state. In addition to providing services, material assistance, and emotional succor they often advocate for the human and social rights of those they represent. Given the cultural, demographic, and social changes that have created the modern world with far longer life spans, larger and older populations, smaller families, increased migration, and more it is unlikely that we could ever return to the ways of life of the past.

In fact, the resurgence of civil society accompanies the emergence of a new post-traditional society that has changed human relationships in fundamental ways that have been described by multiple observers (Angel and Angel 2018; Buman 2000; Giddens 1994b). As we noted in the first chapter, it is possible to view the rise of civil society organizations as reflecting specific social movements, or even a more general movement that embodies demands by ordinary citizens, as well as the previously marginalized and powerless, for a voice in matters that affect their own lives and society more generally. As we have witnessed in many nations around the world, including the storming of the U.S. Capitol by supporters of ex-President Donald Trump on January 6, 2021, those demands for recognition can reflect the sense of alienation by previously dominant racial, political, or other groups who feel they are the victims of globalization, modernization, immigration, and the unfair advantages that have been given to previously subordinate groups.

In Mexico, as in any other nation, such demands and the social movements of which they are a part can only be understood within the political and economic context from which they emerge and function. In Mexico, as in many other nations, that recent context has been defined by neoliberalism and a retreat from the expansion of the welfare state has dominated public policy during the latter decades of the 20th Century and the beginning of the 21st. Neoliberalism reflects an economic and political philosophy that focuses on economic efficiency and aggregate productivity, but progressively undermines the already inadequate governmental supports of many social groups, including workers in certain sectors of the economy, women, Afro-descendants, indigenous peoples, environmentalists, students, and many more. In that context, progressive CSOs reflect an evolving demand for human rights and more direct democracy, one that involves more than just free elections, but also guarantees "constitutional liberalism," a political philosophy and system that rejects autocracy and guarantees individual freedom and autonomy in all areas of life, including public life (Zakaria 1997).

Of course, we must once again emphasize that not all organized activity is progressive in the sense of promoting collective welfare. Paramilitary groups, anti-immigrant parties, fringe parties that espouse conspiratorial theories, cults, and many more are clearly part of civil society with their own non-inclusionary objectives. As part of the increase in civil society activism that has taken place in recent decades, a countermovement or countermovements, perhaps best described by Fareed Zakaria's (1997) concept of "illiberal democracy," have displaced constitutional liberalism in many nations. Illiberal democracy refers to a moral and political program that rejects the basic tenets of constitutional liberalism. Although illiberal democracies allow open elections and referendums, they do not allow citizens any real say concerning important social policies. It is a philosophy that, in conjunction with a growing xenophobic nationalism, looks inward and rejects any sort of cosmopolitan internationalism. Illiberal democracy, with its rejection of intellectual and political cosmopolitanism, and its xenophobic focus on the local, perhaps provides a sense of security to believers, but it bodes ill for greater inclusiveness and the recognition of the unique attributes and rights of other groups and cultures.

The conflict between constitutional liberalism and illiberal democracy makes predictions concerning the future of civil society and the possibilities for the extension of human and social rights, as well as economic, environmental, and cultural rights, impossible. Although a return to the authoritarian and repressive regimes of the past is increasingly unlikely in Latin America and the Caribbean, illiberal democracy raises the possibility that the dynamic extension of civil society could be blunted by other means. Which leads us to caution against any uncritical belief that civil society organizations foster democracy and openness by the simple fact of encouraging collective action. As we have emphasized throughout, the existence of a large number of non-governmental organizations does not in and of itself guarantee the spread of constitutional liberalism. That point cannot be made too forcefully or too often. Many organizations are exclusive and fail to recognize the human and social rights of groups whose members are not like themselves, or with whom they disagree. Nonetheless, as we have argued, given a general disillusionment with grand totalizing philosophies and a loss of faith in the possibilities of revolutionary movements to bring about true democracy and social justice, civil society and the social movements it encourages appear to be among the few viable alternatives. Determining the extent to which civil society in general, and civil society organizations in particular, can make a significant difference represent a major intellectual, practical, and research challenge.

A Diversity of Missions: Service vs. Advocacy

In Mexico, as in most nations, one finds a range of CSOs that differ in size, structure, organization, financing, and membership, but perhaps most importantly they differ in terms of their core missions as we noted above. All of these factors affect their effectiveness in bringing about change and positively impacting individuals' and groups' lives. There are clearly many possible ways of categorizing CSOs based on everything from their structure, the characteristics of their membership, their financing, their relationship to the State and political parties, and more. Our theoretical and empirical classification focused on their missions and the ways in which they frame the issues they address. We also characterized organizations in terms of their degree of focus on service delivery and the material and social support of older individuals, and advocacy, which entails more militant attempts to change the basic rules of the game (Pereira and Angel 2009; Pereira, Angel, and Angel 2007). The first objective reflects a desire to improve the physical and mental quality of older individuals' lives by assuring that they have access to the basic necessities of a dignified existence and encouraging participation with others in the community. The second objective, that of advocacy, focuses on active citizenship. This objective is certainly furthered by voluntary action that addresses the needs of older individuals, but it is also achieved by empowering older individuals themselves to confront the State to demand and defend their basic social and human rights.

One might conceive of these two objectives, service delivery and advocacy, as conflicting, meaning that the more an organization engages in one, the less it can do of the other. In advocating for individuals' rights an organization might alienate State sources of financing. During the dictatorship in Chile, civil society organizations focused on human and political rights could certainly not expect support from the State. On the other hand, depending on how it operates, an organization might engage in both simultaneously, at least to some degree. Any particular CSO or group of CSOs can choose which combination of service delivery and advocacy is optimal in terms of its objectives. In particular historical and political contexts advocacy requires taking an oppositional stance toward the State. In Chile many of those oppositional CSOs had to redefine their missions with the return of democracy (Pereira and Angel 2009). In many cases, oppositional CSOs became subcontractors to the State for the delivery of services to populations in need. Many organizations combine aspects of advocacy and direct service provision, often by providing basic necessities and services, while working to assure that individuals in need receive the services to which they are entitled from the State under existing laws and regulations.

The Problem of Coordination

In the end, our objective was not to determine whether or not CSOs are in principle efficient service delivery mechanisms, or whether they are effective in changing hearts and minds and bringing about structural change. By and large, the latter goal seems unlikely, at least for CSOs operating alone, since few have any real political clout. At most they can motivate citizens to act collectively to further their own interests, or they can join with other organizations to attempt to bring about larger-scale change. One serious shortcoming of CSOs in general, though, is that this sector does not have an organizational or structural mechanism for encouraging cooperation or coordination of group efforts (Gajewski et al. 2011). As numerous as CSOs may be, little of their activity is closely coordinated with that of other organizations. The result can lead to duplication and misdirection of efforts, inefficiencies, and a failure to effectively address major needs (Angel et al. 2012). One might imagine the Allied invasion of Normandy without a Supreme Allied Commander to coordinate the efforts of the British, the Americans, the Canadians, the Australians, and the others involved. Chaos would have reigned and the invasion would likely have been repelled. In major crises, such as the earthquake that struck Haiti in January, 2010 and Hurricane Matthew which devastated the island in October, 2016, the actions of CSOs were widely criticized for being uncoordinated, politicized, and ineffective (Edmonds 2013; Hsu and Schuller 2020). Indeed, observers have long debated whether various outside non-governmental actors have benefitted Haitian development, or whether they have actually been a hindrance (Schuller 2007).

Again, the basic motivation for investigating the range and missions of CSOs in a middle-income country arises from the remarkable growth and the number of such organizations and their reach in terms of the domains in which they operate, largely as the result of weak States and ineffective governments. Only time and experience will allow us to answer questions about their effectiveness. As optimistic as we are concerning the possibilities for civil society to encourage active aging, a pandemic such Covid-19 that has taken a particularly heavy toll among older people, makes it clear that while older individuals may remain active and engaged, they share certain vulnerabilities that accompany aging. It is also clear that in such situations the family cannot provide all of the material, social, and medical support that aging parents require. For better or worse, strangers must assume many of the functions of traditional families. The pandemic reminds us yet again of our basic human interdependence, but it also serves as a stark reminder that we are all dependent on a beneficent and efficient State. CSOs can certainly assist in crises, but as the Haitian experience and other natural and man-made disasters show, they are no substitute for a functioning government. Perhaps in the case of eldercare the solution lies in an intersectoral care system in which each sector has clear responsibilities and in which government institutions, community organizations, families, and, of course, CSOs clearly identify their roles and capacities and communicate openly with one another. Any efficient public action depends on the coordination of key actors.

Too Narrow a Focus?

Whatever the range of forces that are driving the expansion of civil society and CSOs, it is clear that those forces are global and powerful and that they represent many different interests and distinct ideological positions. Whether these organizations, and the social movements of which they are a part, can make a positive difference for humanity as a whole, or for particular groups, will take years to assess. There are many potential pitfalls as well. One major concern is that CSOs and the identity politics which many of these organizations promote represent a potentially disastrous abandonment of political parties and their agendas, particularly those of the center and left (Lilla 2016; Roman 2004; Schlesinger Jr. 1992). Despite widespread disillusionment with collectivist or revolutionary philosophies, it is difficult to imagine how the guarantee of universal human and social rights can be achieved without a powerful political presence. It is quite possible that an excessive focus on local group issues could undermine more collective identities and action, undermining attempts to institutionalize human and social rights. All we can say is that despite any ultimate judgement concerning effectiveness, CSOs appear to be here to stay. A focus on civil society, direct democracy, and a greater focus on human and social rights have superseded totalizing ideologies and brought discourse concerning collective issues back to a human level.

The emergence of greater civil society activity at the very least reflects the maturation of many previous struggles, including the fight for labor rights that were undermined by neoliberalism. It reflects demands by ordinary citizens for improved living conditions. It is fueled by the new overarching human and social rights agenda. It also reflects the struggles of feminist and women's groups that question patriarchal domination, as well as associations of older people that have entered the fight against ageism and various forms of violence directed against older people. It reflects the claims of LBGTQ groups that are struggling to reframe public discourse to recognize the legitimacy, and even the benefits of, the sexual diversity of humanity. It reflects demands by associations of indigenous peoples that have fought for their lands and rights since colonial times. It reflects the struggles of the disabled that have modified the architecture of cities, as well as educational, labor, and other policies. Recognizing human, social, economic, cultural, and environmental rights strengthens the human experience and humanizes societies.

Challenges from Within and Without

Fostering a more direct and participatory democracy clearly represents an ideal. It is quite easy to imagine that active participation in group-related activities inevitably furthers liberal values in the traditional sense of respect for others' cultures and beliefs, their religious and political free-doms, and their basic human rights. As we have stressed throughout our investigation, though, such a view is clearly naïve and ignores the large number of voluntary groups with illiberal objectives. Groups can foster a high degree of solidarity among their members at the same time that they fail to recognize the basic rights of others. Many reject a cosmopolitan perspective that might lead them to reach beyond parochial racial, ethnic, religious, political, or other distinctions in order to achieve a rapprochement with groups who have different values and world views. In that regard, civil society can embody and foster illiberal values as easily as it can inclusive values.

Attempts to foster inclusive or cosmopolitan objectives face other serious challenges as well. Active civic engagement and demands by organizations for their members' basic human and social rights do not take place in closed environments. Group demands for significant social change invari-ably face varying degrees of pushback. Every movement gives rise to countermovements (Meyer and Staggenborg 1996; Mottl 1980; Tilly 1978; Zald and Useem 1987). As recent events in various parts of the world demonstrate, some of those countermovements can be seriously undemocratic and even repressive. Individuals and groups that benefit from the status quo and who fear that they will lose their advantages in any rearrangement of the social order resist, often violently. This stark reality applies at the local level where anti-equal rights amendment groups, anti-affirmative action groups, anti-gay, anti-gun control groups, and many other reactionary groups are common. But it also operates at the level of regional and national politics.

As we discussed in Chapter one, a new post-post-neoliberalism seems to be asserting itself in many nations of the world with the rise of right-wing populist anti-globalization, anti-immigrant, and anti-intellectual parties and political figures. In Europe parties of the center right and especially of the center and far left have begun losing votes at an astonishing pace (Plattner 2019). Among democratic governments in Latin America and the Caribbean, the same polarization occurs. In many places right-wing groups seek to confuse citizens and sometimes ally themselves with pro-gressive positions to gain support and political influence. A politics based on the polarization between cosmopolitan and globalized world views and more local views focused on local identities and culture has replaced a more inclusive political discourse focused on social class and the need for democratic solutions (Case and Deaton 2020; Goodhart 2017). Hopefully that inclusive discourse was not hopelessly naïve.

The Threat to Open Societies

As we discussed in Chapter one, during the 1990s, largely in response to their seriously negative impact on the poor and marginalized, neoliberal policies were weakened, even if they were not totally abandoned, in most Latin American countries (Stiglitz 2008). The resulting shift to the left, referred to as the "Pink Tide," gave greater weight to the needs of those who had been most harmed by neoliberalism. The tide began with Hugo Chávez' 1998 presidential victory in Venezuela and went on to include most Latin American nations (Cameron 2009; Macdonald and Ruckert 2009). Almost inevitably, though, post-neoliberalism gave rise to opposition from defenders of open markets, cuts in social spending, and the rest of the neoliberal agenda. In fact, the neoliberal agenda was not completely abandoned in any nation and still largely defines the dominant economic paradigm in Latin America.

However, recently the situation has taken an ominous turn. The resurgence of populist nationalism in many nations of the world includes significant anti-global, anti-immigrant, and other protectionist policies. Recently Argentina, Brazil, and Chile shifted from left-wing to right-wing administrations (Encarnación 2018), although Argentina has now moved left again. In Ecuador Andrés Arauz, a protégé of populist past president, Rafael Correa, received the largest fraction of votes in the first round of the 2021 presidential election, although the win was not large enough to avoid a second round, which may see a new shift to the left. These shifts clearly reflect voters' exasperation with ongoing governmental shortcomings, including economic inefficiencies and corruption, but they also threaten a potentially significant weakening of attempts to further human and social rights. The broad appeal of populism clearly demonstrates that progressive victories at any level of government and society are always vulnerable to reversals. The human and social rights discourse that has become common in Latin America faces difficult challenges in becoming institutionalized and gaining the force of public opinion and the law.

In Mexico, conservative right-wing forces, as well as transnational investors, favor fiscal austerity measures that threaten programs for the poor. Ironically, though, progressive groups that advocate for the poor today often find themselves marginalized by an administration and strong president who wishes to be the primary benefactor of the poor. In 2018, Andres Manuel López Obrador, the left-of-center candidate who narrowly lost the presidency in 2006 in a contested election, finally became President of Mexico. As one would expect, right-wing and neoliberal forces have attempted to discredit the pro-poor stance of the new administration, which seeks to be effective without purchasing pro-government journalism, or granting favorable contracts for political gain, or undermining the State's energy sovereignty.

Despite the new administration's genuine concern for the poor and older persons, civil society groups, including women's organizations, groups representing the poor and marginalized, indigenous groups, LGBTQ organizations, the homeless, organizations focused on the needs of older people, and others, many of which received funding from previous administrations, are largely ignored. Given this situation, many of these organizations find themselves without support from a government that itself rejects neoliberalism, an ironic situation that has never occurred before. Even with a growing awareness of inequities, full incorporation of various groups has yet to occur. Today, for example, although women serve in the administration, that representation does not guarantee an effective feminist agenda. Violence against women, including murder, remains a serious problem (Lettieri 2021). Without buy-in from civil society organizations of all sorts, the progressive perspective of the current government may be lost, and with it a great deal of political capital could be squandered. To avoid this eventuality, it is necessary to reaffirm and support the work of CSOs whose agendas are based on humanist and progressive principles, even though they may not receive the support of the current administration. Networking and greater communication and cooperation among CSOs is necessary to leverage the potential power of small organizations in order to influence government and to bring about positive change that benefits society as a whole.

CSOs Are Here to Stay

Even as neoliberalism reasserts itself, it is difficult to imagine that new conservative governments will completely undo the progress in extending social rights that has been made, or that they could completely blunt the ongoing human rights discourse. However, events such as the serious collapse of Venezuela's economy, and the crash in oil prices could make that observation seem naïve. On the bright side, though, numerous social movements have changed many individuals' and groups' notions of what is possible and what is right. The groups we have discussed have been mobilized and are not likely to fade back into obscurity and silence. Given the democratic openness of contemporary Latin American societies it seems unlikely that they are in any real danger of reverting to the old regime of stolen elections and open political oppression. Neoliberalism itself requires a national and international openness that would be almost impossible to reverse.

Nonetheless, the spread of democratic elections that has occurred in recent years does not in and of itself guarantee respect for human or social rights. As we have noted, democratic elections do not guarantee that the elected government will respect human or social rights (Plattner 2019; Zakaria 1997). Large-scale social change must begin at a lower level. As we have seen, one of the major objectives of civil society organizations that work in the area of human and social rights is to alter the ways in which oppressed and dominated individuals and groups view the causes of their marginalization, as well as the possibilities for change. Individuals who believe that their subjugated position is a reflection of some divinely mandated order, or that it is in some other way legitimate, are unlikely to demand change. Change requires that those individuals alter their perceptions to view unjust and illegitimate social arrangements rather than fate or destiny as the cause of their misery.

Yet such changed consciousness among the oppressed is insufficient to bring about systemic or structural changes. It is, though, a beginning. A recognition of the power relations that foster and support sexism, racism, ageism, and the stigmatization of the disabled represents a first step toward overcoming them. The disadvantaged and their allies must alter the larger public's perceptions by successfully reframing the causes of inequitable social arrangements, as well as the necessary solutions. The Civil Rights movement's reframing of the issue of racial inequality and segregation in the southern United States during the mid-20th Century is one example. Changing the status quo has always involved altering false consciousness and changing people's acceptance of the current state of affairs as reflecting what is inevitable or even right. Unfortunately, such attempts take time and often suffer serious setbacks.

International Human Rights Conventions

In this closing chapter we must return to a topic we dealt with in Chapter three, in which we reviewed important international conventions on the rights of older people. The growth in the number of conventions dealing with the rights of older people reflects a potential sea change in public perceptions and attitudes toward older persons and their rights and responsibilities as citizens. It also accompanies demands by other groups for greater recognition of their rights. As we mentioned, the Universal Declaration of Human rights (United Nations 1948) affirms the basic rights of all humans so conventions dealing with the needs of specific groups should be unnecessary. Unfortunately, affirmations of general rights that apply to everyone in principle often do little to address the plight of the seriously marginalized. For that reason, demands for new and more forceful affirmations of the rights of older persons have continued, driven largely by civil society organizations that advocate for older persons, and by older people themselves. As we explained, these conventions do not have the force of law, in that they are not binding on the nations that ratify them, except insofar as those nations choose to make the principles expressed in the conventions legally enforceable, something that few have done. These conventions represent what is referred to as "soft law," in that for the most part, they simply state principles that should ideally guide a nation's treatment of older citizens.

Even if they do not immediately result in enforceable laws that protect the rights of older persons and other marginalized groups, though, international conventions can have significant real-world effects. Largely as the result of a long struggle by international social networks and civil society organizations, slavery is no longer legally accepted in any nation, although it may occur in practice (Keck and Sikkink 1998). Serious human rights abuses today draw the attention of civil society organizations such as Amnesty International and Human Rights Watch (Sikkink 2017), and in the case of older individuals from HelpAge International, and HelpAge Latinoamerica, to mention a few. In 2016, again largely in response to pressure from civil society organizations, the United Kingdom dropped its opposition to the proposed United Nations *Convention on the Rights of Older Persons*, becoming one of the first nations to express guarded support (Herro 2019). Supporters of this new U.N. Convention feel that it is needed because the existing conventions, such as the Madrid International Plan of Action on Ageing, and the conventions that followed it are insufficient to guarantee the rights of older persons (Herro 2019). As the nations of the world age rapidly, organizations consisting of older persons and their supporters will no doubt become more active in national and international policy making.

This new convention is only the most recent in a series of agreements related to older persons. As we discussed in Chapter three, Latin America and the Caribbean have been at the forefront of advocacy for and adoption of conventions that affirm the rights of older persons (Montes de Oca et al. 2018). The reasons for the continent's receptivity to such conventions may relate to the more limited old-age welfare states in Latin America than exists in Europe. Older individuals in Mexico and other Latin American nations have been discriminated against and have suffered serious marginalization and poverty (Montes de Oca 2000; Montes de Oca Zavala 2013). In the context of the basic lack of human and political rights, the demand for more formal recognition and redress of the injustices suffered by older persons have resulted in the widely perceived need for such international conventions.

The ratification of conventions that promote the rights of older persons and others are important in and of themselves, but they also reflect the actions of many civil society organizations. Even if the activities of such organizations are not highly coordinated, they represent forces for change that reflect more than the desires of one or even just a few groups. Effective social movements eventually motivate thousands of individuals to act. A major aspect of the dynamics behind the adoption of international conventions is the behind-the-scenes preparatory legwork done by various civil society groups. CSOs have met before each UN Conference on Women to include their agendas and to monitor the implementation of the principles affirmed. CSOs met alongside the major conventions on the rights of older persons in meetings that preceded the official conferences (Santiago de Chile, Tres Ríos, Brasilia, Ypacaraí) (Montes de Oca et al. 2018).

Realistic but Cautious Expectations

As we have noted repeatedly, and what we must continuously keep in mind, is that it is quite easy to romanticize civil society and non-governmental approaches to complex social problems or to overestimate the ability of voluntary collective action to empower the powerless (Giddens 1994a). Local approaches to the care and support of vulnerable individuals are appealing because they appear to be more personal and on a more human scale than services provided by large impersonal bureaucracies (Quadagno, Kail, and Shekha 2012). The rejection of leftist welfare state philosophies that have informed public policy in various countries in recent decades reflects a deep distrust of big government and the welfare state, a large part of which consists of old-age supports (Binstock 2004). Although support for public pensions remains high everywhere, fiscal constraints and frequent economic crises have fueled efforts to control the growth of such public programs. Thatcherism in Great Britain, the Regan revolution in the United States, and new Third Way philosophies in other nations have been accompanied by a growing anti-welfare state rhetoric and the adoption of policies intended to cap or even reduce social expenditures and the responsibility of the state (Andrews 1999; Faux 1999; Stiglitz 2008). Public anti-welfare state sentiment and neoliberal social and economic policies have serious implications for the material and social welfare of individuals with limited resources including women, racialized minority groups, and older people (Angel and Angel 1997; Angel and Angel 2009).

There can be little doubt that older people benefit from programs that provide companionship and opportunities for engagement with others (Hood et al. 2018; Krause 2006). The data are clear that isolation, disconnectedness, and loneliness represent health risks (Cornwell and Waite 2009; National Institute on Aging 2019). Evidence from programs in the U.S. clearly demonstrates the benefits of intensive social engagement and support for older individuals in the community (Hansen and Hewitt 2012). Yet there are serious dangers in placing too much hope in the ability of local communities and organizations to provide all of the supports that older citizens need. In the United States Social Security and Medicare are fundamental and indispensable support programs without which millions of older individuals would fall into poverty and be denied the medical care they need. In Mexico medical care coverage for low-income older individuals from the *Instituto Nacional de Salud para el Bienestar* (INSABI), and the non-contributory pensions upon which most older Mexicans rely are indispensable. As we attempt to mobilize family and local resources for the care of older people, we confront the very real danger that the supposed superiority of non-governmental approaches will be used to justify excessive and harmful cuts to state-sponsored and funded programs. The most vulnerable would be the biggest losers. The life-long labor force disadvantages faced by older Mexicans and minority Americans leaves them particularly dependent on publicly funded programs in old age. If an unrealistic belief in the support capacities of local organizations and community groups were to encourage reductions in funding for formal services the results could be disastrous.

As appealing and non-controversial as civil society approaches to dealing with human needs might seem at first glance, then, there are serious criticisms of CSOs and the non-governmental approach generally that potentially apply to civil society solutions to dealing with older people or human and social rights more generally. In the area of development and assistance to poor countries CSOs have been criticized for often being too apolitical and unwilling or unable to deal with basic social structural factors that account for the powerlessness and exclusion of particular groups. They can, in fact, be seen as part of the neoliberal agenda, the objective of which is privatizing (or refamilising) what are in fact public responsibilities (Clarke 1998; Sangeeta 2004; Srinivas 2009). International development CSOs are criticized for an excessively narrow focus on specific projects and fostering dependency rather than furthering self-sufficiency and sustainability (Edmonds 2013; Sangeeta 2004). They are criticized for being too accountable to their funders and less concerned with the perspectives of those they supposedly intend to help.

As we noted earlier, CSOs and the civil society focus more generally are also criticized for their often narrow and excessive focus on subgroups defined in terms of gender, race, ethnicity, disability status, specific illnesses, and more. An excessively narrow focus on particular subgroups or problem areas can undermine efforts to address collective political issues (Schlesinger Jr. 1992). Supporters of the international labor movement, for example, continue to believe that the major locus of disadvantage and struggle in the world that in principle unifies workers in developed and developing nations lies in the conflict between labor and capital. From this perspective an excessive focus on gender, race, or other narrow identities undermines the possibility for the sort of collective political action necessary to better the lot of ordinary citizens (Roman 2004). Whatever the merits of the various criticisms of civil society, it seems clear that the core danger to the interests of older people lies in the potential justification of the devolution of State responsibilities for income support and health care, or drastic reductions in funding for such programs, on the basis of the supposed availability and superiority of local non-governmental approaches.

We end by returning to the organizing theme of the entire presentation, the evolving discourse in which social rights are seen as an integral component of more general human rights. While basic civil and political rights were granted to ever larger segments of the populations of the developed world during the 19th and 20th Centuries, basic social rights remain contested even as the modern welfare state has become the norm. In many traditional and conservative nations cultural norms and formal social policy look to the family for the material and instrumental support of dependent family members, including aging parents (Esping-Andersen 1990; Esping-Andrsen 2010). In Latin America and the Caribbean, the family continues to serve as the basic social welfare provider for the care and support of aging parents. Although Latin American nations have been leaders in adopting international conventions that affirm the social and human rights of older individuals, as we noted, many of these conventions affirm an older person's right to be cared for by his or her family, if there are family members able to do so. Such a proposition clearly furthers the refamilisation of the support of older parents. Yet, as we have argued, demographic, economic, and social changes have greatly altered the family's ability to serve in that role, even in highly familistic cultures such as those of Latin America and the Caribbean. Smaller families, lower fertility, increasing divorce rates, the migration of children away from their parents' communities, and the need for women to work means that the family-based old-age support system of previous eras is being seriously strained.

Given this changing eldercare environment greater defamilisation of care and support seems inevitable (Esping-Andrsen 2010). Yet in low and middle-income countries such defamilisation faces serious barriers. While the affluent social democratic States of northern Europe can afford generous and extensive welfare states, low and middle-income nations face serious fiscal limitations to what they can offer. Given the seriousness of the problem of poverty among older people, over forty nations have adopted some form of non-contributory pension. In Mexico approximately 60% of the population over 65 depends on such non-employment-based pensions. As the population of Mexico and other nations age financing such extensive support systems, even if the basic pension amount remains minimal, will present major challenges. It is in this context that the potential role of CSOs becomes more important. In addition to enhancing the quality of life of older individuals with few resources who are at elevated risk of isolation and loneliness, these organizations can potentially empower older individuals to act as effective agents who can demand their basic social and human rights.

Despite our concern for a lack of coordination, one of the appealing characteristics of civil society and civil society organizations is the diversity of objectives and groups they include. These organizations do not reflect a common ideological perspective as is often the case with political parties or highly focused social movements. CSOs reflect a wide range of interests and values that we must better understand, both in terms of their specific objectives and in their ideological and practical use of human and financial resources. That heterogeneity is both the sector's major strength, but also its potential major weakness in that diversity and the identity politics it fosters can preclude necessary collective action. We end with the observation that a major dimension of a redefined civil society is its specific attention to gender and women's issues, to the needs of indigenous groups, racialized minorities, and others and its growing affirmation of and struggle for human rights, not only in discourse but in practice. This new consciousness of diversity requires a greater understanding of the intersectionality of various characteristics that place certain individuals and groups at particularly elevated risk of marginality. The challenges posed by aging, as well as the new consciousness of active aging, have been added to the ongoing campaign for health, security, and human dignity. The challenge has been made all the more obvious by the ongoing Covid-19 pandemic that has disproportionately affected older individuals in situations in which they have limited resources and little access to care. Ultimately, the core task is to identify best practices in the role of civil society and CSOs in the defense of human and social rights.

References

Andrews, Geoff. 1999. "New Left and New Labour." *Soundings* 13:14–24.

Angel, Ronald J., and Jacqueline L. Angel. 1997. *Who Will Care for Us? Aging and Long-Term Care in Multicultural America*. New York, NY: New York University Press.

Angel, Ronald J., and Jacqueline L. Angel. 2009. *Hispanic Families at Risk: The New Economy, Work, and the Welfare State*. New York, NY: Springer.

Angel, Ronald J., and Jacqueline L. Angel. 2018. *Family, Intergenerational Solidarity, and Post-Traditional Society*. New York, NY: Routledge.

Angel, Ronald J., Holly Bell, Julie Beausoleil, and Laura Lein. 2012. *Community Lost: The State, Civil Society, and Displaced Survivors of Hurricane Katrina*. New York, NY: Cambridge University Press.

Binstock, Robert H. 2004. "Advocacy in an Era of Neoconservatism: Responses of National Aging Organizations." *Generations* 28 (1):49–54.

Buman, Zygmunt. 2000. *Liquid Modernity*. Cambridge, UK: Polity Press.

De Tocqueville, Alexis. 2000 (1835,1840). *Democracy in America*. Translated and edited by Harvey G. Mansfield and Delba Winthrop. Chicago, IL: University of Chicago Press.

Cameron, Maxwell A. 2009. "Latin America's Left Turns: Beyond Good and Bad." *Third World Quarterly* 30 (2):331–347.

Case, Anne, and Angus Deaton. 2020. *Deaths of Despair and the Future of Capitalism*. Princeton, NJ: Princeton University Press.

Clarke, Gerard. 1998. "Non-governmental Organizations (NGOs) and Politics in the Developing World." *Political Studies* 46 (1):36.

Cornwell, Erin York, and Linda J. Waite. 2009. "Social Disconnectedness, Perceived Isolation, and Health among Older Adults." *Journal of Health and Social Behavior* 50 (1):31–48.

Edmonds, Kevin. 2013. "Beyond Good Intentions: The Structural Limitations of NGOs in Haiti." *Critical Sociology* 39:439–452.

Edwards, Michael. 2014. *Civil Society*. Cambridge, UK: Polity Press.

Ehrenberg, John. 2011. "The History of Civil Society Ideas." Pp. 15–28 in *The Oxford Handbook of Civil Society*, edited by Michael Edwards. New York, NY: Oxford University Press.

Encarnación, Omar G. 2018. "The Rise and Fall of the Latin American Left: Conservatives now Control Latin America's Leading Economies, but the Region's Leftists Can still Look to Uruguay for Direction." *The Nation*. Retrieved 8/19/2019 from https://www.thenation.com/article/the-ebb-and-flo w-of-latin-americas-pink-tide/.

Esping-Andersen, Gøsta. 1990. *The Three Worlds of Welfare Capitalism*. Princeton, NJ: Princeton University Press.

Esping-Andersen, Gøsta. 2010. "Prologue: What Does it Mean to Break with Bismarck?" Pp. 13–18 in *A Long Goodbye to Bismarck? The Politics of Welfare Reform in Continental Europe*, edited by Bruno Palier. Amsterdam: Amsterdam University Press.

Faux, Jeff. 1999. "Lost on the Third Way." *Dissent* 46 (2):67–76.

Gajewski, Stephanie, Holly Bell, Laura Lein, and Ronald J. Angel. 2011. "Complexity and Instability: The Response of Nongovernmental Organizations to the Recovery of Hurricane Katrina Survivors in a Host Community." *Nonprofit and Voluntary Sector Quarterly* 40:389–403.

Giddens, Anthony. 1994a. *Beyond Left and Right: The Future of Radical Politics*. Oxford, UK: Polity Press.

Giddens, Anthony. 1994b. "Living in a Post-Traditional Society." Pp. 56–109 in *Reflexive Modernization: Politics, Tradition and Aesthetics in the Modern Social Order*, edited by Ulrich Beck, Anthony Giddens, and Scott Lash. Malden, MA: Polity Press.

Goodhart, David. 2017. *The Road to Somewhere: The Populist Revolt and the Future of Politics*. London, UK: Hurst & Company.

Grzybowski, Candido. 2000. "We NGOs: A Controversial Way of Being and Acting." *Development in Practice* 10 (3–4):436–444.

Hansen, Jennie Chin, and Maureen Hewitt. 2012. "PACE Provides a Sense of Belonging for Elders." *Generations* 36 (1):37–43.

Herro, Annie. 2019. "Advocating a UN Convention on the Rights of Older Persons in the United Kingdom: The Case for a Radical Flank." *Journal of Human Rights Practice* 11 (1):132–150.

Hood, Sula, Yvonne Yueh-Feng Lu, Kristen Jenkins, Ellen R. Brown, Joyce Beaven, Steve A. Brown, Hugh C. Hendrie, and Mary Guerriero Austrom. 2018. "Exploration of Perceived Psychosocial Benefits of Senior Companion Program Participation among Urban-Dwelling, Low-Income Older Adult Women Volunteers." *Innovation in Aging* 2 (2):1–12.

Hsu, Kaiting Jessica, and Mark Schuller. 2020. "Humanitarian Aid and Local Power Structures: Lessons from Haiti's 'Shadow Disaster'." *Disasters*. Retreived 4/22/2020 from https://onlinelibrary.wiley.com/doi/abs/10.1111/disa.12380.

Keck, Margaret, and Kathryn Sikkink. 1998. *Activists beyond Borders: Advocacy Networks in International Politics*. Ithaca, NY: Cornell University Press.

Krause, Neal. 2006. "Social Relationships in Later Life." Pp. 181–200 in *Handbook of Aging and the Social Sciences*, edited by Robert H. Binstock and Linda K. George. New York, NY: Academic Press.

Lettieri, Michael. 2021. *Violence against Women in Mexico: A Report on Recent Trends in Femicide in Baja California, Sinaloa and Veracruz*. San Diego, CA: University of San Diego, KROC School Trans-Border Institute.

Lilla, Marc. 2016. "The End of Identity Liberalism." P. SR1, November 19, *New York Times*. Opinion Piece, Retrieved 6/12/2019 from https://www.nytimes.com/2016/11/20/opinion/sunday/the-end-of-identity-liberalism.html.

Macdonald, Laura, and Arne Ruckert. 2009. "Post-Neoliberalism in the Americas: An Introduction." Pp. 1–18 in *Post-Neoliberalism in the Americas*, edited by Laura Macdonald and Arne Ruckert. London, UK: Palgrave Macmillan.

Meyer, David S., and Suzanne Staggenborg. 1996. "Movements, Counter-movements, and the Structure of Political Opportunity." *American Journal of Sociology* 101 (6):1628–1660.

Montes de Oca, Verónica. 2000. "Experiencia institucional y situación social de los ancianos en la ciudad de México." Pp. 419–456 in *Las políticas sociales en México al fin del milenio. Descentralizaíon, disenño y gestión*, edited by Rolando Cordera and Alicia Ziccardi. Mexico City: Coordinación de Humanidades/Facultad de Economia/Miguel Angel Porrúa.

Montes de Oca, Verónica, Mariana Paredes, Vicente Rodríguez, and Sagrario Garay. 2018. "Older Persons and Human Rights in Latin America and the Caribbean." *International Journal on Ageing in Developing Countries* 2 (2):149–164.

Montes de Oca Zavala, Verónica. 2013. "La discriminación hacia la vejez en la ciudad de México: contrastes sociolpoliticos y jurídicos a nivel nacional y local." *Revista Perspectivas Sociales/Social Perspectives* 15 (1):47–80.

Mottl, Tahi L. 1980. "The Analysis of Countermovements." *Social Problems* 27 (5):620–635.

National Institute on Aging. 2019. "Social Isolation, Loneliness in Older People Pose Health Risks." National Institute on Aging. Retrieved 10/16/2019 from https://www.nia.nih.gov/news/social-isolation-loneliness-older-people-pose-health-risks.

Pereira, Javier, and Ronald Angel. 2009. "From Adversary to Ally: The Evolution of Non-Governmental Organizations in the Context of Health Reform in Santiago and Montevideo." Pp. 97–111 in *Social Inequality and Public Health*, edited by Salvatore Babones. Bristol, UK: Policy Press.

Pereira, Javier, Ronald J. Angel, and Jacqueline L. Angel. 2007. "A Case Study of the Elder Care Functions of a Chilean Non-Governmental Organization." *Social Science and Medicine* 64:2096–2106.

Plattner, Marc F. 2019. "Illiberal Democracy and the Struggle on the Right." *Journal of Democracy* 30 (1):5–19.

Quadagno, Jill, Bill Lennox Kail, and K. Russell Shekha. 2012. "Welfare States: Protecting or Risking Old Age." Pp. 321–332 in *Handbook of Sociology of Aging*, edited by Richard A.Settersten Jr. and Jacqueline L. Angel. New York, NY: Springer.

Roman, Joseph. 2004. "The Trade Union Solution or the NGO Problem? The Global Fight for Labour Rights." *Development in Practice* 14 (1 & 2):100–109.

Sangeeta, Kamat. 2004. "The Privatization of Public Interest: Theorizing NGO Discourse in a Neoliberal Era." *Review of International Political Economy* 11:155–176.

Schlesinger Jr., Arthur. 1992. *The Disuniting of America*. New York, NY: Norton.

Schuller, Mark. 2007. "Invasion or Infusion? Understanding the Role of NGOs in Contemporary Haiti." *Journal of Haitian Studies* 13 (2):96–119.

Sikkink, Kathryn. 2017. *Evidence for Hope: Making Human Rights Work in the 21st Century*. Princeton, NJ: Princeton University Press.

Srinivas, Nidhi. 2009. "Against NGOs?: A Critical Perspective on Nongovernmental Action." *Nonprofit and Voluntary Sector Quarterly* 38 (4):614–626.

Stiglitz, Joseph E. 2008. "Is There a Post-Washington Consensus?" Pp. 41–56 in *The Washington Consensus Reconsidered: Towards a New Global Governance*, edited by Narcís Serra and Joseph E. Stiglitz. New York, NY: Oxford University Press.

Tilly, Charles. 1978. *From Mobilization to Revolution*. Reading, MA: Addison-Wesley.

United Nations. 1948. "Universal Declaration of Human Rights." Retrieved 7/22/2019 from https://www.un.org/en/universal-declaration-human-rights/index.html.

Zakaria, Fareed. 1997. "The Rise of Illiberal Democracy." *Foreign Affairs* 76 (6):22–43.

Zald, Mayer N., and Bert Useem. 1987. "Movement and Countermovement Interaction: Mobilization, Tactics, and State Involvement." Pp. 247–271 in *Social Movements in an Organizational Society*, edited by Mayer N. Zald and John D. McCarthy. New Brunswick, NJ: Transaction.

The Study
A Grounded Theoretical Approach

Our classification and description of civil society organizations (CSOs) is based on a convenience sample contacted between 2016 and 2019 in four Mexican states: Jalisco, Nuevo León, Oaxaca, Yucatán, and Mexico City. In the state of Jalisco, we carried out eleven interviews in Guadalajara, Zapopan, and Tlaquepaque; in Nuevo León we conducted ten interviews with organizations in Monterrey; in Oaxaca we contacted ten organizations in Oaxaca de Juarez, Juchitán, and Unión Hidalgo; in Mérida, Yucatán we conducted eleven interviews; and in Mexico City we interviewed thirty-five organizations. In addition, we conducted five focus groups: four in Mexico City and one in Monterrey. The data collection was motivated by the growing importance of secular and faith-based non-governmental organizations in Mexico and all of Latin America and the Caribbean, and of the growing response of these organizations to the problems of a rapidly aging and resource-poor population. Unfortunately, no complete listing of civil society organizations whose missions focus wholly or partially on the problems of older people exists. Our selection, therefore was based on our established contacts and information gathered from the internet and other sources.

Our experience with civil society in Mexico allowed us to select organizations that based on our professional judgement are largely mainstream in terms of their advocacy and service delivery roles related to older individuals. Our data collection approach can be characterized as a version of grounded theory in that it is inductive. We began with very general theories of what civil society organizations do, how they frame the issues they address, and how their ability to act is constrained by political, economic, and political forces. We did not, though, begin with specific hypotheses. Our approach was motivated by a general lack of knowledge of any aspect of these organizations' approach to the needs of older persons. A few qualitative studies have been carried out in Mexico, but no systematic overview of the role of such organizations in advocacy for or service provision to older persons exists.

Data collection was based on personal interviews with staff members of these organizations as well as individual participants. The interview

DOI: 10.4324/9781003205609-10

protocol was informed by the five focus groups that were part of the initial conceptual phase of the study. The analysis in this book represents a description of these organizations and the political, economic, and social contexts in which they function. That context reflects historical forces related to the labor movement in Mexico and the social movements and protests that took place in a highly corporatist and clientelistic State in which a single political party, the Partido Revolucionario Institucional (PRI), dominated for decades. We focus on the social construction of the institutions' eldercare and advocacy missions as expressed by the actions of individuals and groups.

The specific CSOs were selected based on access, and the nature of their functions related to older adults. Given Mexico City's dominance, a large fraction of our interviews and four of the five focus groups were conducted there. The institutions we contacted in Mexico City are located in different alcaldías (boroughs), which vary in terms of their socioeconomic profiles, their average levels of education, and the need profiles of their populations. Nine groups were identified in the alcaldías of Iztapalapa, Gustavo A. Madero, Coyoacán, Benito Juárez, Tlalpan, and Cuauhtémoc. Socioeconomically, these neighborhoods vary from medium high, to medium low and low. The composition of the organizations we contacted vary in terms of the age and sex of their membership. Most were mixed in terms of gender, although certain organizations were predominantly male, while others were predominantly female. As we described in the analysis, these gender differences have significant implications for the organization's objectives and effectiveness.

Interviews followed a semi-structured format. The general themes of the interview are listed below. The interviewer asked about each topic and the respondent structured his or her response in terms of his or her own understanding of the question. Informed consent was obtained for all interviews and focus groups, which were conducted at their organizational locations. Our analyses are based on eighty interviews and the five focus groups. Interviews and focus group discussions were transcribed and coded thematically using ATLAS.ti qualitative analysis software. The interpretation of the narrative material is guided by a general social constructivist theoretical framework that emphasizes the relational and historical character of all aspects of social reality. From this perspective individual and organizational behavior and ideology reflect rational actions that are influenced by historical, political, economic, linguistic, and cultural factors. The objective was to develop some initial sense of those structures. Translation from Spanish to English was carried out by the investigators.

Theoretical Population

The theoretical population about which we wish to make inferences consists of all fairly formally organized groups whose sole or partial objective is to advocate for or provide services and support to older individuals. We excluded informal groups such as neighborhood associations or other groups that lack any aspect of organizational structure such as manager, staff, or other administrative personnel. Nonetheless, our theoretical population comprises a large range of organizations. It includes civil society organizations (CSOs), both religious and secular, unions with active participation of older members, government agencies with ties to civil society, associations linked to local governments that deal with aging issues, religious groups, and even private companies that address the specialized needs of specific groups of elderly individuals.

Operational Sample

The study is based on a purposive sample collected using expert judgement and a snowball approach. The sample was intended to include a wide range of organizations that advocate for or provide services to older individuals in different socioeconomic, social, and cultural contexts. The older individuals who receive services in these organizations differ in age, gender, indigenous status, average educational level, occupational history, union experience, and previous social activism. As we note in the analyses, the characteristics of their memberships structure the manner in which the organizations frame their missions and they influence an organization's degree of activism and the nature of the activities it engages in.

The Political Environment at the State Level

The actions of these organizations are clearly influenced by the political environments in which they operate. Those differ significantly among states and municipalities. At the time of our interviews different political parties were in office in the various states. In the state of Jalisco the Partido Acción Nacional (PAN), a traditionally conservative party, was in power. In Nuevo León the independent Partido Ciudadano held office. This party rejects traditional party affiliations and proposes new initiatives related to the economy, the environment, and other public issues. At the time of the study the party promoted citizen initiatives, but maintained a pro-business stance and an overall conservative approach. The party's perspective reflects Monterrey's economic and social dynamism. In Mexico City the Partido de la Revolución Democrática (PRD), a left-of-center party, was dominant. In Oaxaca the Partido Revolucionario Institucional (PRI), the party that has dominated Mexico for the majority of its modern history, held office; in Yucatán as in Jalisco the PAN was in charge. Given the major political, as well as economic and cultural differences among Mexican states, our intent was to insure a sufficiently broad view of active aging in various political contexts even though we were unable to interview in all states.

Time Frame of the Study

The study was carried out between April 2016 and October 2019.

Major Thematic Areas Covered in the Semi-structured Interview

The interviews were semi-structured and included staff, volunteers, and participants in the various organizations. All interviews followed the same basic format in which the interviewer touched upon the following topics. Of course, staff and participants' perspectives were often different, but as an inductive exploratory approach we wished to focus broadly on certain basic themes. All interviewees provided informed consent in accordance with the ethical guidelines established by UNAM. Respondents often focused on one or more of the topics over others and the interviewers allowed the respondent to interpret the probes and to answer as they wished using their own terms. The general topical areas included:

- Origin of the group or organization.
- Characteristics of participants, including sex, age, education, family status, work history, previous political or social movement activity; their motivation for and type of participation; their beliefs about the benefits and obstacles to participation.
- Type of activities engaged in as participants.
- Sources of financing and government support; efforts to recruit participants and obtain resources.
- The respondent's concept of old age and active aging; discussion of what the organization or group does to foster active aging and citizenship.
- Perceptions of the reality of aging in Mexico.
- Knowledge about the various international and more local conventions and laws concerning human rights, especially those that apply to older people.
- The role of women in the group.
- Knowledge and opinions concerning the role of gender at the individual and societal levels.

Data Analysis

The interviews were on average two and a half hours long. They were transcribed by the interviewers and translated selectively by the investigators. The material was coded on the basis of thematic content as identified by the investigators and archived using the ATLAS.ti qualitative data analysis program.

The Specific Organizations Contacted and Interviewed in each City

State of Jalisco: In the cities Guadalajara, Zapopan, and Tlaquepaque we conducted eleven interviews with individuals 30–72 years old. These included the following individuals identified by their initials and age, as well as their organization:

- Entre hermanos. Fundación Oportunidades A.C.: C. C. (72 years old), Director in charge of strategic planning and communication for the foundation and A.C. (51 years old).
- Fundación años de Plata A.C.: J. G. (32 years old), President of the foundation.
- Jalisciense Association for the Protection of Lepers A.C.: R. G. (51 years old), Administrator of the association.
- Networks of friendly cities with the elderly in Guadalajara: R. G. (56 years old) Project Leader.
- Geronto-Geriatrics Society of Jalisco (SOGEJAL): M. S. (57 years old), gerontologist and President of the society.
- Plenitud y Demencias A.C.: I. B. (30 years old), teacher in gerontology.
- Voluntariado Estamos Contigo.: G. M. and A. M. Administrator and Manager.
- Casa Loyola: C. A. Administrator.
- Juan Pablo II Nursing Home: M. M., S. V. and A. C. Administrators and Manager.

State of Nuevo León: In the city of Monterrey, we conducted ten interviews and one focus group. These were with the following individuals and organizations:

- Pastoral del Hermano Mayor: H. A. Administrator.
- Retirados de la Cervecería Cuauhtémoc: O. J. Administrator and Manager.
- Gericare, A.C.: B. D., Administrator and Manager.
- Elderly Wellness Foundation: F. A., Administrator and Manager.
- Regional Center for the Study of the Elderly: R. S., Director.
- Great People House: RV, Administrator and Manager.
- National Institute for the Family (INFAMILIA): D. I., Director.
- University for the Elderly of the Autonomous University of Nuevo León: L. S. (58 years old), Director.
- Ama y Trasciende Association, Older Adults in Action (AMA): M. F. and M. G., Activist Leaders.
- Luis Elizondo Asylum: BM, Manager.
- Unión de Posesionarios Tierra y Libertad, Monterrey. E. D., Activist

State of Oaxaca: In the cities of Oaxaca de Juárez, Juchitán, and Unión Hidalgo we conducted ten interviews with the following individuals and organizations:

- Councilor for Human Rights and Gender Equity: B. G., Staff Member.
- Ombudsman for Human Rights of the people of Oaxaca: J. S., Staff Member.
- Human Rights Directorate of the municipality of Oaxaca de Juárez (DDHMOHJ): S. C., Staff Member.
- Universidad del Adulto Mayor: M. J. and R. L., Staff Members.
- Atención a Adultos Mayores DIF Oaxaca: M. M. (we were granted permission to conduct the interview, but not to record it).
- Jubilados y Pensionados de la CNTE Oaxaca: J. P., Manager.
- Museo Textil de Oaxaca: A. S. and S. M., Staff Members.
- Comité Melendre: G. G., Manager.
- Un corazón por Unión: S. P. and O. G., Gerontologist and Manager.
- Colectivo Binni Cubi: J. A., Activist.

State of Yucatán: We conducted eleven interviews in the city of Mérida. These included the following:

- La Felicidad Comienza A.C.: R. P., Founder; R. S., Physician.
- Departamento de Atención al Adulto Mayor del DIF: S. P.
- Centro Integral para la Plenitud del Adulto Mayor "Renacer": V. C., Gerontologist; M. D., Coordinator.
- Instituto Nacional de las Personas Adultas Mayores (INAPAM): E. J., Coordinator.
- Club Social para Adultos Mayores Nova Vida Platino: G. R., Owner.
- Luna Nueva. Residencia para Adultos Mayores: G. R., Owner.
- Instituto Geriátrico Mexicano A.C.: I. R., Director.
- DIF estatal Encargado de Programa de Adultos Mayores: A. M., Staff Member.
- Jubilados y Pensionados del ISSTEY (seguridad social del estado de Yucatán): B. S., Centro para Jubilados y Pensionados Manager.
- Asociación de Jubilados y Pensionados de la CFE de Yucatán: J. E. and C. N., Founders.
- Movimiento de adultos mayores de Yucatán: R. M. C., Activist.

Mexico City: We conducted thirty-five interviews and four focus groups in the boroughs of Gustavo A. Madero, Iztapalapa, Tlalpan, Benito Juárez, Coyoacán, and Cuauhtémoc. These individuals and organizations consisted of the following:

Retirees and Pensioners of the Institute of Social Security and Services for State Workers (PISSSTE). The age range of the people interviewed was 70–79 years:

- A. B. (71 years old), representative of the organization.
- J. M. (79 years old), participant.
- J. R. (70 years old), Metro Balderas of the ISSSTE, member of the commission.
- M. P. (79 years old), Retirees and Pensioners Dr. La Vista, participant.
- M. P. (77 years old), Retired from Route 100, participant.
- S. M. (72 years old), participant.
- V. S. (79 years old), participant.
- Focus group (S. M., M. P., J. M., and J. R. R.).

Retirees of the National Coordinator of Education Workers (JPCNTE): Focus Group (six participants)

Retirees and Pensioners of the Mexican Union of Electricians (JPSME). The age range of the people interviewed was 57–68 years:

- J. L. (58 years old).
- J. A. (66 years old), participant.
- M. D. (57 years old), participant.
- R. S. (68 years old), participant.
- S. M. (62 years old), participant.
- Focus group (S. M., M D., J. L., and R. S.).

Retirees of the UNAM academics "Pioneers in Creativity and Freedom" (PICRELI). The age range of the people interviewed was 73–79 years:

- C. L. (78 years old), retired.
- C. H. (74 years old), retired.
- O. V. (74 years old), retired.
- S. C. (79 years old), retired.
- V. M. (73 years old), retired.
- M. B. (74 years old), retired.
- H. A. (74 years old), retired.

Fundación de Mano amigo a mano anciana I.A.P.:

- M. B., representative of the foundation.
- O. L. (40 years old), physician.

Granito de Arena A.C.:

- P. R. (56 years old), Director of the Foundation.

Amanecer Veracruzano:

- M. H.
- E. (68 years old).
- R. L. (78 years old).
- J. (83 years old).
- T. D. (79 years old).
- M. G.
- Focus group (J., T., T. (82 years old), C. (72 years old), R., and G. (75 years old)).

RENUEVA Group:

- E. B. (66 years old), pensioner.
- S.G. (72 years old).
- M. Z.
- A. G. (67 years old).
- A. S. (68 years old), coordinator of the Active Aging course.
- A. S. (65 years old).

Ajusco Human Rights Committee:

A.F. (75 years old).

Index

Page numbers in italics refer to figures. Page numbers in bold refer to tables.